Psychiatry P.R.N.

Psychiatry P.R.N.

Principles, **R**eality, **N**ext Steps

SECOND EDITION

Edited by

Sarah Stringer
Laurence Church
Roxanne Keynejad
Juliet Hurn

With illustrations by

Darcy Muenchrath
Helen Potschisvili
Mao Fong Lim

OXFORD
UNIVERSITY PRESS

OXFORD
UNIVERSITY PRESS

Great Clarendon Street, Oxford, OX2 6DP,
United Kingdom

Oxford University Press is a department of the University of Oxford.
It furthers the University's objective of excellence in research, scholarship,
and education by publishing worldwide. Oxford is a registered trade mark of
Oxford University Press in the UK and in certain other countries

© Oxford University Press 2020

The moral rights of the authors have been asserted

First Edition published in 2009
Second Edition published in 2020

Impression: 2

All rights reserved. No part of this publication may be reproduced, stored in
a retrieval system, or transmitted, in any form or by any means, without the
prior permission in writing of Oxford University Press, or as expressly permitted
by law, by licence or under terms agreed with the appropriate reprographics
rights organization. Enquiries concerning reproduction outside the scope of the
above should be sent to the Rights Department, Oxford University Press, at the
address above

You must not circulate this work in any other form
and you must impose this same condition on any acquirer

Published in the United States of America by Oxford University Press
198 Madison Avenue, New York, NY 10016, United States of America

British Library Cataloguing in Publication Data

Data available

Library of Congress Control Number: 2019957787

ISBN 978-0-19-880608-0

Printed and bound by
CPI Group (UK) Ltd, Croydon, CR0 4YY

Oxford University Press makes no representation, express or implied, that the
drug dosages in this book are correct. Readers must therefore always check
the product information and clinical procedures with the most up-to-date
published product information and data sheets provided by the manufacturers
and the most recent codes of conduct and safety regulations. The authors and
the publishers do not accept responsibility or legal liability for any errors in the
text or for the misuse or misapplication of material in this work. Except where
otherwise stated, drug dosages and recommendations are for the non-pregnant
adult who is not breast-feeding

Links to third party websites are provided by Oxford in good faith and
for information only. Oxford disclaims any responsibility for the materials
contained in any third party website referenced in this work.

Cure sometimes, relieve often, comfort always.

From the 15th-century French proverb,
Guérir quelquefois, soulager souvent, consoler toujours.

SS: *To my greatest loves, Beth and Arthur.*
LC: *With all my love to Monica, Ben, and Millie. Thank you all my family, friends and those who have worked with me - staff, patients and carers.*
RK: *For my childhood friend, Sophie Rhodes, who taught me much, and who is greatly missed.*
JH: *With thanks to the patients, students, and colleagues who have taught me so much.*

FOREWORD

I first came across *Psychiatry P.R.N.* in 2012. While at the Royal College of Psychiatrists International Congress in Liverpool, I had attended a workshop on Extreme Psychiatry, a course developed to teach communication skills to medical students. This was a course with a difference, loved by students, many of whom were drawn to careers in psychiatry as a result of what they learnt. When I heard that a book had been developed from this teaching, I had to get hold of a copy.

Psychiatry P.R.N. did not disappoint. A world away from the rather dry academic texts that I studied as a student and trainee psychiatrist, I quickly realized it was special. There are many textbooks of psychiatry, but this one stood out as being interesting, colourful, vivid, and compassionate. It made the dry facts—and Vincent van Gogh—come alive and gave many practical tips that students or junior doctors could actually use when meeting people with mental illness. Over the years, it's become a favourite of medical students, but after 10 years, it needed a shake up—and this is what Sarah, Laurence, Juliet, and Roxanne have done with the second edition. All the facts are updated and reflect new research; practical tips have been rewritten with the editors' further years in clinical practice; there are now role plays in every chapter, to help with clinical and OSCE revision; and the Next Steps reflect the challenges regularly faced in the Foundation Years by many doctors. The illustrations are fun and engaging, and there is clever use of novels and films to help learning and to inspire the next generation of psychiatrists.

Since becoming President of the Royal College in 2017, I've been involved in many initiatives to attract the best and brightest doctors into psychiatry. People with mental illness deserve nothing less! I hope that *Psychiatry P.R.N.* catches the eye and the imagination of medical students and junior doctors who are excellent communicators, sharp and creative thinkers, and compassionate human beings—and nudges them into considering a career in psychiatry. But beyond that, I hope that this book helps all doctors understand mental health problems and be able to speak to people in distress—mental health is everyone's business.

Professor Wendy Burn
President, Royal College of Psychiatrists

PREFACE

Part 1: Overview in Psychiatry

Psychiatry is all about stories. Listing symptoms is all very well, but you can only really help people with mental distress if you understand *who* they are, *where* they're coming from, and *why* they're struggling *now*—you'll do this by drawing out their life stories. With this in mind, *Psychiatry P.R.N.* opens with the psychiatric assessment and formulation of the great painter, Vincent van Gogh, at the time when he cut off his earlobe, in 1888. We hope this brings the process of assessment to life and helps you understand and remember how to structure your history, mental state examination, and formulation.

We'd recommend you start with Vincent (Chapter 1), and read the rest of the Overview in Psychiatry (Chapters 2–6) at least once before beginning your psychiatry placement. This should give you the skills, knowledge, and confidence you need to make a good start. You can then delve into Part 2, as it suits you best.

Part 2: Clinical conditions: Principles, Reality, Next steps

You'll often see the abbreviation *PRN* on drug charts. It stands for *pro re nata* ('as needed'). We've written *Psychiatry P.R.N.* to try to help you access the right type, amount, and depth of information, *as and when you need it* (rather than overloading you with everything at once). Every chapter covers a different topic, and is divided into PRN: Principles, Reality, and Next Steps.

Principles are the key facts for each topic, presented as succinctly and comprehensively as possible.

The *Reality* section then helps you understand how to talk to someone with this mental health problem. It provides general tips and example interview questions. We've included role-plays to illustrate different conditions; you may find them useful as practice for clinical work or for your practical exams, the Objective Structured Clinical Examinations (OSCEs).

Finally, the *Next Steps* section provides common clinical scenarios you'll encounter as a new doctor (e.g. Foundation Year 1 or 2). Whatever your job, you'll see people with mental health problems, and find you can help them more effectively when you address these difficulties *alongside* their medical or surgical problems.

Wherever you see this icon, we're trying to bring risk issues to your attention.

This icon denotes practical tips, interesting facts, or ideas that may help you understand what it's like to experience mental health problems.

At the end of each chapter, we've included a selection of interesting 'extras' about the condition:

- Movie buff: films
- Book shelf: novels and biographies
- Footlights: plays
- Journal club: key papers
- Resources: links to useful websites and charities

The illustrations in the book will have fans and critics, but we hope the material is memorable and thought-provoking—for both camps. As with all of the content in the book, the illustrative material is designed to help you understand mental illness. At no stage has it been our intention to take a reductionist approach, nor to stereotype any particular group. Some of the drawings may be a little disturbing, but then the lived experience of psychiatric illness often falls into the same category.

Some drawings in the book are designed as a sort of visual mnemonic—to help you think and remember. Other drawings depict clinical signs, and/or are designed to be suggestive of the experience of a particular condition, e.g. withdrawal from opiates. Photographs have been carefully selected to illustrate things you may not have seen before, such as illicit drugs, histopathology, or brain imaging.

We hope you enjoy this book.

Sarah Stringer,
Laurence Church,
Roxanne Keynejad, and
Juliet Hurn

ACKNOWLEDGEMENTS

Contributors

Penny Brown (Chapter 22, Forensic psychiatry)
Roxanne Keynejad (Chapter 7, A career in psychiatry)

Illustrations

Mao Fong Lim
Darcy Muenchrath
Helen Potschisvili

Clinical photographs

TicTac Communications Limited (drug photographs)

Expert advisors

Frankie Anderson (organic)
Charley Baker (culture)
Hannah Campling (Vincent van Gogh)
Mujtaba Husain (medically unexplained symptoms)
Shivani Patel (child and adolescent psychiatry)
Trevor Shine (substance misuse)
Jennifer Taylor (organic: Creutzfeldt–Jakob disease)

Medical student

George Vaughan (depression and exercise)

CONTENTS

Abbreviations	xiv
Contributors to the first edition	xvii
Ancillary Resource Centre	xviii

Part 1 Overview in Psychiatry

1. Psychiatric assessment	1
2. Safety	17
3. Essential interview skills	19
4. How to succeed in psychiatry OSCEs	24
5. Classification and diagnosis	27
6. Mental health and the law	29
7. A career in psychiatry	31

Part 2 Clinical Conditions: Principles, Reality, Next Steps

8. Affective disorders	33
9. Self-harm and suicide	61
10. Psychotic disorders	77
11. Substance use disorders	101
12. Organic psychiatry	127
13. Old age psychiatry	149
14. Anxiety disorders	167
15. Medically unexplained symptoms	189
16. Eating disorders	199
17. Conditions related to sexual health	213
18. Perinatal psychiatry	223
19. Intellectual disability	231
20. Child and adolescent psychiatry	243
21. Personality disorders	257
22. Forensic psychiatry	269

Appendix: True/false question answers	277
Index	279

ABBREVIATIONS

5-HT	5-hydroxytryptamine	CJD	Creutzfeldt–Jakob disease
AA	Alcoholics Anonymous	CJS	criminal justice system
AAC	augmentative and alternative communication	CMHT	community mental health team
ABC	antecedent, behaviour, consequence	CNS	central nervous system
ABV	alcohol by volume	CO_2	carbon dioxide
ACE-III	Addenbrooke's cognitive examination	CRP	C-reactive protein
AChEI	acetylcholinesterase inhibitor	CRT	cognitive remediation therapy
ACT	acceptance and commitment therapy	CSF	cerebrospinal fluid
AD	Alzheimer disease	CSBD	compulsive sexual behaviour disorder
ADHD	attention deficit hyperactivity disorder	CT	computed tomography
ADI	autism diagnostic interview	CVA	cerebrovascular accident
ADLs	activities of daily living	CXR	chest X-ray
AIDS	acquired immune deficiency syndrome	DA	dopamine
ALP	alkaline phosphatase	DBT	dialectical behavioural therapy
AMHP	approved mental health professional	DJ	disc jockey
AN	anorexia nervosa	DLB	dementia due to Lewy body disease
APP	amyloid precursor protein	DSM	Diagnostic and Statistical Manual of Mental Disorders
ARC	Ancillary Resource Centre		
ARFID	avoidant/restrictive food intake disorder	DTs	delirium tremens
ARMS	at-risk mental state	DUP	duration of untreated psychosis
ASD	autism spectrum disorder	DVLA	Driver and Vehicle Licensing Agency
AUDIT	Alcohol Use Disorders Identification Test	DVT	deep vein thrombosis
BA	behavioural activation	ECG	electrocardiogram
BBV	blood-borne virus	ECT	electroconvulsive therapy
BDD	body dysmorphic disorder	ED	emergency department *or* erectile dysfunction
BDI	Beck depression inventory	EE	expressed emotion
BED	binge eating disorder	EEG	electroencephalography
BEN	benign ethnic neutropenia	EMI	elderly mentally infirm
BILD	British Institute of Learning Disabilities	ENT	ear, nose, and throat
BMI	body mass index	EPSE	extrapyramidal side effect
BN	bulimia nervosa	ESR	erythrocyte sedimentation rate
BP	blood pressure	EUPD	emotionally unstable personality disorder
BPAD	bipolar affective disorder	FBC	full blood count
BPSD	behavioural and psychological symptoms of dementia	FCMHT	forensic community mental health team
		FEP	first-episode psychosis
BSE	bovine spongiform encephalopathy	FGA	first-generation antipsychotic
Ca^{2+}	calcium	FLS	frontal lobe syndrome
CAM	Confusion Assessment Method	FPT	focal psychodynamic therapy
CAT	cognitive analytical therapy	FSAD	female sexual arousal dysfunction
CAMHS	child and adolescent mental health services	FSH	follicle-stimulating hormone
CBD	cannabidiol	FTD	frontotemporal dementia
CBG	capillary blood glucose	FY	foundation year
CBT	cognitive behavioural therapy	GABA	gamma aminobutyric acid
CBT-ED	eating disorder-focused cognitive behavioural therapy	GAD	generalized anxiety disorder
		GBH	grievous bodily harm
CDD	conduct/dissocial disorder	GBL	gamma-butyrolactone
CFS	chronic fatigue syndrome	GGT	gamma-glutamyltransferase
CIWA	Clinical Institute Withdrawal Assessment for Alcohol	GHB	gamma-hydroxybutyrate
		GI	gastrointestinal

GMC	General Medical Council	MSE	mental state examination
GP	general practitioner	MSU	mid-stream specimen of urine
HADS	hospital anxiety and depression scale	MUS	medically unexplained symptoms
HAD	HIV-associated dementia	Na$^+$	sodium
HAND	HIV-associated neurocognitive disorder	NA	Narcotics Anonymous *or* noradrenaline
Hb	haemoglobin	NAC	*N*-acetylcysteine
HbA1c	glycated haemoglobin	NAPQI	*N*-acetyl-p-benzoquinone imine
HD	Huntington disease	NAT	negative automatic thought
HIV	human immunodeficiency virus	NFT	neurofibrillary tangle
HR	heart rate	NMDA	*N*-methyl-D-aspartate
HSDD	hypoactive sexual desire dysfunction	NPH	normal pressure hydrocephalus
HTT	home treatment team	NPS	novel psychoactive substances
ICD	International Classification of Diseases	NSAID	non-steroidal anti-inflammatory drug
ID	intellectual disability *or* identification	OCD	obsessive–compulsive disorder
IM	intramuscular(ly)	ODD	oppositional defiant disorder
IMCA	independent mental capacity advocate	OSCE	objective structured clinical examination
IPSRT	interpersonal and social rhythm therapy	OSFED	other specified feeding or eating disorder
IPT	interpersonal therapy	OT	occupational therapist
IQ	intelligence quotient	PANDAS	paediatric autoimmune neuropsychiatric disorder associated with streptococcal infection
IV	intravenous		
IVF	*in vitro* fertilization	PCP	phencyclidine
K$^+$	potassium	PCS	post-concussion syndrome
KS	Korsakoff syndrome	PD	Parkinson disease *or* personality disorder
LCQ	logical curious question	PET	positron emission tomography
LD	learning disability	PhD	doctor of philosophy
LFTs	liver function tests	PHQ-9	patient health questionnaire
LGBT (Q, I, A)	lesbian, gay, bisexual, transgender (queer/questioning, intersex, asexual)	PND	postnatal depression
		PO	*per os* (orally)
		PO$_4^{3-}$	phosphate
LH	luteinizing hormone	PPD	postpartum depression
LPA	Lasting Power of Attorney	PPP	postpartum psychosis
LSD	lysergic acid diethylamide	PrP	prion protein
MAO	monoamine oxidase	PTSD	post-traumatic stress disorder
MAOI	monoamine oxidase inhibitor	QTc	corrected QT interval
M-ACE	mini-Addenbrooke's cognitive examination	RCPsych	Royal College of Psychiatrists
MARSIPAN	management of really sick patients with anorexia nervosa	RMN	registered mental health nurse
		RR	respiratory rate
MBCT	mindfulness-based cognitive therapy	rTMS	repetitive transcranial magnetic stimulation
MBT	mentalization-based therapy	SaO$_2$	oxygen saturation
MBU	mother and baby unit	SCRA	synthetic cannabinoid receptor agonist
MCA	Mental Capacity Act	SD	standard deviation
MCV	mean corpuscular volume	SGA	second-generation antipsychotic
MDMA	3,4-methylenedioxymethamphetamine	SLE	systemic lupus erythematosus
ME	myalgic encephalomyelitis	SNP	single nucleotide polymorphism
MHA	Mental Health Act	SNRI	serotonin and noradrenaline reuptake inhibitor
MHOA	mental health of older adults	SpO$_2$	peripheral capillary oxygen saturation
MI	motivational interviewing *or* myocardial infarction	SPPD	sexual pain-penetration disorder
MMR	measles, mumps, rubella	SSB	safety seeking behaviour
MMSE	Mini Mental State Examination	SSRI	selective serotonin reuptake inhibitor
MOCA	Montreal Cognitive Assessment	SUSS	sit up–squat–stand
MP	Member of Parliament	TB	tuberculosis
MRCPsych	membership of the Royal College of Psychiatrists	TBI	traumatic brain injury
MRI	magnetic resonance imaging	TC	therapeutic community
MS	multiple sclerosis	TCA	tricyclic antidepressant

TFTs	thyroid function test	UK	United Kingdom
TGA	transient global amnesia	UKDILAS	UK Drugs in Lactation Advisory Service
THC	tetrahydrocannabinol	UKTIS	The UK Teratology Information Service
TIA	transient ischaemic attack	UTI	urinary tract infection
TLE	temporal lobe epilepsy	VD	vascular dementia
TSE	transmissible spongiform encephalopathy	VGKC	voltage-gated potassium channel
TV	television	VMA	vanillylmandelic acid
U&Es	urea and electrolytes	WCC	white cell count
UDS	urinary drug screen	WRAP	Wellness Recovery Action Plan

CONTRIBUTORS TO THE FIRST EDITION

Martin Baggaley
Charley Baker (literary advisor)
Ajay Bhatnagar
Michelle Butterworth
Sarah Cader
Laurence Church (editor; all 'Next Steps')
Hazel Claydon
Phillip Collins
Mazen Daher
Susan Davison (editor)
Mark N. Haddad
Matthew Hagger
Jennifer Haworth
Juliet Hurn
Noreen Jakeman
Laura Jones
Alex Liakos
Maurice Lipsedge (editor)
Greg Lydall
Amy E. Manley
Jack Nathan
Dimitrios Paschos
Thomas Pollak
Alice M. Roberts
Saman Saidi
Naveen Sharma

Anna Streeruwitz
Sarah Stringer (editor; all 'Reality' sections)
Janet Treasure
Deborah A. Woodman
Sheena Webb

Artists

Risk factor drawings by Ayesha Lodhia
Clinical signs drawings by Darcy Muenchrath
Chapter opening drawings by Helen Potschisvili

Video team

Production

Laurence Church—executive producer
Jessica Hart, Shanika Nayagam, and Sam Saidi—assistant producers
Sam Saidi and Sarah Stringer—screenwriters

Actors

PTSD: Richard Tate (Alfred Keane) and Daniel Furmedge (self)
Depression: Jenny Howe (Mary Knight) and Gemma McCulloch (self)
Suicide: Vishal Bhavsar (Amit Patel) and Anneke Van Mol (self)

ANCILLARY RESOURCE CENTRE

www.oup.com/uk/stringer2e

OSCE marksheet

An OSCE marksheet is hosted online which you can download and adapt to mark any OSCE in the book. It covers the points we feel are necessary in any psychiatric interview, and has space for you to record key symptoms for the diagnosis you're exploring. Nobody will expect you to 'tick off' every possible symptom when seeing someone in a short interview, but it's a good idea to try to cover key symptoms, as well as touching on symptoms from different domains. For example, in depression, it would be important to cover the core symptoms (mood, enjoyment, ± energy) as well as some biological (e.g. sleep, appetite) and cognitive (e.g. guilt, hopelessness) symptoms. You may find it helpful to annotate the mark scheme as you read *Psychiatry P.R.N.*, building your own bank of mark schemes for when you practice role plays. Assessment criteria vary depending on your university and year of study, so our marksheet is provided for general reference only—check local guidelines.

Also online is the '*Take me with you*' guide to assessment, which can be downloaded, along with instructions on how to perform and mark the MSE.

The 'Take me with you' guide to assessment

This is available for you to download to help jog your memory when interviewing people. It'll help you remember all the subheadings of the psychiatric history and mental state examination.

Videos

We've filmed three clinical scenarios, and provided some written feedback and suggestions for dealing with the patients' questions and worries. We hope that you and your lecturers will find the clips form useful preparation for seminars and, in particular, that they help you feel more confident, ahead of placements. The interviews depicted are designed to be realistic, not perfect, so should provoke some useful tutorial discussion.

Clips are dedicated to depression, post-traumatic stress disorder, and assessing risk of self-harm. Lecturer and student preferences guided the choice of topics for these clips.

Self-assessment resources

Each chapter in Part 2 of the book opens with multiple choice questions, to check your existing knowledge and whet your appetite for the chapter. Online, you can find additional self-assessment resources: extended matching questions (EMQs) and single best answers (SBAs) for *all* chapters.

1 PSYCHIATRIC ASSESSMENT

But you people do not understand me, and I am afraid you never will.

Vincent van Gogh[1]

Your first patient

History

Name

Vincent Willem van Gogh.

Date of birth

30 March 1853.

Referral

Vincent van Gogh (**Figure 1.1**) was brought to Hotel Dieu Hospital, Arles, by police on 24 December 1888. The police were contacted following an incident the previous night when Vincent threatened his friend, Paul Gauguin, with an open straight razor. He fled the scene and later reappeared at a brothel on Rue du Bout d'Arles, asking to see a maid named Gabrielle. He handed her his severed left ear, saying, 'Guard this object very carefully'. He then left. Police discovered blood-soaked towels near the bottom of the stairs in his house, and found Vincent unconscious in his bedroom, bleeding from the wound.

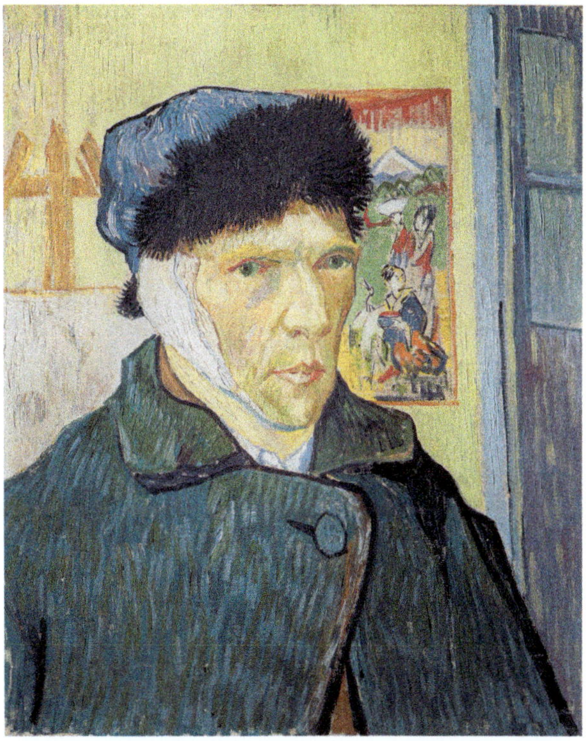

Presenting complaint

'I am having frightful ideas . . . I fear that God has abandoned me.'

History of presenting complaint

Vincent reports that for the past month, he has been aware of God punishing him. Although he denies hearing God speaking, he says he receives divine 'communications' that only he can understand. He won't elaborate further.

Vincent says that his thoughts have become confused over the past month, their volume increasing to the point that 'the noise inside has become unbearable'. He reports not needing to eat, sleeping 2–3 hours a night, and having to work constantly 'to regain God's favour' through art.

Vincent says that his mood has changed as quickly as his thoughts for the past month. He is unable to identify a cause for this change but refers to Paul Gauguin's 'impending treachery'. He provides no explanation for cutting off his ear, saying it was 'quite personal'.

FIGURE 1.1 *Self Portrait with Bandaged Ear*, 1889 (oil on canvas) by Vincent van Gogh (1853–1890).
Ian Dagnall/Alamy Stock Photo

Past psychiatric history

He describes two previous depressive episodes, each lasting a few months. The first followed rejection by a woman in London. The second followed dismissal as an evangelist in Belgium, when he was 25. He did not see a doctor, but his family attempted to arrange inpatient admission twice. After both episodes, Vincent recalls periods of immense energy and productivity, pursuing both religion and art with great intensity, while needing less sleep.

Past medical history

Vincent has suffered gastrointestinal irritability throughout adult life; no cause has been identified. His medical notes mention 'epilepsy' without details. At the age of 29, he needed inpatient treatment for gonorrhoea in The Hague.

Medication history

No prescribed medications.
No known drug allergies.

Family history

Vincent's mother, Anna Cornelia, is still alive. His father, a preacher, died 3 years ago and he is the eldest of six surviving siblings (**Figure 1.2**). His mother delivered a stillborn boy, also named Vincent Willem, exactly 1 year before his birth: Vincent believes that his name is cursed. There is no family history of mental illness, though his siblings, Theo, Willemina and Cornelius, are described as 'sensitive'.

Personal history

Birth and early development

Vincent was born in Groot-Zundert, Holland. His mother experienced an unremarkable pregnancy and labour. There were no delays in reaching developmental milestones. The doctors were concerned about craniofacial asymmetry and his parents described him as a clumsy, quiet and thoughtful child.

Family background and early childhood

Vincent described himself as a moody child, often disobedient, with few friends. He had an early interest in flowers, birds, and insects, but preferred to play alone. His younger brother (Theo) was his closest friend and he felt distant from his parents and other siblings.

Education

He was taught by a governess until he was 12 and then attended boarding school until starting middle school in Tilburg. His attendance was satisfactory but he did not excel in any subject, including art.

Occupation

Vincent worked for his uncle as an art dealer's apprentice from the age of 16, travelling to Brixton, London for work. He then returned to Britain at the age of 23, as a supply teacher in Ramsgate. He tried to study theology, but failed the exams. At 25, he took a post as a missionary in Belgium, but was dismissed for not maintaining a sufficiently tidy appearance. Aged 27, he started painting in Brussels. He has been living and working as an artist in Antwerp, Neunen, Paris, and The Hague for the past 8 years. He reports little financial success from his art and is largely supported by his brother, Theo.

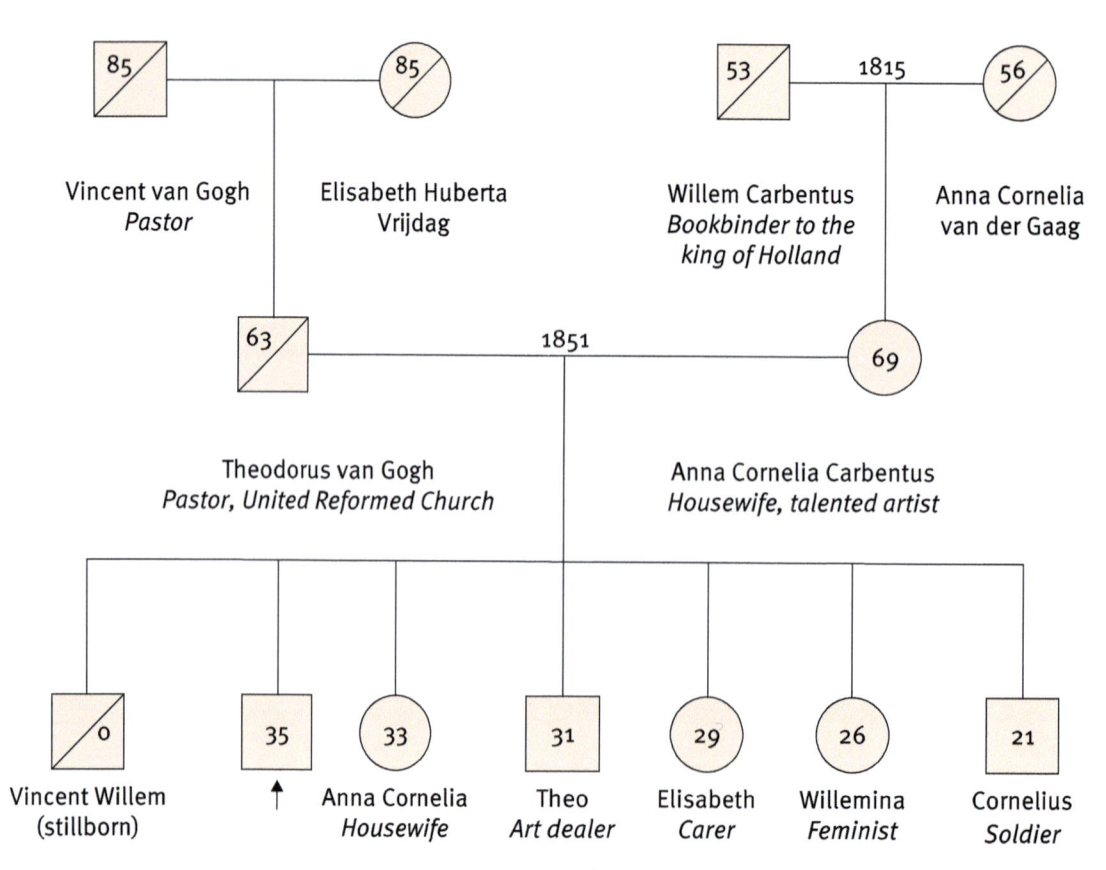

FIGURE 1.2 Vincent van Gogh's genogram

Psychosexual/relationships

Vincent reports two experiences of unrequited love during his twenties, in London and Etten. He intentionally burned his hand with a lamp after the second rejection (by his cousin). His first significant relationship was at 28, with Sien, a former prostitute. She was pregnant when they met and she had problems with alcohol. The relationship ended after about 1 year, following pressure from his family.

Vincent's second significant relationship was with a neighbour, Margot: he proposed to her after she attempted suicide but they did not marry. He saw prostitutes in Arles frequently, whom he describes as his 'sisters of mercy'. He has had less contact with them recently due to reduced libido. Recently, he has been in a close relationship with Gabrielle, a maid in a brothel.

Substance use

Alcohol

He reports drinking alcohol daily to 'stun' himself when 'the storm inside gets too loud'. Without alcohol he shakes, sweats, and craves a drink. He needs increasing amounts of alcohol: he is currently drinking 1.5 bottles of red wine a day.

Vincent has drunk beer and wine in moderation since his late teens. For the past 2 months he has been drinking in the mornings, leading Paul Gauguin to criticize his drinking; this makes him feel guilty and angry. He has never tried to abstain but has thought about cutting down. He recognizes having lost control of his drinking and reports frequent blackouts when intoxicated. He has had fights with Paul Gauguin which he has not remembered and has been barred from several Arles inns for aggressive behaviour.

Smoking

He has smoked a pipe since his teens and is now using 15g of tobacco per day.

Other substances

Vincent admits to occasionally chewing lead-based paints, and sipping turpentine; he does not offer reasons for this.

Forensic history

He denies any criminal convictions, but can be aggressive when intoxicated.

Premorbid personality

Vincent describes being prone to long periods of low mood in adolescence but says he was 'not quite miserable'. He describes himself as hard-working and a loner. He often feels overwhelmed by setbacks, struggling to get back on track afterwards. He enjoys travel, frequently moving between cities. He has a strong Christian faith and believes passionately in social justice. He gave up most of his possessions to work among the poor in Belgium as an evangelist, and sees himself as producing art 'for the people'.

Social history

Vincent's brother, Theo, provides emotional and financial support. Despite offering practical help, his mother can make disparaging remarks about his behaviour, which she considers odd. He moved to Arles in February 1888, to establish a 'southern school' of artists in southern France. He has been sharing 'The Yellow House' with the Parisian artist Paul Gauguin for the past 9 weeks. There has been a mixed reception from the Arles community; Vincent thinks that they view him as an eccentric.

Collateral history from Paul Gauguin, with Vincent's consent

Paul reports that over the past 9 weeks Vincent has been increasingly irritable, unpredictably aggressive, and talking to himself. He has been preoccupied with religious matters, speaking of profound meanings in his paintings which are not obvious to others. Vincent has not been sleeping much, and has been eating poorly, drinking heavily, and painting continuously. In the past month, Vincent has produced over 25 paintings, which he considers his best to date.

Paul reports unresponsive episodes which Vincent cannot recall afterwards. These are associated with shaking and loss of motor control, or apparent sleepwalking. Paul thinks his own intention to leave Arles may have affected Vincent, who he thinks is 'terrified' of living alone. Paul suggests Vincent cut off his ear to emulate the Arles practice where victorious bullfighters cut off a bull's ear for their beloved.

Mental state examination (MSE)

Appearance and behaviour

Gaunt, white man with red hair and beard, his head bandaged; bloodstains over his left ear.[2] Appropriately dressed in blue cap with fur trim and matching coat. Appears poorly kempt, with sallow skin, unshaven, and a strong smell of alcohol. Smokes a pipe nervously throughout the interview. Has difficulty maintaining eye contact and is frequently distracted by objects in the room, including a vase of sunflowers. Noted whispering to himself throughout the interview, apparently responding to someone or something. He looks tense, pacing the room agitatedly for 10 minutes. Although not keen to engage, no evidence of aggression.

Speech
Pressure of speech. Volume varies from a whisper to a shout, when agitated. Tone switches between irritable, gloomy, and excited. Vincent complains that he 'cannot keep up' with his thoughts and finds their speed distressing. Evident flight of ideas, with rapid changes in topic. Fluent French, with Dutch accent.

Mood
Subjectively: 'Black, black as the night!' Objectively: Labile, switching rapidly between euphoria, tearfulness, and irritability.

Thought
Predominant religious themes, although specific beliefs unclear. Repeats that God 'has forsaken me', which is communicated to him through everyday objects. At one point says 'I am in the Garden of Gethsemane'. Persecutory delusions regarding Paul Gauguin: believes conspiring against him with other Parisian artists. Will not elaborate on their alleged plans but cannot be convinced of their innocence. Reports no thoughts of self-harm. When asked about his ear, replies, 'That affair is over now'. Denies thoughts of harming others, including Paul Gauguin.

Perception
Denies illusions or hallucinations in any modality. Whispers to himself as though responding to auditory hallucinations. Probable visual hallucinations: eyes repeatedly tracking unseen stimulus around the room.

Cognition
Fully oriented to time and place; further cognitive exam not carried out.

Insight
Partial insight into his condition. Admits feeling unwell from a 'malady of the soul' inflicted by God. Agrees to admission and to accept medication but believes that medicines cannot 'undo God's doing'.

To be continued . . .

Psychiatric assessment

Assessments in psychiatry can seem overwhelming at first: they are longer, more detailed, and have more subsections than in other specialties. Vincent's assessment offers a vivid example of how to structure a psychiatric history and mental state examination, demonstrating where to place information gathered during an assessment.

The exact division of information in the history and MSE isn't set in stone, reflecting the challenge of summarizing someone's entire life into simple categories. The most important thing is to *listen* to the person's story, to understand why *this* person is experiencing *this* problem at *this* time. Your assessment should lead readers through the information, formulating your conclusion as you go. Just as maths exams say 'Show your working', your assessment should provide all the information needed to justify your differential diagnosis, and bring the person to life.

History

Referral
Set the scene with the person's name, age, gender, and ethnicity. Explain how they presented to the hospital or clinic, and whether admission was voluntary ('informal') or compulsory (e.g. under a section of the Mental Health Act in England and Wales).

Presenting complaint
Use the person's own words—it keeps their story fresh and avoids misinterpreting their presentation from the start. Useful questions might be:

- What brought you into hospital today?
- Have you had any problems recently? Can you tell me about them?

History of presenting complaint
Describing the period leading up to admission, explore the presenting complaint(s), or problem(s), as for any history. This might be a worry, mood, delusion, (e.g. 'The government is spying on me'), hallucination (e.g. 'I hear people talking about me'), physical ailment, or social problem.

Use 'NOTEPAD' to ensure that you include:

- **N**ature of problem.
- **O**nset.
- **T**riggers.
- **E**xacerbating/relieving factors.
- **P**rogression (improving, worsening, or staying the same; intermittent or continuous).
- **A**ssociated symptoms.
- **D**isability (effect on life).

Before finishing, summarize the person's presenting complaint and ask:

- Is there anything else I should know?

💡 **Associated symptoms are guided by *your* knowledge. Patients may not know that depression is associated with insomnia and hopelessness, so ask *specific* questions.**

Past psychiatric history

Ask about previous contact with mental health services, symptoms treated by their general practitioner (GP), and times of stress or depression which they handled without medical input.

- Has anything like this ever happened before?
- Have you had any stress-related problems before?

Find out when past episodes occurred, how long they lasted, and whether they required admission to hospital or use of the Mental Health Act. Note diagnoses and treatments, highlighting treatments that helped. Always check for previous risks while unwell (self-harm, self-neglect, suicide attempts, violence or neglect of children or vulnerable adults).

Past medical history

List past and present physical health problems:

- Physical symptoms may relate to the presenting complaint (e.g. hyperthyroidism can cause anxiety, multiple sclerosis can cause depression).
- People with mental health problems are at increased risk of certain physical problems (e.g. diabetes secondary to antipsychotic medication or lifestyle factors).

Medication history

List current medications, both prescribed and over-the-counter. Always note drug allergies and side effects. Ask about previous psychiatric medications, and why they were stopped.

Family history

Drawing a genogram *with* the person is the clearest way to obtain a family history. For each relative, include:

- Name, age, and occupation.
- Any mental health problems.
- Physical health problems.
- Age of death and cause.

> Genograms are tricky at first, but quickly become easier with practice.

Personal history

This is the person's life story. At first, include as much detail as possible in each section, practising how to ask questions and order information. With experience, you can act more like a biographer, focusing on headline events that directly relate to the presenting complaint.

Birth and early development

Unless assessing a child or someone with a neurodevelopmental or neurological disorder, it's usually enough to ask:

- Do you know if there were any problems with your mother's pregnancy and your birth?
- When did you start walking and talking?

Generally, if they don't know much about this, they were probably 'normal' (i.e. full-term spontaneous vaginal delivery reaching milestones at average ages). If there *were* problems, find out details, including:

- Prematurity.
- Labour complications/birth trauma/interventions, e.g. Caesarean section.
- Time in special care/delayed discharge.
- Paediatric follow-up.

Family background and early childhood

Record periods of serious or prolonged illness, separation from parents, and neglect or abuse.

- What was it like growing up in your family?
- What were your parents and siblings like? How did you get on?
- Was early childhood a happy time?
- Did anything traumatic happen?

Education

This section provides lots of information about personality and social skills, and some indication of intelligence. Note age and level of achievement on leaving education, e.g. number of qualifications and grades:

- What was school like for you?
- Did you have any problems at school?

Also explore specific issues:

- Did you have close friends?
- What were they like?
- Were you shy?
- Were you bullied?
- Did you ever get in trouble for things like bullying or playing truant?
- How did you get on with teachers?
- Were you near the top, middle, or bottom of the class?

Occupation

Chronologically list the person's jobs, including durations and reasons for leaving, e.g. promotion/

resignation/dismissal. Did they enjoy working? Look for trends, e.g. numerous brief jobs ending with arguments. This may say something about their interpersonal relationships or response to authority.

Psychosexual/relationships

List relationships chronologically, using common sense to determine the level of detail. Which was their longest relationship? What happened? Have they noticed any patterns?

- Age of first intercourse.
- Sexual orientation.
- Quality of relationships, e.g. abusive, supportive.
- Marriages, civil partnerships, cohabiting, or otherwise.

If currently in a relationship, ask about duration, partner's name and occupation, and whether they are content. Check for any sexual problems.

Substance use

Ask about past and present drug, alcohol, and cigarette use. Check when they first tried each drug individually, tracking their pattern of use forward from that point. Ask about route of administration and amount used, including changes over time. Look for features suggesting *dependence*, e.g. withdrawal symptoms, increasing use (tolerance). Note attempted abstinence and formal detoxifications. Check for associated physical symptoms, e.g. hepatitis, withdrawal seizures.

Forensic history

This covers offending behaviour:

- Have you ever been in trouble with the police?

List offences, noting serious convictions and sentences. Clearly record details of violent or sex offences. Find out whether they were committed while unwell, and think about symptoms which might increase risk, e.g. persecutory delusions can lead a person to carry a weapon for self-protection. Consider offences linked to the person's diagnosis, e.g. theft to fund addiction.

> 💡 It's worth asking if they have ever broken the law without being caught.

Social history

The social history is the person's *current* day-to-day situation. It should cover:

- Housing type (rented/owned/homeless/hostel) and who they live with.
- Finances, including welfare benefits.
- Current employment/training.
- Activities and interests.
- Carer responsibilities.
- Social network.

Premorbid personality

Ask explicitly *what the person was like* before they became unwell, in addition to their personal history.

- Before all this happened, what kind of person were you (e.g. Anxious? Easy-going? Sociable? Shy?)?
- How would your friends describe you?
- How do you cope under pressure?
- Do you have any views that you hold strongly? Are you religious?

> 💡 **Always check for final points:**
> - **Is there anything we haven't covered that you think I should know?**
> - **Have we missed anything important?**

Collateral history

Information from someone who knows the person well is useful—especially if the patient can't or won't talk to you, or has limited insight into how their behaviour or personality have changed. You need consent to actively contact their family or friends, as doing so may disclose a hospital admission of which they were not aware. If a relative approaches *you* (e.g. on the ward), listening to them doesn't breach confidentiality, you just can't *tell* them anything without the patient's permission. If collateral historians don't want the person to know what they have said, document the information in a separate part of their notes—consider the potential impact on their relationships if they access their notes in future.

> 💡 Don't *assume* that collateral histories are always accurate. Some people *may* give misleading or deliberately false information.

Mental state examination

Past psychopathology belongs in the history; if *you* observe it, put it in the MSE. Like cardiovascular or neurological examinations, your MSE describes *your* findings after history-taking. In an abdominal examination, you wouldn't report jaundice if the person wasn't yellow—even if you knew they had liver disease or looked jaundiced yesterday. Likewise, don't mention hallucinations in your MSE unless you observe the patient hallucinating or they describe *current* hallucinations. Many symptoms fluctuate. It's crucial to document the presence *or absence* of symptoms on examination, to enable accurate monitoring of a person's recovery or deterioration. If your MSE doesn't report psychopathology described in a recent history, note this clearly, to ensure that it isn't overlooked (e.g. 'No hallucinations elicited in any modality, in contrast to history provided'). Often, your history relies on the person's own words; your MSE allows you to *label* symptoms you've identified.

The MSE follows a set of structured headings:

- Appearance and behaviour.
- Speech.
- Mood.
- Thought.
- Perception.
- Cognition.
- Insight.

💡 You'll collect most of the information for your MSE while taking a history; if the person spent the last hour outlining a complex conspiracy against them, *don't* ask all over again just because you're 'now doing' the MSE. Instead, write details about their delusions under 'Thought'.

💡 Remember, your MSE is subjective: it's *your* assessment. Write your *own* impression but bear cultural differences in mind. What you find 'disinhibited' might be an appropriate expression of distress for another culture. Keep language factual, but non-judgemental.

Appearance and behaviour

Imagine you're watching a film with the sound off. Include everything you can describe under appearance and behaviour (plus smells, if relevant). A good description highlights diagnostic clues. Anyone who had read it could easily identify your patient.

General appearance

Start with age, gender, build, and ethnicity. Then note (if relevant):

- Hair, make-up, clothing.
- Physical features, e.g. gait, sensory aids, body habitus.
- Scars, piercings, tattoos.
- Self-care: well-kempt or self-neglecting, e.g. dishevelled, stained clothing, malodorous.

Clothing deserves special mention if inappropriate (e.g. shorts in winter) or striking. Sometimes it reflects underlying mood, e.g. dark clothes in depression; garish clothes in mania. Very loose or tight clothing may indicate recent weight change.

Behaviour

- Facial expression, e.g. smiling, scowling, fearful.
- Eye contact, e.g. responsive/staring/downcast/avoidant/distracted.
- Posture, e.g. hunched shoulders.
- Activity level: overactive/underactive.
- Describe *what* they're doing, e.g. pacing/standing motionless.
- Movement speed may be slowed (motor retardation) in depression or speeded up in mania.
- Rapport: does the person relate to you in a withdrawn/cold/polite/friendly/rude/guarded (suspicious, or deliberately withholding information) manner? A disinhibited person may be over-familiar, invading your personal space.

Other movements

- Extrapyramidal side effects can result from antipsychotics (see p. 87). Mention their absence or report:
  - Akathisia: internal restlessness, causing fidgety movements, especially of legs.
  - Parkinsonism: shuffling gait, 'pill rolling' hand tremor, slowed movements, rigidity.
  - Tardive dyskinesia: rhythmic involuntary movements of the face, limbs, and trunk, e.g. grimacing, chewing.
- Repetitive movements:
  - Mannerisms: appear goal-directed, e.g. sweeping hair from face.
  - Stereotypies: *not* goal-directed, e.g. flicking fingers at air.
  - Tics: purposeless, involuntary movements involving a group of muscles, e.g. blinking.
  - Compulsions: irresistible rituals, e.g. hand-washing.
- Catatonia: rare presentations of abnormal mobility, e.g. 'waxy flexibility' (see p. 85).

Other

- Responding to (suspected) hallucinations, e.g. looking intently at 'nothing', talking to an unseen person.
- Smells, e.g. body odour, urine, alcohol.

Speech

Everyone's speech can be described in terms of:

- **Rate:** fast, slow, normal.
- **Volume:** loud, soft, normal, e.g. shouting, whispering.
- **Tone:** the emotional quality of speech, e.g. sarcastic, angry, glum, calm, neutral. Loss of prosody (the natural lilt and stresses in sentences) produces monotonous speech.
- **Flow:** speech may be spontaneous, or only when prompted; hesitant, or with long pauses before answers; garrulous and uninterruptible.

Because of the overlap between them, speech and thought are difficult to separate: speech is our window to the person's thoughts. Think of speech as a train and thoughts as passengers.

- Train speed: the rate of speech.
- Number of passengers: abundance of thoughts.
- Route: the way that thoughts progress, linking from one idea to the next.

Therefore, normal speech and thought would be a train travelling at normal speed, reasonably full of passengers. The train takes a logical route from station A to station B.

In *formal thought disorder*, the route is disrupted in various ways: the *form* of thought (and speech) is abnormal, independent of the *content* of the thoughts. The train can drive too quickly or too slowly (increased or decreased rate of speech and underlying thoughts). It can also:

- Drive too fast, while overcrowded with passengers. This is *pressure of speech*, reflecting underlying *pressure of thought*. It feels like machine-gun fire and is hard to interrupt. It is usually seen in mania.
- Drive slowly with few passengers. This is *poverty of speech*, reflecting underlying *poverty of thought*, usually seen in depression.
- Stop without warning and throw passengers off. This is *thought block*: complete emptying of the mind of thoughts, shown by sudden halts in speech. It's sometimes seen in schizophrenia.

With normal speed and passengers, a train can still make an unnecessary lengthy detour, via minor, peripheral stations, finally reaching station B at last. This is *circumstantial speech*, reflecting *over-inclusive thinking* which adds excessive details and sub-clauses to every point.

While overcrowded and speeding, a train can make sudden detours, quickly passing through unexpected stations. This is *flight of ideas*. The route is understandable, because there's a reason for each detour. Ideas may be linked normally, or through *clang associations* (rhyming connections, e.g. bang, sang) or puns (playing on words with the same sounds but different meanings, e.g. tire, tyre). Often in flight of ideas, new thoughts arise from cues in the room. The original route to station B is abandoned when new passengers join the train; this keeps happening, so the intended destination is never reached. This is commonly seen in mania.

Derailment may occur if the train leaves the tracks, reaching a set of unintended destinations not obviously connected by railway lines. This may happen in schizophrenia and is difficult to follow, since speech is muddled, without understandable connections between thoughts. Derailment is also called *knight's move thinking*—because of the knight's indirect path in chess—or *loosening of association*.

Neologisms (made-up words or standard words given an idiosyncratic meaning) are also seen.

Although the train would usually progress from station B to station C, in *perseveration* it becomes stuck at station B. Answers to questions are repeated inappropriately, e.g.:

> **You:** What's your name?
> **Elvis:** Elvis.
> **Y:** How old are you?
> **E:** Elvis.

This usually occurs in organic states (e.g. dementia).

The following neurological symptoms should be noted in your MSE, but aren't features of thought disorder:

- Dysarthria—impaired articulation.
- Dysphasia—impaired comprehension or generation of language, due to brain injury.

💡 In *word salad*, words are so disconnected that sentences lack all meaning, e.g. 'Limerick and alter prep lemon enlist if light subsonic thrum ginger'.

Mood

Mood and affect can be used synonymously, e.g. 'affective disorders' are disorders of mood. Technically, mood is the person's pervasive, sustained experience (their 'climate') and affect is their momentary changing state (the current 'weather'). Divide this section into:

- **Subjective:** how the *person* says they feel, in their own words.
- **Objective:** what *you think* about their emotional state, e.g. low, elated, irritable, anxious. As well as describing a general *mood*, comment on its variability:
  - Labile—changeable affect, e.g. flitting between anger, tears, laughter (like weather switching between sunshine and showers).
  - Flattened/blunted—lack of normal affective variability.

Affect is *incongruent* if the person's report doesn't match their presentation, e.g. they giggle while saying they feel depressed. If the person's affect varies appropriately during the conversation and is neither particularly 'up' nor 'down' you can write, 'Reactive and *euthymic*'.

💡 **Save symptoms of depression (e.g. appetite, sleep) for the history.**

1 Psychiatric Assessment

Thought

The *content* of thought is the person's *beliefs* and *ideas*. Give verbatim examples or fully describe the content of any delusions.

> 💡 **Even if there is nothing 'abnormal' about the person's thought content, you need to record something! What are they thinking about?**

Preoccupations and worries

Preoccupations are recurrent thoughts which the person is able to put aside. *Worries* are similar, but cause feelings of anxiety or tension.

- What kinds of things do you worry about?
- What's on your mind?

Delusions

A delusion is a fixed (usually false) belief, held despite rational argument or evidence to the contrary. It can't be fully explained by the person's cultural, religious, or educational background. Occasionally, the belief is true, but coincidentally, since the reasoning behind it is faulty, e.g. a person with delusional jealousy might (rightly) believe that their partner's cheating, but when asked how they know, might say it's because their partner burned the dinner.

Delusions feel as real as any other thought. If you were *deluded* that you were a medical student, this belief would feel as real as the belief you currently have that you *are* a medical student. No one could convince you otherwise because you would *know* it was true, and other people's disbelief would annoy you. This makes asking about delusions a sensitive subject! Fortunately, delusions generally relate to things that are important to the person, so often come up in conversation. Listen sensitively and explore anything unusual, non-judgementally.

> 💡 **Be alert to evasive replies from someone who's guarded: be curious but respectful.**

> 💡 *See p. 93 for tips on asking about delusions.*

True *primary delusions* are rare. They arise completely 'out of the blue' in someone without any prior symptoms. You're *much* more likely to encounter *secondary delusions*, which follow another symptom, such as an altered mood, or a hallucination (e.g. after hearing disembodied voices, the person starts believing they're being followed). *Systematized delusions* occur when delusions grow and build on each other, into an elaborate delusional system. See **Table 1.1** for types of delusions.

TABLE 1.1 Types of delusions

Type	Absolutely believing that . . .	Example
Grandiose	You're extremely special/important/powerful	'I'm rich and famous'
Persecutory	Others are persecuting/targeting/harming you	'They're spying on me'
Hypochondriacal	You have a specific illness	'I have cancer' (despite no evidence)
Nihilistic	Something vitally important is absent	'I'm dead/my organs are rotting'
Of guilt	You've committed a sin/crime	'I murdered that guy'
Of reference	Objects/events/actions have a very special meaning for you	'The news is about me', 'cars are arranged as messages'
Of infidelity	Your partner is unfaithful	'They're cheating, I just *know* it!'
Amorous/erotomanic	Someone is in love with you	'Prince William's my boyfriend'
Of control/passivity	Your movements, sensations, emotions, or impulses are directly controlled by outside forces	See p. 82
Of thought interference: *Thought withdrawal*	Someone/something is removing thoughts from your head	See p. 82
Thought insertion	Thoughts are being placed into your mind	
Thought broadcast	Your thoughts are audible to others	

Psychiatric assessment

💡 *Paranoid* is an umbrella term, meaning something relates to the self. *Technically*, all delusions are paranoid: they all refer to the person, somehow. Paranoid delusions *officially* include persecutory, grandiose, jealous, and erotomanic delusions. Nevertheless, when people say they feel 'paranoid', they're usually talking about persecutory beliefs.

Partial delusions are like delusions but not held quite as firmly—the person acknowledges some doubt (partial conviction). They include 'nearly' delusional beliefs building up to a psychotic episode, and delusions that are weakening during recovery. With close questioning, someone with a partial delusion would accept the possibility their belief *could* be wrong, e.g. that their imagination could be playing tricks on them.

Overvalued ideas

These are reasonable ideas, pursued beyond the bounds of reason. The person's life revolves around the idea, to the point that it causes distress to them or others. For example, you might, reasonably, become annoyed that your neighbour fills their front garden with gnomes, believing they 'make the neighbourhood look cheap'. It's *not* reasonable, though, to quit medical school to sue your neighbour and finally destroy the gnomes with a hammer! Your overvalued idea is that the gnomes make the neighbourhood look cheap.

Obsessions

These are recurrent, unwanted intrusive thoughts, images, or impulses which enter the person's mind, despite attempts to resist them. Deep down, the thought is known to be irrational, *unlike* a delusion, where it's absolutely believed to be true. Obsessions are also recognized as the person's own thoughts; they don't come from an outside source (unlike thought insertion).

Obsessions are unpleasant, and make the person feel acutely uncomfortable or anxious. They often have taboo themes, like contamination, violence, sex, or religion, e.g. 'I've got HIV'. This discomfort can often be relieved or 'neutralized' by a compulsion. *Compulsions* are repeated, stereotyped, superficially purposeful rituals that the person feels compelled to perform. They may be resisted, since the person knows that they are senseless. Compulsions can be actions (e.g. hand-washing) or thoughts (e.g. counting) but are mentioned here because of their relationship to obsessions. If you observe compulsions during your assessment, note them under Appearance and Behaviour.

- Do any thoughts keep coming into your head, even though you try to block them out?
- Some people have rituals that they need to do in a specific way. Do you do anything like that?

Thoughts of harm

Ask *everyone* about thoughts of harming themselves or others. Document all thoughts with full details of any plans, e.g. preparations, method, timing, victim. (See p. 71 and p. 273.)

Perception

Perception relates to the person's sensory world. Explore all five modalities; if unremarkable, you can state 'No illusions or hallucinations in any modality'.

Illusions

An illusion is the *misperception* of a real, external stimulus. People are more likely to make perceptual mistakes when they're drowsy, unable to attend to the stimulus, very upset, or can't see or hear clearly (e.g. someone who's scared of spiders could mistake a shadow for a spider after waking at night without their glasses). We all experience illusions, but they're especially common in delirium (where consciousness is clouded).

Hallucinations

A hallucination is a perception in the *absence* of an external stimulus, e.g. hearing a voice when no one has spoken. Hallucinations feel as real as any other perception, so don't ask 'Do you have hallucinations?' (Instead, see p. 94 for tips on asking about hallucinations.)

Check all modalities:

- **Auditory**, e.g. music, voices.
- **Visual**, e.g. flashes, animals.
- **Touch:**
  - **Tactile:** superficial sensations on, or just below, the skin, e.g. of being scratched.
  - **Deep:** internal sensations, e.g. of the liver being twisted and pulled within the belly.
- **Olfactory**, e.g. smelling smoke.
- **Gustatory**, e.g. tasting 'poison' in food.

Voices may be in the first person (speaking as 'I' / 'me'), second person (addressing the person directly as 'you') or third person (talking *about* the person, referring to 'him/her'). Voices particularly suggestive of schizophrenia discuss or argue about the person, give a running commentary of their actions, or say their thoughts aloud (*thought echo*). Always describe the person's experience, e.g. 'second-person auditory hallucinations of an unfamiliar man shouting, 'Your mum's a prostitute!'.

Many people have experienced hallucinations, usually briefly, e.g. on waking (*hypnopompic hallucinations*),

1 Psychiatric Assessment

falling asleep (*hypnagogic hallucinations*), or following bereavement (e.g. hearing the deceased speaking). Auditory hallucinations are the commonest modality in psychosis; visual hallucinations are particularly associated with organic conditions, including delirium and dementia.

Depersonalization and derealization

These are unnerving feelings of unreality, which you may have experienced when tired or anxious. They occur in many disorders.

- **Depersonalization:** the *person* feels unreal—detached, numb, or emotionally distant.
  - Do you ever feel as if you aren't quite real?
- **Derealization:** the *world* feels unreal, e.g. 'like a film set'.
  - Do you ever feel as if the world around you isn't quite real?

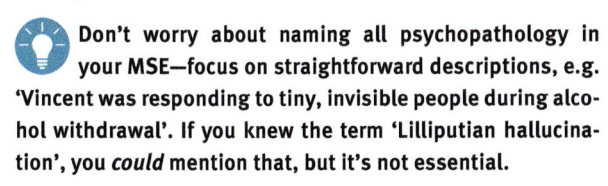

💡 Don't worry about naming all psychopathology in your MSE—focus on straightforward descriptions, e.g. 'Vincent was responding to tiny, invisible people during alcohol withdrawal'. If you knew the term 'Lilliputian hallucination', you *could* mention that, but it's not essential.

Cognition

Cognition is the umbrella term covering thinking and remembering. It includes orientation, attention, concentration, language, and memory, all of which are affected by the person's level of consciousness. By the time you've taken the history, you'll have a reasonable understanding of the person's general cognitive functioning. If they're alert and gave a clear, detailed, and accurate history, it's reasonable to note that attention, concentration, and memory were grossly intact. Orientation to time, place, and person may be clear from the history, although to be certain, you might briefly check these. Perform a cognitive examination, e.g. Mini-Addenbrooke's Cognitive Examination (M-ACE) or Mini Mental State Examination (MMSE), if you have any concerns.

💡 You can find the M-ACE on p. 144.

Insight

Generally used to mean a person's awareness of their mental health problems, insight is never simply *present* or *absent*; it has different levels:

- Awareness that others are concerned by their symptoms or behaviour.
  - Do your friends think you're your usual self?
- Agreement that there's a problem.
  - Do you think there's anything wrong at the moment?
  - Is this normal for you? How are you different to usual?
- Recognition of *mental* health problems (e.g. not attributing them to physical illness).
  - What do you think is causing this? Could it be stress? Or mental health problems?
- Awareness that symptoms require treatment.
  - Do you think that treatment could help?
  - Would you be happy to try some treatment?

Insight can be partial, e.g. someone may not believe they are unwell, but still take medication because they think it satisfies the Mafia, stopping their persecution. It's common to deny having mental health problems. A person attending the emergency department in crisis may have some awareness of relapsing without being fully conscious.

Final thought

A *full* assessment includes a physical examination. Always take a chaperone, and remember that many people don't want repeated physical examinations by students.

Formulation

The formulation includes the case synopsis (most important points from the history and examination), differential diagnosis, risk assessment, aetiology, investigations, management, and prognosis.

Case synopsis

- Background information: name, age, occupation, ethnicity, marital status.
- Summary of current episode.
- Relevant history.
- Examination:
  - Salient features of MSE.
  - Important physical findings, e.g. hemiparesis, jaundice.

Differential diagnosis

Start with your *preferred diagnosis* and then list other differentials, from most to least likely. For each, add reasons for and against the diagnosis. Keep the list short and don't show off by naming rare or eponymous conditions unless certain you're right! Always consider organic (physical health) causes for symptoms, and remember that a person may have more than one diagnosis, e.g. schizophrenia and alcohol dependence.

TABLE 1.2 Factors influencing risk

Current factors	History
• Current mental state, e.g. command hallucinations, persecutory delusions, passivity	• History of self-harm and suicide attempts
• Stated intent/threats to harm someone	• History of violence to others
• Concerns expressed by family/carers	• Past psychiatric history
• Disengagement from services/non-concordance with medication	
• Drug and alcohol use	
• Weapon carrying	
• Social isolation	
• Homelessness	

Risk assessment

Every psychiatric assessment includes consideration of risks posed by the person to themselves or others, whether through intentional injury or neglect (**Table 1.2**). You may state whether you consider each risk to be low, moderate, or high.

Aetiology

From your history and MSE, consider possible *biopsychosocial* causes of the person's difficulties. *Predisposing* factors make people vulnerable to a disorder; *precipitating* factors trigger an episode; perpetuating factors maintain symptoms and may prevent recovery. A grid can structure this material (**Table 1.3**).

Social and psychological factors are often intermingled, e.g. redundancy (a social problem) has a psychological impact. The same factor can both precipitate and perpetuate an episode, and not every 'box' is always filled.

Investigations

We use investigations to exclude physical causes of the presenting complaint (e.g. hypothyroidism causing depression). Review the person's general physical health, and request baseline measures before starting medications:

- Biological, e.g. blood tests, ECG, neuroimaging.
- Psychological, e.g. symptom rating scales, neuropsychological testing.
- Social, e.g. collateral history, GP records.

Management

Management is equally biopsychosocial, i.e. *holistic*: medication is not prescribed in isolation. Consider immediate, medium-term, and long-term treatment—again, a grid helps (**Table 1.4**).

Prognosis

Give your opinion on the person's prognosis, both for their current episode and long term. Include strengths in the person's favour as well as challenges to recovery.

Formulation: Vincent Van Gogh

Case synopsis

Vincent van Gogh is a 35-year-old, single, white Dutch artist. The police brought him to hospital on 24/12/1888 after he threatened a friend with a razor, before cutting off his left ear and giving it to a female acquaintance. He struggles to explain his actions but mentions 'frightful ideas' and being forsaken by God. Over the past 9 weeks, Vincent became increasingly agitated, painting continuously. He describes divine 'communications' and feeling punished by God for the past month. He reports racing, confused thoughts, labile mood, reduced appetite and libido, and sleeping 3 hours per

TABLE 1.3 Aetiology example for depression

	Biological	Psychological	Social
Predisposing	Genetics Family history	Premorbid personality	Childhood abuse
Precipitating	Substance use	Feeling helpless	Recent bereavement
Perpetuating	Untreated pain	Cognitive distortions, e.g. pessimism	Lack of support network

TABLE 1.4 Management example

	Biological	Psychological	Social
Immediate	Alcohol detoxification	Psychoeducation	Hospital admission
Medium term	Regular medication	Cognitive behavioural therapy (CBT)	Assist with benefits
Long term	Improve physical health through diet and lifestyle change	Psychodynamic psychotherapy	Gradual return to work

night. Possible triggers include breakdown of his friendship with Paul Gauguin, exacerbated by alcohol, lead paint, and turpentine misuse.

Vincent has a history of two previous episodes of depression following losses, neither of which was treated. Each was followed by elevated energy and creativity. He self-harmed once before, burning his hand (aged 28). He was treated for gonorrhoea at 29 and has a history of possible seizures.

On MSE, he was unkempt, distracted, and agitated, with labile affect, responding to apparent visual and auditory hallucinations. Vincent showed pressure of speech and flight of ideas. He was preoccupied with religious themes and persecutory delusions regarding a conspiracy by Parisian artists.

Physical examination noted an amputated left earlobe, with a sutured wound, free from signs of infection.

Differential diagnosis

Bipolar affective disorder (BPAD)

- **Current episode mixed affective (see p. 45).**
  - *For*: mixed affective state, in the context of previous depressive episodes and possible hypomania. Depressive symptoms: low mood, appetite, libido, and mood-congruent delusion of punishment by God. Manic symptoms: reduced need for sleep, increased creative energy, and flight of ideas.
  - *Against*: organic aetiology still to be excluded.
  - *Severity*: severe, as psychotic symptoms (hallucinations and delusions) are present.

Organic disorders

- **Temporal lobe epilepsy (TLE):**
  - *For:* history of probable seizures. Affective and psychotic symptoms are common in TLE.
  - *Against*: unclear description of seizures.
- **Neurosyphilis ('general paresis'):**
  - *For:* history of sexually transmitted disease and known relationships with commercial sex workers. Neurosyphilis can present with seizures and affective symptoms.
  - *Against:* no symptoms or signs of syphilis on examination, e.g. Argyll–Robertson pupil, tremor, leg weakness, cognitive impairment. Symptoms develop 10–20 years after infection.
- **Lead encephalopathy:**
  - *For:* chewing lead-based paint. Seizures, hallucinations, abdominal pain, irritability, and affective symptoms.
  - *Against:* no confusion, vomiting, ataxia, or peripheral weakness.

Substance use disorder

- **Comorbid alcohol dependence/harmful use of other substances:**
  - *For*: features of dependence syndrome—tolerance, withdrawal, craving, loss of control, and use despite harm. Consumes paint and turpentine.
  - *Against:* no evidence of salience or reinstatement after abstinence. No definite harm from paint/turpentine.
- **Delirium tremens:**
  - *For:* chronic alcohol excess and hallucinations.
  - *Against:* neither tremulous nor disoriented.
- **Alcoholic hallucinosis:**
  - *For*: chronic alcohol excess and hallucinations.
  - *Against:* affective symptoms.

Schizoaffective disorder

  - *For*: psychotic *and* affective symptoms together.
  - *Against*: affective symptoms predate psychotic symptoms.

Risk assessment

Although Vincent denies thoughts of harm to himself or others, he is at *high* risk of both, having recently cut off his earlobe and threatened a friend. Continued excessive substance use increases his risk of impulsive acts; he has a history of aggression when intoxicated.

TABLE 1.5 Aetiology—Vincent van Gogh

	Biological	Psychological	Social
Predisposing	Neurodevelopmental abnormalities (craniofacial asymmetry, clumsiness)	Low self-esteem secondary to recurrent rejection History of depression Possible attachment problems with mother, born 1 year after stillborn brother	Financial hardship and reliance on brother Lack of artistic recognition
Precipitating	Substance use Sleep deprivation	Threatened loss of friendship	Social rejection in Arles Critical family (mother)
Perpetuating	Substance use Sleep deprivation	Fear of public humiliation	Isolation

Aetiology

See **Table 1.5**.

Investigations

1. Blood tests: FBC, U&Es, LFTs, TFTs, and lead levels.
2. Blood-borne virus screen, syphilis serology, and genital swab.
3. Consider neuroimaging: recent history of 'seizures' with hallucinations.
4. Electroencephalogram (EEG).
5. Collateral history: Theo van Gogh and Gabrielle.

Management

See **Table 1.6**.

In the short term, inpatient admission will reduce the risk of self-harm, access to weapons, and contact with at-risk individuals. Vincent should be observed by ward staff for psychotic symptoms. Longer term, treatment of his underlying illness and follow-up by a community mental health team will reduce risk.

Prognosis

In the short term, Vincent's prognosis is good, since he's accepting medication, is abstinent from substances, has a supportive brother, and has strong interests and abilities in art and theology. He's at risk of relapse long-term, especially given his prior episodes. Concordance with medication will improve his prognosis, although comorbid substance misuse, being male, a poor employment history, and psychotic symptoms are poor

TABLE 1.6 Management—Vincent van Gogh

	Biological	Psychological	Social
Immediate	Alcohol detoxification Medical ± plastic surgery review of earlobe	Reassurance Carer support (Theo)	Inpatient admission Support alcohol abstinence
Medium term	Refer to physicians if lead poisoning/syphilis/epilepsy confirmed Mood stabilizer (e.g. lithium)	Education and motivational interviewing for substance misuse Cognitive behavioural therapy Safe-sex education	Alcoholics Anonymous Accommodation support (risk of eviction) Reconnect with church network
Long term	Monitor for mood stabilizer side effects	Psychodynamic psychotherapy, e.g. explore issues relating to loss of stillborn brother	Social skills training for relationships Support to exhibit art/return to education

prognostic indicators. He is at high risk of future self-harm and suicide attempts.

Follow-up information

Vincent was diagnosed with epilepsy by Dr Felix Rey, at Hotel Dieu Hospital. He was prescribed potassium bromide (a popular anti-epileptic at the time), which seemed beneficial, short term. Gauguin returned to Paris and never saw Vincent again. After discharge, Vincent suffered numerous psychotic relapses, probably precipitated by continued substance use. In 1889, he admitted himself to an asylum in St Rémy, where he remained for a year, suffering at least three further relapses. He produced 300 works of art, including *Starry Night*. On 27 July 1890, Vincent shot himself in the chest, in a field outside Auvers. He died at home, 2 days later, with Theo by his side; his artwork received little recognition during his lifetime.

Over 30 diagnoses have been proposed for Vincent's presentation, including BPAD, schizophrenia, neurosyphilis, lead poisoning, Ménière disease, and acute intermittent porphyria.

Although there was no family history of mental illness at the time of his admission, members of his family developed psychiatric disorders after his death.

- Theo died in 1891 at the Medical Institution for the Insane following a 'mental and physical collapse,' possibly due to syphilis.
- Willemina (sister) may have suffered schizophrenia. She was institutionalized and died in an asylum in 1941.
- Cornelius (brother) was a soldier, officially killed in action in 1900. Unconfirmed reports claim that he committed suicide.

Movie buff
At Eternity's Gate (2018).
Loving Vincent (2017).
Vincent and Theo (1990).

Book shelf
Gayford, M. (2006) *The Yellow House: Van Gogh, Gauguin and Nine Turbulent Weeks in Arles*.
Murphy, B. (2016) *Van Gogh's Ear: The True Story*.
Sims, A. (1988) *Symptoms in the Mind: An Introduction to Descriptive Psychopathology*.
Tralbaut, M.E. (1959) *Van Gogh: A Pictorial Biography*.

Notes

The information contained in Vincent's assessment is drawn from several sources, particularly *The Illness of Vincent van Gogh* (Blumer 2002) and *The Yellow House* (Gayford 2006). Vincent's views on his alcohol consumption have been elaborated to show symptoms of alcohol dependence.

1. *The Complete Letters of Van Gogh: With Reproductions of All the Drawings in the Correspondence.* (Thames and Hudson Ltd 1958).
2. Vincent drew himself in a mirror, so his *right* ear looks bandaged.

The 'Take me with you' guide to assessment

History
- Background information
- 'Presenting complaint'
- History of presenting complaint
- Past psychiatric history
- Past medical history
- Medication history
- Family history
- Personal history
  - Birth and early development
  - Family background and early childhood
  - Education
  - Occupation
  - Psychosexual/relationships
- Substance misuse
- Forensic history
- Social history
- Premorbid personality
- Collateral history

Mental state examination (MSE)
- Appearance and behaviour
- Speech:
  - Rate
  - Volume
  - Tone
  - Flow
- Mood:
  - Subjective
  - Objective
- Thought:
  - Preoccupations and worries
  - Delusions
  - Overvalued ideas
  - Obsessions
  - Thoughts of harm
- Perception:
  - Illusions
  - Hallucinations
  - Depersonalization and derealization
- Cognition—see M-ACE (p. 143–4).
- Insight

2 SAFETY

Students sometimes worry they'll be attacked during psychiatric placements. In reality, very few people with mental health problems are aggressive and even fewer would target a medical student. Nonetheless, maximize your safety by reading this chapter before you start at a hospital or community mental health team (CMHT).

1. Dress code

Wear practical and non-provocative clothing—nothing tight, short, or revealing. Anything around your neck could be grabbed or pulled, so avoid ties, scarves, and necklaces; wear your ID badge at your belt, or on a 'quick release' lanyard with three break points.

2. Stick together

Don't interview alone. Working in pairs lets you seek help easily if feeling uncomfortable. Mixed-sex pairings mean you always have a chaperone for sensitive issues, e.g. discussing sexual abuse.

3. Work with staff

Introduce yourself to medical and nursing staff; they can't support you if they don't know you exist. Ask them to show you around the ward or CMHT, noting exits, and asking how their alarm system works (e.g. personal alarms, wall alarms). When choosing people to interview, ask:

- Who'd be good for me to talk to?
- How have they been today?
- Is there anything I should know before seeing them?
- What's their risk history?

Make sure a supportive staff member knows *who* you're interviewing, *where* you'll be, and *how long* you expect to take; ask them to check on you intermittently. Borrow a personal alarm if available.

4. Prepare the room

Choose an interview room with a window in the door so that staff can see you. Remove potential weapons (e.g. snooker cues) and arrange chairs beforehand:

- Locate the alarm(s).
- Sit nearest the door and within reach of an alarm.
- Ensure you both have a clear path to the door.
- Keep 'personal space' between chairs. Sitting too close heightens tension and places you within grabbing distance.

! **Don't arm people with scalding liquids—stick to offering cold drinks or put plenty of cold milk in cups of tea!**

5. No drink or drugs

Don't interview anyone you suspect is intoxicated: drugs and alcohol increase the risk of aggression.

6. Behave yourself

Courtesy is essential and helps you stay safe:

- Gain consent to interview, explaining that it's voluntary and they can stop at any time.
- Seek permission before taking notes. Stop writing if it makes someone suspicious or uncomfortable.
- Never laugh at someone, argue, or dismiss their beliefs.
- Respect culture, religion, age, gender, and sexuality.
- Make 'appropriate' eye contact (staring is threatening; avoidant eye contact looks disinterested).
- Don't intimidate: question gently and use calm body language.

7. Read the signs

Most aggression is preceded by *warning* signs. If you spot any of these, calmly and politely end the interview, thanking the person for speaking to you or suggesting you take a break. If they're unhappy about something, offer to address this for them by speaking to nursing staff.

- Verbal warnings:
    - Tone: angry, sarcastic, threatening, rude.
    - Volume: shouting *or* prolonged silence.

- Abuse: swearing or insults.
- Direct threats, e.g. 'I'll hit you in a minute!' (Take these seriously!)
• Physical warnings:
  - Fast breathing, sweating, facial reddening/blanching, dilated pupils.
  - Prolonged staring, frowning.
  - Gritted teeth, clenched fists, trembling, agitation.
  - Pacing or entering your personal space.
  - Violent gestures, e.g. pounding the table, jabbing fingers at you.

8. Trust your gut

Always take your instincts seriously. If you *feel* unsafe (even if you don't know why), end the interview (as mentioned earlier) and leave. Your safety is more important than any history. If you feel threatened, press the alarm to call staff.

9. De-escalation and escape

While exiting or resolving mild hostility . . .
Do:

- Keep your tone and body language calm—no sudden movements.
- Give the person space.
- Apologize if you've upset them, e.g. 'Sorry, I didn't phrase that very well. What I meant was . . .'
- Empathize with them, e.g. 'It sounds like you feel frustrated about . . .'
- Back out (never turn your back on a threatening person).
- Tell staff immediately.

Don't:

- Say 'Calm down!' (This is paradoxically inflammatory—it implies that you think they're *unreasonably* angry).
- Get closer or touch them.
- Try to defuse the situation with humour.
- Mirror (see p. 20) confrontational body language, e.g. by 'squaring up' to someone who stands up, putting your hands on your hips or balling your fists.

If someone stands aggressively, put space between you and stand slightly to their side, shoulder-on, keeping your hands visible and below your waist. This makes you a smaller target, is less confrontational, and lets you back out more easily.

10. In the unlikely event of being assaulted

- Shout, press alarms: staff will sprint to help you.
- Get away.
- Let a doctor fully assess and treat any wounds.
- Complete an incident form.
- Contact the consultant(s) responsible for you and the person concerned, to debrief and gain support.
- Inform your clinical tutor and/or the psychiatry placement lead.
- Take the day off.
- In the very unlikely event of a serious assault, clinical staff will contact the police.
- Seek further support as needed, e.g. university counselling service.

❗ **Never get involved with restraint situations; staff usually have decades of experience and specialist training in verbal 'de-escalation' and managing aggression. Get out of the way, clearing potential weapons and ushering others away.**

3 ESSENTIAL INTERVIEW SKILLS

Psychiatry is brilliant. You're privileged to hear the most interesting, poignant, and inspiring stories. 'Taking a history' is simply helping someone tell their story. It takes excellent communication skills, curiosity, and empathy.

We focus here on the skills you'll need during clinical placements (Chapter 4 covers exam skills). Nurses or doctors can suggest patients for you to approach in wards/clinics. They'll know who's happy to talk, and help you avoid anyone too unwell for you to assess. They usually know how the person likes to be addressed (although always check anyway).

Introductions

Starting out

Nobody *has* to talk to you, so you need to 'sell' it. Don't ask to 'clerk' someone or 'take a history'—it's meaningless to non-medics. Be friendly, confident, and courteous:

- Smile and make eye contact.
- Use their name.
- Introduce yourself.
- Explain why you want to talk.

For example:

> **You:** Ms Jones? Hello, my name's *[name]*. I'm a medical student working with Dr Singh; she said you might talk to me. Is that OK?
>
> **Ms Jones:** What about?
>
> **You:** I'd like to hear about how you came into hospital, and how this admission's been for you. I'm learning to be a doctor, so it would be really helpful.
>
> **Ms Jones:** Sure.
>
> **You:** Thank you. Do you prefer being called Ms Jones, or something else?
>
> **Ms Jones:** Mary is fine.
>
> **You:** Mary it is.

If they don't want to talk, be gracious, and leave it open, e.g. 'No problem. I'm here all week, in case you feel like talking another day.' Some people will talk once they've seen you around, or heard from others that you're ok.

💡 **Offer to help busy staff with ward activities, e.g. music or walking groups. People may feel more comfortable talking after getting to know you better.**

💡 **Some people love handshakes, others can't bear them, e.g. due to arthritis (pain), obsessive–compulsive disorder (perceived contamination), or their cultural background. If you *do* shake, shake well! Perfect yours with a friend, avoiding forceful crunches *or* limp, clammy shakes.**

Comfort and privacy

Speak somewhere private, but let them bring a friend or relative if they like. Move chairs so they're at 90 degrees (facing head-on feels antagonistic, while side-on limits eye contact). Be aware of personal space and how comfortable the distance feels; if they lean or shuffle backwards, you're too close, so back off.

Active listening

Hearing is relatively passive. Listening is an *active* process: you need to *do* something to make it happen. Active listening means fully, thoughtfully concentrating on someone, so you really understand them; it's a way of saying, 'your experience matters to me.' Many people think they're listening when sounds bounce off their eardrums, and may unconsciously employ *anti-listening* techniques (**Box 3.1**) suggesting they don't want to listen.

💡 ***Really* listen to someone today without doing anything else. How's this different from your 'normal' listening? What happens?**

BOX 3.1 Anti-listening techniques with 'translations'

- *Wriggling/fidgeting*—My bladder's *so* full right now.
- *Rushing*—I've something much more important to do.
- *Crossed arms/legs*—Why are you still talking?
- *Slouching*—Boring, boring, boring!
- *Interrupting*—Yeah, whatever.
- *Blank facial expression*—Hmm . . . Spaghetti for dinner?
- *Staring eye contact*—We should fight. I'd definitely win.
- *Writing notes constantly*—Secrets! Not *for* you! *About* you.

Silence

It's hard to listen when two people speak at once, especially if you're one of them. Be quiet, giving the person space to talk. Make intermittent 'listening noises' (*uh-huh/mmm*) and interested facial expressions, so they know you're paying attention.

Don't fear silences, or fill them with questions. Being comfortable with silence lets the person set the pace of the interview, and shows you're confident, and unafraid of difficult subjects. Sometimes, letting a silence last a moment longer than normal can help people open up.

Body language

Show you're listening, friendly, and interested:

- Sit still.
- Lean forward, slightly.
- Use open body language (don't hunch up, or draw in/cross your arms and legs).
- Make eye contact/be ready to meet their gaze if they look up).
- Nod intermittently (to show understanding/agreement).
- Wear an interested expression.

Sit *comfortably* so you don't keep wriggling into new 'listening poses' every few minutes. Although crossed legs can look 'closed', cross them if that's how you're most comfortable—just point your body *towards* the person to show interest.

Making notes keeps your history accurate but can ruin eye contact and rapport. *Ask* whether you can take notes, explaining that you don't want to forget anything important. Only write key points/quotations—you'll naturally remember more if you're listening attentively.

> When people get on well, they unconsciously *mirror* (copy) each other's movements. Deliberately mirroring someone *very subtly* can build rapport.

> Tilting your head to one side *very slightly* lets the speaker know you're listening.

> Be aware: *excessive* nodding, eye contact, and leaning forward can make you look scary.

Ask questions

Style

Questions can be:

- **Closed:** require a brief answer.
  - For example, *Are you Italian? Where are you from?*
- **Open:** encourage people to talk freely.
  - For example, *Why? How? What happened? Can you tell me more about that?*

Start the interview with a relevant open question, e.g.:

- *How were things before you came into hospital?*
- *I don't know why you came to hospital. Could you tell me what happened?*

Now, settle back and listen.

Don't avoid closed questions—they're useful for clarifying important details, but problematic when 'fired' at people, or used like a checklist, e.g.:

You: Was your pain sharp?
Pete: No.
You: Did it burn?
Pete: No.
You: Was it crushing?
Pete: Yes.
You: Did it get worse with breathing in?
Pete: No.
You: With exercise?
Pete: Um . . . No?
You: Was it in the middle of your chest?
Pete: Yes.
You: Have you had it before?
Pete: Yes.
You: Were you short of breath?
Pete: Yes.
You: Did it improve with GTN [glyceryl trinitrate]?
Pete: With what?
You: That medicine in your hand.
Pete: My spray?
You: Yes. Your GTN spray. Did it get better with GTN?
Pete: Nope.

This feels clumsy and uncaring (**Figure 3.1**).

> Try using the *question funnel*. Start with
> an open question or two, before using
> closed questions
> to 'funnel'
> answers
> down
> like
> this
> .

FIGURE 3.1 Question funnel

20   3 Essential Interview Skills

For example:

> **You:** What happened? *[Open]*
>
> **Pete:** I ran upstairs and the pain came on suddenly—crushing me, like someone sitting on my chest, right here *[clenches fist over central chest]*. I couldn't breathe. I was terrified! The pain spread into my jaw and down my left arm. It was just like the last time I had a heart attack. I wanted to get my spray, but it was downstairs, and when I moved, the pain got worse.
>
> **You:** That sounds frightening. How long did it last? *[Closed]*
>
> **Pete:** Half an hour.
>
> **You:** Did you notice anything else? *[Closed]*
>
> **Pete:** Um . . . I was really sweaty.
>
> **You:** Did you feel sick? *[Closed]*
>
> **Pete:** Yes.

Start a new funnel with each new, major topic.

Linkages

Jumping around the history feels awkward. To ensure the person feels heard, link your questions to what they're talking about, e.g.:

> **Mary:** I've been anxious for 2 months.
>
> **You:** Did anything happen 2 months ago? *[Link duration to triggers]*

> **Pete:** I only sleep for 3 hours a night.
>
> **You:** That sounds exhausting. Are you tired? *[Link insomnia to fatigue]*

With a little creativity, you can link most things. You can also gently redirect the interview this way without seeming pushy.

Logical, curious questions

It's easy to worry so much about remembering the 'right' questions, that you forget the *obvious* ones. If a friend said they'd been followed home, you wouldn't—even as a medical student—immediately ask if they'd taken drugs! Your curiosity would spark a logical sequence of questions to understand their story. Taking a psychiatric history is no different, it's just that you're alert to the psychiatric *significance* of the answers, e.g.:

> **Abdul:** *[Slamming door behind him]* I'm being followed!
>
> **You:** Who by?
>
> **Abdul:** A Secret Service guy!
>
> **You:** Why would the Secret Service follow *you*?
>
> **Abdul:** Because I know stuff I shouldn't.
>
> **You:** What stuff?
>
> **Abdul:** About the Illuminati taking over . . .
>
> **You:** How'd you know that?
>
> **Abdul:** I've heard them!
>
> **You:** Heard them?
>
> **Abdul:** Through their bugging device.
>
> **You:** Wow. Tell me exactly what's going on.

Don't overthink things—just listen carefully and ask the next logical, curious question.

People often scatter clues as they talk. If you interrupt their flow to jump in and grab the clue (e.g. 'You did *what* to his grandmother?'), they may feel annoyed, or afraid to answer. Instead, log the clue, wait for the right moment, and calmly redirect the conversation later (e.g. 'You mentioned something about his grandmother?').

Build rapport

People often describe their favourite doctor as having a great 'bedside manner'—otherwise known as *rapport*, or the *ability to get on with people*. It's a combination of good communication skills and your personality. It's why you must be yourself, and retain your individuality. Be professional and polite at all times, but don't let 'being on your best behaviour' make you bland; people want to be looked after by people, not robots, see **Boxes 3.2 and 3.3** for some further advice.

Empathize

One of the reasons people don't want robots as doctors is that robots can't empathize. Empathy isn't feeling *sorry* for someone, but is sometimes described as 'walking in someone else's shoes'. It's trying to imagine what it's like to be in their position, and letting them know that you *get it*. Empathy has three steps:

- **Absorb the story.** Often, you'll have to read between the lines, using context and body language to work

---

BOX 3.2 Useful echolalia

Softly echoing back the person's last words can nudge them to elaborate, without interrupting their flow, e.g.:

Mary: They made it impossible for me.

You: *They . . .?*

Pete: My wife was always up to no good.

You: *Up to no good . . .?*

> **BOX 3.3 Questions to avoid**
>
> - **Multi-barrelled questions** squash two or more questions together.
>   - People generally only answer the first or last question in the bundle.
>   - For example, 'Have you had trouble sleeping or eating more or less than usual, or are you suicidal and a bit tired?'
> - **Leading questions** strongly suggest the answer you want/expect.
>   - People usually give the expected answer, even if it's inaccurate.
>   - For example, 'You're *not* suicidal, are you?'

out how they're feeling, e.g. if they're tearful, they're communicating sadness, even if they *say* they're fine.

- **Imagine how the person is feeling.** If you're *not* naturally intuitive, take a moment in every interview to wonder, 'How would *I* feel if this happened to me?'
- **Show that you *get it*.** You can empathize in your head all you like, but if you don't *communicate* this, people will think you're cold and distant.

To show empathy, you might lean forward, shuffle your chair closer to show solidarity, or speak more quietly about sensitive issues. Speak softly while holding eye contact—this is no time to look shifty. Try not to worry about your precise words: the key is *how* you say it, and *meaning* it. Listen to yourself when friends tell you about something upsetting. What do you say? Gather these phrases and use them clinically. As long as they're not full of expletives, they're probably the most genuine things to say.

💡 **Check your empathy face. You may be surprised to find you look cross/confused/constipated, not concerned!** Put your face through its paces while looking in a mirror: imagine a friend told you they'd bought a puppy . . . that's sick . . . Now recovered . . . Now been run over . . . Now it's died. Don't overdo it, but *do* react. Sometimes raised eyebrows or a frown are enough.

💡 **Empathy isn't just about sadness. It includes laughing with someone and smiling when they're happy or proud.**

Sometimes there's a moment when it feels natural to reassure or offer comfort through touch. People won't spontaneously combust if you do, and there are definitely times when touching someone is the perfect response. *However*, touching can feel uncomfortable, upsetting, even traumatic. *Don't* touch if:

- *You'd* feel uncomfortable.
- *They'd* probably feel uncomfortable (e.g. history of abuse or assault; their culture doesn't sanction touching between men and women).
- You're *unsure* if it's OK.
- You'd *stop or have to explain* yourself, if their partner/ your consultant walked in.

If it feels appropriate, you could, e.g. gently place your hand on their arm or back when they're tearful. Be sensitive: if they flinch or shrink back, stop, apologize, and give them space.

💡 **When watching films, your imagination's switched on to understand the characters' feelings. If you don't want your feelings to overwhelm you, you can switch off your imagination and distance yourself by turning your attention to something easier (e.g. wondering how long the zombies spent in make-up). As doctors, we sometimes need to switch off to prevent feeling overwhelmed. But if we never switch *on*, other people make no emotional sense—affecting bedside manner and our enjoyment of medicine. Switch *on* whenever possible.**

Reflect

This is a powerful rapport-building tool, as it shows you've listened, and puts your understanding of the situation into words. It's not hard, either—just paraphrase what the person has said (now and then—not constantly!).

> **Mary:** . . . Then everyone laughed at me. I felt so embarrassed! When I told my boyfriend, he laughed too.
> **You:** You felt humiliated?
> **Mary:** Exactly. That's exactly how it felt.

Try using a slightly uncertain tone for reflections, as you're not *telling* someone what they think, but checking you've understood.

Validate

Look for the good in everyone, and let them know what you find, as it raises self-esteem, and builds rapport; do it once an interview and people will feel better for talking to you. Simply say what you like, respect, or value about them, e.g.:

- That took guts!
- You're incredibly patient.
- You've been through a huge amount.

This is especially important when people have mental health problems, as they may not get a lot of praise or validation.

Close

Interviews that limp to a standstill or end abruptly can ruin an otherwise brilliant conversation. Try to signpost that you're coming to the end, by summarizing and asking for questions and concerns, before saying goodbye.

Summarize

Don't say, 'I'd like to summarize'—you'd never say that in real life! Also, don't repeat *everything*. The skill is in mentioning the main things, drawing together the story so far, e.g.:

- Let me check I've got this right. You've been low since Jake left, 3 months ago. You're tired, can't enjoy anything, and have problems sleeping and eating. You feel really guilty and hopeless about returning to work. Is that right?

They can then agree, correct, or expand on your summary. It lets the other person know you've been listening, checks you've understood, and jogs your memory for anything important you've forgotten.

> **Everyone goes blank or 'dries up' sometimes. Rescue an awkward silence by summarizing: it often restarts the conversation.**

Check

Before ending, check for questions and concerns. Highlight important areas you've missed.

> **You:** So, we've talked a lot about your heart attack. Is there anything you'd like to ask me?
>
> **Pete:** Are these tablets alright with my diabetes?
>
> **You:** *[I forgot to check past medical history!]* That's a good question. First, tell me about your diabetes . . .
>
> *[Later]*
>
> **You:** Is there anything else worrying you?
>
> **Pete:** Have you been secretly filming me?
>
> **You:** No. Why do you ask?

Work within your limitations. If you don't know the answer, say so (only offer to find out if you plan to do so). Simply hearing someone's worries can be therapeutic; don't feel you have to solve them.

Say goodbye

Don't just wander off!

- Thank them for their time.
- Say goodbye. Smile, make eye contact!

4 HOW TO SUCCEED IN PSYCHIATRY OSCEs

Objective structured clinical examinations (OSCEs) are the practical exams many medical schools use to assess clinical skills. They're a circuit of tasks or 'stations', e.g. examinations, history-taking, catheterization. In psychiatric stations, you'll usually interview an actor, who's playing a patient or carer. Although details differ between universities, the following tips will help, wherever you are.

Beforehand

1. Get 'real-life' feedback before it's too late

It's not ideal to discover *during* an OSCE that your 'bedside manner' is universally hated, and a sophisticated form of psychological torture. Identify and fix problems beforehand:

- Speak to as many patients as you can: they're your experts. Afterwards, *ask them* how you did, and how you could improve.
- Pair up with another student. Take turns observing and giving feedback on each other's assessment skills.
- Ask health professionals to give feedback whenever they've seen you with patients.

Change, according to feedback, especially if there are recurring themes.

2. University rules

Beforehand, check:

- Examination format, e.g. timings, rules, rest/double-length stations.
- How instructions are presented. The task (e.g. '*Take a psychosis history*') may be the first line, or follow a long clinical summary.
- Whether examiners ask questions, e.g. differential diagnosis, risk assessment.

3. Practise

Ask if tutors can provide 'mock' OSCEs, and use the role-plays in the 'Reality' sections of this book to practise stations with friends:

- Take turns to interview, examine, give feedback, and act (playing the patient offers valuable insights).
- Plan for likely OSCEs: think how you'd structure them, and write down key questions/points.
- Time stations accurately to make them realistic, and develop an instinct for station length.
- Do multiple stations, to practise switching between tasks and learning to move on from a 'bad' station.
- Get used to being watched by a few peers, so a single examiner won't intimidate you.
- Exams are noisy. So you're not distracted on the day, practise with the radio or TV on in the background.
- Get someone to film you. Watch yourself to spot strengths and weaknesses (and justify your new smartphone).

During exams

1. Outside the station

Each station can be a thrilling surprise if you enter without reading the brief. It's less exciting to follow the instructions, but you'll be more likely to pass. Carefully read the vignette outside the station, e.g.:

You're a final year medical student in general practice. Greg Pearce is a 19-year-old apprentice. He's attended because his parents are worried he's stressed at college. The GP asks you to take a psychosis history.'

Identify the task (*psychosis history*), then read the rest of the story. When there's lots of information, this helps you pick out the task-relevant points. *Ideally*, while waiting, plan the main areas you'll cover. If you go blank, don't panic:

- Learn the person's name *[Greg Pearce]*.
- Memorize their reason for attending *[parents worried]*.
- Gather clues *[college stress]*.
- Prepare your introduction and first question.

2. Introduce yourself

Every introduction = [Check the person's name] + ['Hello, my name is . . .'] + [Your status].

You: Mr Pearce? Hello, my name is *[full name]*. I'm a *[year]* medical student.
Greg: Hi. Call me Greg.

Smile, make eye contact, and sit down *while* introducing yourself. Don't stand over someone who's already seated—you'll seem nervous, or intimidating.

3. Gain consent

Succinctly gain consent, e.g.:

You: Your GP's asked me to speak to you before you see her, to find out more about why you've come in. Is that OK with you?
Greg: Yeah.

Greg's agreed to talk, so don't expand on consent (or confidentiality) at this point.

4. Ask a *relevant* open question

Don't waste time with:

- *Why have you come today?* (You already know this.)
- *How are you?* (Pleasant but vague.)

Instead, use the vignette to ask a *relevant* open question, focusing the interview without closing it down, e.g.:

- I understand your parents are worried about you. Why are they worried?
- I was told you're having a stressful time at college. What's been happening?

A good open question lets the other person talk. You can simply relax, listen—and breathe!

5. Have a conversation

The best histories are conversations. Chapter 3 covers these skills in detail. Essentially:

- Listen attentively.
- Ask questions.
- Build rapport.

For information-giving stations, see **Box 4.1**.

6. Structure

Explore the presenting complaint to identify potential diagnoses. Then ask about:

- Key symptoms (build the diagnostic picture).

BOX 4.1 Information-giving stations

- Don't give a non-stop lecture!
  - Check what they *already* know.
  - Check what they *want* to know.
- Pitch information at their level, avoid medical jargon, and ask them to say if they don't understand anything.
- *Chunk and check*: give a small chunk of information, then check it's been understood before offering the next chunk.
- Draw simple explanatory diagrams if helpful.
- Ask for questions and worries.
- Help retention by summarizing, offering written information, and follow-up meetings.
- NB: always gain the patient's permission before explaining things to their friends or relatives.

- Symptoms that suggest/exclude differential diagnoses (test whether your primary diagnosis is correct).
- Effect on life.
- Coping strategies.
- Risk.
- Brief background history as appropriate (e.g. past psychiatric history).

Explore the other person's *agenda* (what *they* want to talk about). Then find ways to *link* it to *your* agenda (psychiatric history) so questions feel relevant. For example, if Greg wants to talk about college, and you want to explore psychotic symptoms, ask:

- How do other staff/students treat you? (*Paranoia*)
- Do they talk about you? (*Auditory hallucinations*)

💡 If someone *keeps* saying the same—seemingly random—word or phrase, you've got a 'stuck record' (e.g. Greg keeps mentioning 'sore eyes'). Explore this as soon as possible: it's usually an essential point, and you won't move forward until you've understood it (e.g. spies have put cameras in Greg's eyes).

7. Do it for real

Be yourself. Take your personality into every station: if you're an empathic person, it'll shine through, and win over the actor and examiner. Don't 'act' or adopt a different persona—you'll seem wooden or insincere.

Believe that the actor *is* a patient and *really* experiencing everything they say, or you'll underperform. Do what you'd do in a real clinical situation, e.g. show concern, offer to find information leaflets. (Don't *mime* handing over invisible tissues or leaflets. It looks silly.)

💡 **If you find empathy difficult, or exam nerves make it hard to empathize, discuss this with your clinical or educational supervisor.**

8. Know your limits

Your university is training *safe* future doctors, not *perfect* future doctors. If you're working within your limitations, you've nothing to worry about. So if you don't know the answer to a question, say so and offer to find out. This shows confidence, which relaxes patients *and* examiners.

9. Endings

You'll usually have a warning (e.g. bell), 1–2 minutes before the station ends. If the examiner asks you anything, turn to face them, make eye contact, speak clearly, and answer precisely (rambling off topic wastes valuable time). Then thank them and turn back to the patient.

Draw things to a close. Cover anything *critical* (e.g. suicide risk in depression), before:

- Summarizing.
- Asking for questions/concerns (address them if possible).
- Thanking the patient.
- Smiling, saying goodbye, and leaving calmly.

Don't leave early. A full psychiatric history easily takes an hour, so there will *always* be more to ask, and marks to gain. In some universities, you *can't* exit early, and may be prevented from leaving (then having to sit in awkward silence).

10. Move on

Each station is a fresh challenge. No matter how badly things go, never dwell on a previous station. Remember: unless you enter the next station with a black eye and bloody nose, your new examiner won't suspect a thing.

5 CLASSIFICATION AND DIAGNOSIS

Diagnostic systems

Psychiatry has two main diagnostic classification systems (**Table 5.1**):

- International Classification of Diseases (ICD).
- Diagnostic and Statistical Manual of Mental Disorders (DSM).

Both rely largely on *categorical* classification: criteria indicate whether someone does or doesn't have the disorder. The current versions also make increasing use of the *dimensional* approach, in which a scale shows 'how much' someone is affected by a symptom or disorder. This reflects the idea that many illnesses (e.g. affective and psychotic disorders) aren't discrete entities, but part of a continuum from 'normal' to 'pathological', with complex, shared aetiologies. This approach is more nuanced, but also time-consuming and harder to standardize.

Advantages

- Diagnoses are useful shorthand for complex illness concepts, helping patients and professionals share an understanding of the problem. This can validate symptoms and offers a way forward, essentially saying, 'Your problems are important and we can help you, because we've seen them before'.
- Diagnoses let professionals focus research, share clinical experiences, and build an evidence base for treatment.

Disadvantages

- Diagnostic 'labels' can be unhelpful: once 'stuck onto' people, they can feel difficult to 'peel off' and may lead to stigma and misunderstanding.
- The *validity* of diagnostic categories is continually debated, especially as there aren't biological markers to 'prove' the diagnosis, e.g. a blood test for schizophrenia.
- Given the diversity of psychiatric presentations, and widely different cultural 'norms', diagnoses may not be applied *reliably* between professionals, i.e. different doctors may give the same person different diagnoses.
- The DSM has been particularly criticized for 'medicalizing' normal distress and behaviour, allegedly in response to pressure from health insurance companies and the pharmaceutical industry.

Clinical compromise

Although you'll become skilled at diagnostic 'pattern recognition', don't get carried away with it. Diagnoses can't convey anyone's unique experience, no matter how similar their symptoms might seem to those of someone with the same diagnosis. Always keep an open mind, remembering that symptoms of one condition may be caused by something else, e.g. anxiety symptoms may be due to an anxiety disorder, *or* an organic state (e.g. dementia, hyperthyroidism, alcohol withdrawal), depression, psychosis, or personality disorder.

Also remember that *unusual* experiences aren't necessarily *abnormal* experiences, and that *symptoms without disability or distress don't need a diagnosis*. For example, hearing voices is relatively common in the general population, and may even feel comforting; diagnosing 'psychosis' could distress and stigmatize, without bringing

TABLE 5.1 ICD versus DSM

	ICD	DSM
Current version	ICD-10 ICD-11 will be used from 2022	DSM-5
Developed by	World Health Organization (WHO)	American Psychiatric Association (APA)
Use	Official world classification, for all health workers.	North American classification, mostly for psychiatrists.
Scope	All medical disorders	Mental health only
Categorization method	Matches descriptions to broad diagnostic guidelines	Definitive inclusion and exclusion criteria

any benefits. Normalize rather than medicalize where possible, and consider:

- *Utility*—diagnosis must be useful, ideally helping you *and* the patient make sense of a problem.
- *Humility*—believe it possible you may be wrong.
- *Humanity*—diagnosis is never more important than the person.

> **Nobody should be defined by illness; don't refer to people by their diagnoses, e.g. *a schizophrenic*: this is a *person* who *has* schizophrenia.**

Book shelf
Groopman, J. (2008) *How Doctors Think*: a Harvard professor of medicine considers the cognitive errors that doctors make in misdiagnosis.

6 MENTAL HEALTH AND THE LAW

Most psychiatric care is provided with consent, as a person thinks they need it. People also have the right to *refuse* healthcare and treatment, unless (a) their refusal could harm them or someone else, or (b) they don't have the ability to consent to treatment. In these cases, clinicians may need to legally enforce healthcare. In England and Wales, key laws are:

- Mental Health Act 1983, amended 2007.
- Mental Capacity Act 2005.

💡 **Scotland uses the *Mental Health (Care and Treatment) (Scotland) Act 2003* and Northern Ireland uses the *Mental Health (Northern Ireland) Order 1986*.**

Mental health act

The Mental Health Act (MHA) enables the compulsory healthcare of people suffering from a '*mental disorder*' (defined broadly, as 'any disorder or disability of the mind') which poses a risk to their health, safety, or to others. Since overriding someone's autonomy is a serious decision, the MHA is not used lightly, and features safeguards to protect the person's human rights. Being detained in hospital can be very distressing: staff need to forge therapeutic, trusting relationships with the person, despite aspects of their care being against their wishes. The Act's guiding principles reflect this: detention is a last resort when there is no safe, less restrictive alternative (e.g. voluntary admission or care at home); patients and carers must be respected; and the purpose of treatment should be clearly explained. The MHA has numerous *sections* (parts of the law for particular situations): see **Table 6.1** for the ones you might encounter. Remember:

- Durations are *maximum* lengths of detention: the person is often discharged or the section rescinded (ended) before that time passes.
- Sections *don't* cover treatment of *physical* health problems (*unless* they're directly causing or resulting from the mental disorder).
- The MHA contains many checks to prevent human rights abuses, e.g.:
  - Three independent assessors must *all* agree to S2 or S3 (if one disagrees, there's no section).
  - The person's 'nearest relative' (spouse/adult child/parent/sibling) can request their discharge from S2 or S3 *or* object to S3 (preventing it).
  - The person can appeal S2 and S3, with (free) representation by a solicitor, at an independent tribunal or hospital managers' hearing.

💡 **Using the law to force someone to come into hospital or accept treatment is a major decision. How would *you* feel if a doctor placed you in hospital and made you take medication against your will?**

Mental capacity act

Mental capacity is the ability to make decisions; people are presumed to have it unless there are reasons to suspect otherwise. Mental capacity is *decision specific:* it's assessed separately for *each* decision. *All* health professionals can assess capacity—not just psychiatrists. To 'have capacity' to make a specific decision, the person must be able to:

- **Understand** information relevant to the decision (e.g. pros and cons of an operation).
- **Retain** that information.
- **Use or weigh** that information to make their decision (e.g. risks versus benefits).
- **Communicate** their decision (through speech/sign language/other means).

Someone lacks capacity (under the Mental Capacity Act (MCA)) to make a particular decision at a particular time if they lack *any* of these abilities as a direct consequence of a '*disorder of mind or brain*'. When someone *temporarily* lacks capacity, it should be frequently reassessed. People should be supported to make decisions by providing understandable information and helping them to communicate. Also, making seemingly *unwise* decisions doesn't necessarily mean that someone lacks capacity.

The MCA is used primarily for physical healthcare decisions, allowing professionals to act in the person's *best interests*, e.g. giving antibiotics when the person is too confused to consent. These steps:

- Are those *least restrictive* of rights and freedoms.

TABLE 6.1 Key MHA sections

Section	Purpose	Maximum duration	Staff involved
2	Admission for assessment ± treatment	28 days	• 2 registered doctors (1 with prior knowledge of the person where possible, at least 1 'Section 12 approved'[a]) • AMHP[b]
3	Admission for treatment	6 months (can be renewed)	As for S2
4	Emergency admission	72 hours	• 1 doctor • 1 AMHP
5(2)	Holding order for a person already admitted to an inpatient ward to allow full MHA assessment	72 hours	1 doctor (with at least 1 year's clinical experience).
5(4)	As for S5(2)	6 hours	1 registered mental health/learning disability nurse.
17(a)	*Community Treatment Order (CTO)*: places conditions on someone discharged from S3, e.g. requirement to meet health professionals/take medication. Power to *recall* someone to hospital	6 months (can be renewed)	• AMHP • 'Responsible clinician' (usually consultant psychiatrist, occasionally a non-medical senior practitioner)
135	Warrant: allows entry to a property to remove someone suffering from a mental disorder, if at risk	24 hours	• AMHP • Doctor • Police officer
136	Power to remove someone appearing to suffer from a mental disorder from a public place to a place of safety	24 hours	Police officer

[a] 'S12 approved' doctors have expertise in diagnosing and treating mental disorders; they're usually psychiatrists or GPs. [b] AMHPs are approved mental health professionals, commonly social workers.

- Allow as much participation as possible in decision-making (e.g. providing a specially trained, independent advocate).
- Take the person's beliefs (if known) into account.
- Consider the views of involved people (e.g. relatives).

The MCA allows people to make *advance decisions* while they have capacity, describing specific treatments they wouldn't want if they lacked capacity in future (e.g. refusing life-prolonging treatment following an illness from which they're unlikely to recover).

Deprivation of Liberty Safeguards (DoLS) are an MCA subsection used to legally keep someone in hospital (or a care home), for necessary care. These are likely to be replaced by the Liberty Protection Safeguards.

For a practical example of capacity assessment, see p. 164.

7 A CAREER IN PSYCHIATRY

Are you reading my mind? Is that the same as psychology? Do you have a couch in your office?

These are a few of the questions you may be asked in parties/taxis/aeroplanes, should you choose this most varied and inspiring career path. We love our jobs—but just what *exactly* do we do?

💡 A wealth of up-to-date, high-quality information about psychiatry careers is available from the Royal College of Psychiatrists: www.rcpsych.ac.uk/discoverpsychiatry/acareerinpsychiatry.aspx

lasting 4–6 years in the UK). Following this, they usually complete the **UK Foundation Programme** of 'FY1' and 'FY2' years, in which they rotate through 4-month posts in medical, surgical, psychiatric, or community specialties. In FY2, doctors apply for 'core training', which lasts 3 years in psychiatry. During **core psychiatry training**, doctors rotate through (usually) 6-month posts in different psychiatric subspecialties, while attending weekly teaching (including lectures, training courses, reflective practice groups, journal clubs, and case presentations).

Medical school and core training

Every psychiatrist is a medical doctor first, i.e. a bachelor of medicine and surgery (an undergraduate degree

Higher training and beyond

Membership of the Royal College of Psychiatrists (MRCPsych), the postgraduate qualification required

---

BOX 7.1 Why choose psychiatry?

This is a personal choice and varies from person to person. There are lots of reasons to consider becoming a psychiatrist and we hope many of them are evident in this book. Here are a few of our reasons:

SS: I've always loved hearing people's stories and pictured myself as a GP, until I did a GP post as a junior doctor. I found my favourite patients were people with mental health problems: I looked forward to seeing them and they kept choosing to see *me*. My first week in psychiatry taught me that the starting point for helping people recover was making a connection through listening and understanding their stories; this was something I was good at *and* really enjoyed. I've had recurrent depression myself since I was a medical student, and it's taught me a huge amount, particularly about suffering and the difference doctors can make when they combine knowledge with empathy and compassion. Psychiatry gives me the space, time, and skills to try to make that difference every day.

LC: I always knew that I wanted to be a doctor. Although I didn't have any doctors in my family I was drawn to helping people and applying science. After qualifying, I remember some pivotal surgical night shifts, talking and listening to particular patients as I re-sited IV cannulas and took blood tests. It became clear to me that I wouldn't be the doctor operating on their cancer but the one talking to them about their fears or recognizing their depression: an equally valuable role and one that I was better suited to. I've never looked back since choosing psychiatry and patients sometimes tell me that I have saved their life.

RK: My first degree was in psychology with philosophy. I applied to graduate-entry medicine after a neuropsychology module made me rethink everything I knew about the brain. I was drawn to psychiatry at medical school but was interested in obstetrics and gynaecology too. During the foundation programme, I realized how much I enjoy working with a team to conduct comprehensive, holistic assessments, to implement the most constructive management plan. I also enjoy the diversity of our work, the interface with physical healthcare and social support services, and the chance to provide hope when people are at their lowest ebb. Core training maintains your medical skills and combining it with research and teaching means every day is a chance to make things better. I'm now doing a PhD in perinatal psychiatry, so all that obstetrics and gynaecology paid off after all!

JH: I was first drawn to psychiatry because I was fascinated by the relationship between the brain and psychiatric symptoms: how could a change in the anatomy or chemistry 'up there' lead to a person hearing an alien voice or becoming convinced they were being watched? How did all those unique personal factors precipitating their illness fit in? Psychiatry attracts a range of people because it can be approached on such a variety of levels; beyond the clinical it's truly multidisciplinary, involving education, philosophy, ethics, and law. Whether you're moved by personal narratives, psychopharmacology, child development, social justice, or magnetic resonance imaging (MRI) scans, psychiatry may be the specialty for you. I gain great satisfaction from trying to help people who are often marginalized by their illnesses, I enjoy supporting their families and friends, and I love the rough and tumble of a varied, demanding, and eye-opening job.

to progress further, is obtained by passing written examinations (Papers A and B) and a practical, OSCE-style examination (the 'Clinical Assessment of Skills and Competencies' (CASC)). With membership, core trainees may apply for **higher training** in a subspecialty, which lasts 3–5 more years. Subspecialties currently include *general adult, old age, child and adolescent, forensic, intellectual disability psychiatry* and *medical psychotherapy*. Within general adult psychiatry, there are further 'endorsements' available, in areas such as *liaison, rehabilitation, addictions psychiatry*. Training can be extended to pursue research, fellowships (e.g. in medical education, leadership, or management), for maternity/paternity leave, or to work less than full-time.

Psychiatrists work in a wide range of settings. This, combined with the range of subspecialties, makes it a hugely diverse career. For example, a general adult psychiatrist could work in an inpatient perinatal mother and baby unit, a community home treatment team, a personality disorders therapeutic community, or an eating disorders ward.

What next?

We recommend getting experience through student selected components (SSCs), electives, summer schools, joining or setting up a university psychiatry society, taster weeks, foundation doctor posts, and joining the RCPsych as a student associate. We chose psychiatry for different reasons and we all love it, many years on (**Box 7.1**). Lots of people enter the specialty later in their careers, so it's never too late. If you like this book, you might just like psychiatry, too!

8 Affective Disorders

True or false?

Answers on p. 277

1. Mood fluctuations are commonly pathological in humans.
2. Childhood adversity is associated with depression in adulthood.
3. Antidepressants reduce overall levels of central monoamines.
4. Cyclothymic disorder is a type of bipolar affective disorder.
5. Pseudodementia is a presentation of depression.
6. Antidepressant treatment should continue for 1 month after a first depressive episode.
7. Hypothyroidism is a side effect of lithium.
8. Psychosis alongside affective symptoms is common.
9. Loss of libido is a core symptom of depression.
10. Depression resulting from organic causes is rare.

Contents

Principles
Introduction
Epidemiology
Aetiology
- Genetics
- Childhood and life experiences
- Stressful life events
- Organic causes

Theories
- Behavioural and cognitive theories
- Psychoanalytic theories
- Neurochemical theories
- Neuroendocrine abnormalities
- Neuroanatomical abnormalities

Depression
- Clinical presentation
- Differential diagnosis
- Investigations
- Management
- Prognosis

Mania and bipolar affective disorder
- Clinical presentation
- Differential diagnosis
- Investigations
- Management
- Prognosis

Reality: depression
General approach: tips, tricks, and cautionary tales
The interview
- Depression history
- Depression with psychotic symptoms history

Reality: mania
General approach: tips, tricks, and cautionary tales
The interview
- Manic episode history

Next steps
Poor recovery post myocardial infarction
- Differential diagnosis
- Preparation
- Assessment
- Management

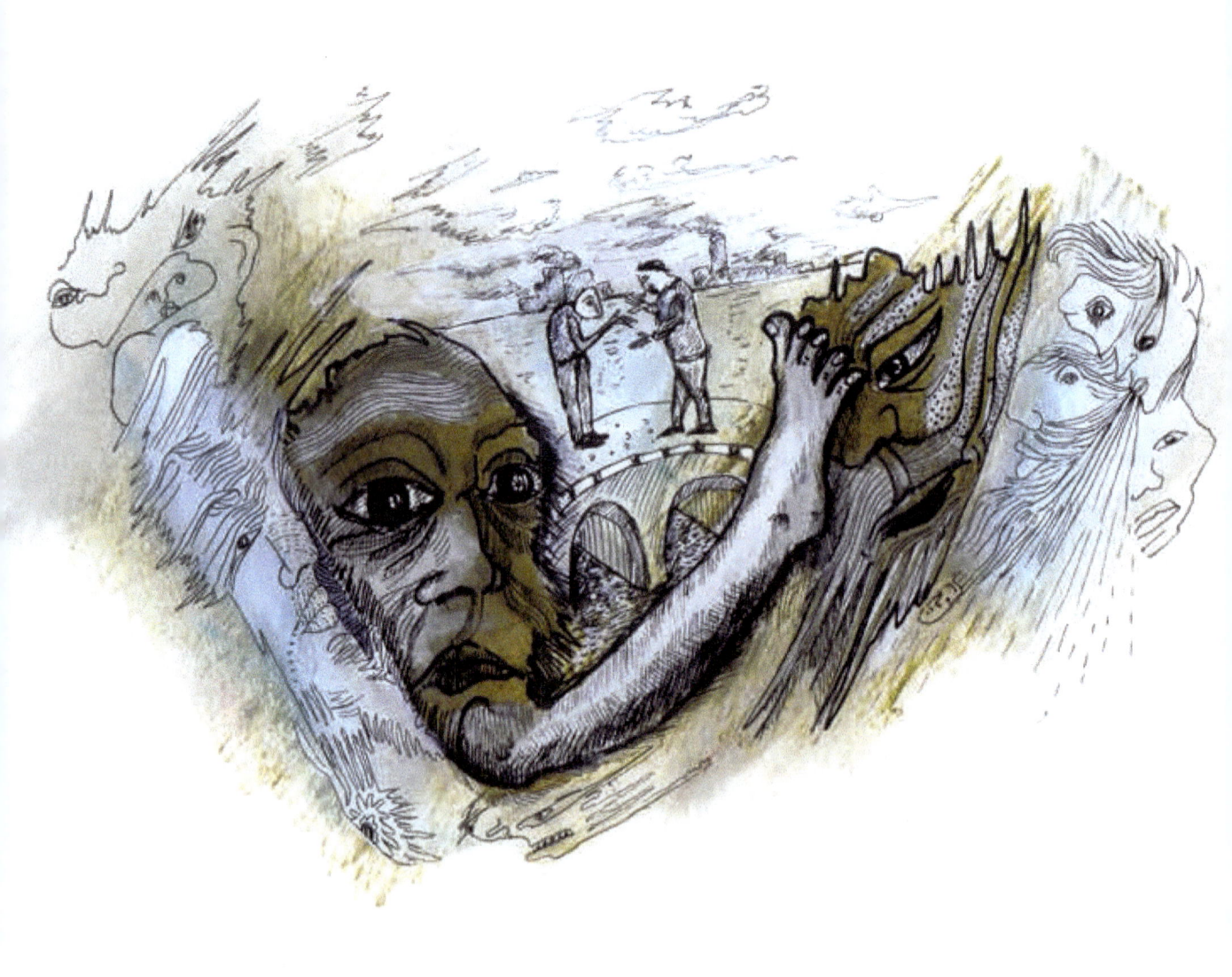

PRINCIPLES

> Dementors are among the foulest creatures that walk this earth. They infest the darkest, filthiest places, they glory in decay and despair, they drain peace, hope and happiness out of the air around them. Even Muggles feel their presence, though they can't see them. Get too near a Dementor and every good feeling, every happy memory, will be sucked out of you.
>
> J.K. Rowling, *Harry Potter and the Prisoner of Azkaban*[1]

> The fast ideas are far too fast, and there are far too many; overwhelming confusion replaces clarity. Memory goes. Humor and absorption on friends' faces are replaced by fear and concern. Everything previously moving with the grain is now against—you are irritable, angry, frightened, uncontrollable, and enmeshed totally in the blackest caves of the mind.
>
> Kay Redfield Jamison, *An Unquiet Mind: A Memoir of Moods and Madness*[2]

Introduction

Moods fluctuate as part of normal human experience, but mood (affective) *disorders* are illnesses where mood is excessively high (hypomania/mania) or low (depression). People often use 'depression' to describe a transient, healthy feeling of sadness. However, clinical depression is no more like feeling sad than falling in love is like having a crush. J.K. Rowling's metaphor of Dementors describes her experience of depression. Likewise, Jamison's depiction of mania is very different from the normal experience of happiness.

Although some people only experience a single affective episode, mood disorders generally run a relapsing and remitting course. In *unipolar* illness, the person experiences episodes of depression. In *bipolar affective disorder* (BPAD), they have episodes of mania *or* of mania *and* depression. Where 'depression' is used in this chapter, it means unipolar depression.

Epidemiology

Depression is the leading cause of disability worldwide. It's more common than BPAD and affects twice as many women as men (**Table 8.1**).

Aetiology

Genetics

Mood disorders are influenced by genetic and environmental factors. *Heritability* is an estimate of how much variation of a phenotype (e.g. depression) in a population results from genetic variation. Heritability estimates suggest greater heritability of BPAD, with depression more related to environmental factors (**Table 8.1**). As with most psychiatric disorders, mood disorder inheritance is *polygenic*: contributed by many alleles, each of which exerts a small effect.

There's overlap between the inheritance of affective disorders: relatives of people with depression have a higher risk of depression, while relatives of people with BPAD have a greater risk of both BPAD *and* depression. The genetic contribution to mood disorders is supported by twin concordance rates and adoption research. Large-scale studies have also shown genetic overlap between BPAD and schizophrenia, leading some researchers to advocate for *dimensional*

Table 8.1 Epidemiology and heritability of depression and BPAD

	Depression	BPAD
Female:male ratio	2:1	1:1
Lifetime prevalence[a]	16.6%	3.9%
Heritability[b]	35–50%	80–90%

Data from: (a) Kessler, R.C., et al. (2005) Lifetime prevalence and age-of-onset distributions of DSM-IV disorders in the National Comorbidity Survey Replication (NCS-R). *Archives of General Psychiatry*, **62**, 593–602; (b) McGuffin, P., et al. (2003) The heritability of bipolar affective disorder and the genetic relationship to unipolar depression. *Archives of General Psychiatry*, **60**, 497–502.

rather than *categorical* approaches to classification (see p. 27).

Childhood and life experiences

Childhood adversity, like abuse and neglect, is a risk factor for recurrent and persistent depressive episodes in adulthood, and for treatment resistance. A major study showed high rates of mental health problems in adulthood in Romanian children adopted into the UK after long periods of institutional care. However, one in five of adoptees remained well, despite these experiences, demonstrating *resilience* in a subgroup. Epigenetics research may explain how genes and the environment interact. In adulthood, *vulnerability factors*, including unemployment, lack of a confiding relationship, lower socioeconomic status, and social isolation are associated with increased risk of depression.

Despite the high heritability estimate of BPAD, childhood maltreatment is associated with greater BPAD severity and comorbidity and more frequent relapses and suicide attempts than in people without childhood abuse.

> 💡 Depression can occur without an obvious trigger, especially with a strong family history. This can be particularly difficult to cope with, as sufferers (and carers) may think there's 'nothing to be sad about'.

Stressful life events

Life events can cause depressive episodes and have been classified according to their degree of stressfulness (**Box 8.1**).

'Loss events' are particularly important triggers for depression. Loss includes a range of experiences beyond bereavement, including loss of role (e.g. in retirement) and loss of autonomy (e.g. following hospital admission). Both negative and positive life events can precipitate mania, although in established BPAD, environmental triggers are less important. Childbirth, sleep deprivation, and flying across time zones can all trigger manic episodes.

> 💡 Although depression may be 'understandable' (e.g. following a stressful life event), this doesn't mean it doesn't need treatment.

Organic causes

Physical illness and chronic pain can influence someone's quality of life, predisposing them to depression. Physical illnesses may also cause depression through shared aetiology (e.g. Cushing syndrome, hypothyroidism, stroke, Parkinson disease, multiple sclerosis, and hyperparathyroidism). Some medications cause depression (e.g. beta-blockers), as can substance misuse (e.g. alcohol, cocaine).

Mania can be caused by physical disorders such as Cushing syndrome, head injury, or multiple sclerosis. Steroids, antidepressants, and stimulants can all trigger mania.

Theories

Behavioural and cognitive theories

The *learned helplessness* model of depression was developed from observations that dogs punished with repeated, unavoidable electric shocks *gave up* trying to escape, even when free to leave. Maier and Seligman (1976) argued that depressed people learn they can't change their situation, leading them to give up.

Beck's model of depression informs cognitive behavioural therapy (CBT). It shows how negative thinking can depress mood, generating negative thoughts, creating a downward spiral. He proposed a negative *cognitive triad* of views on the self, the world, and the future in depression (**Figure 8.1**) and a positive triad in mania.

Psychoanalytic theories

Psychoanalysis holds that early experiences, particularly the quality of early relationships, predispose people to depression. Problems in work and relationships are thought to re-evoke early life losses. Depression can be understood as a harsh internal judge ('superego') bullying a helpless self ('ego') into despair. Mania can be considered an unconscious self-defence against depression, by denying vulnerability.

Neurochemical theories

The *monoamine hypothesis* proposes that depression entails a deficiency in brain monoamine neurotransmitters:

BOX 8.1 The Holmes–Rahe Social Adjustment Scale (1967)

1. Death of spouse.
2. Divorce.
3. Marital separation.
4. Jail term.
5. Death of a close relative.

Reprinted from *Journal of Psychosomatic Research*, **11**(2), Holmes T.H and Rahe R.H., 'The Social Readjustment Rating Scale', pp. 213–218. Copyright © 1967, with permission from Elsevier Inc. https://doi.org/10.1016/0022-3999(67)90010-4.

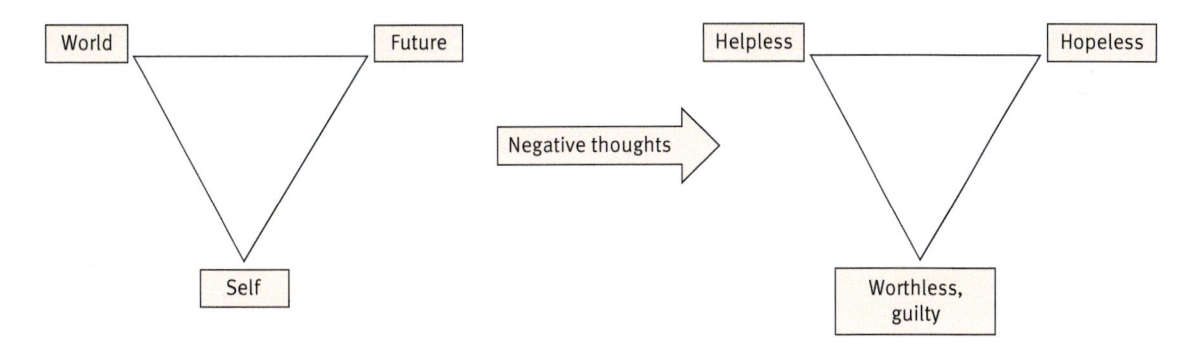

FIGURE 8.1 Beck's negative cognitive triad in depression

- **Serotonin** (5-hydroxytryptamine; 5-HT) affects mood, sleep, appetite, and memory.
- **Noradrenaline** (NA) affects mood and energy.
- **Dopamine** (DA) affects psychomotor activity and motivation.

Observations supporting the monoamine hypothesis include:

- Most antidepressants increase 5-HT and NA levels (**Figure 8.2**).
- Medications that deplete monoamines (e.g. reserpine) cause depression.
- In depression there is:
  - Reduced plasma tryptophan (a 5-HT precursor).
  - Reduced cerebrospinal fluid homovanillic acid (a dopamine metabolite).
- Positron emission tomography (PET) studies show reduced 5-HT transporter binding sites in the midbrain and amygdala and decreased availability of 5-HT receptors in many brain areas.
- Degeneration of dopamine striatal projections in Parkinson disease is associated with depression.

The *mechanism* of monoamine dysfunction in depression is unclear and may be a 'downstream' effect of other abnormalities. More recent studies suggest potential contributions from other neurotransmitters (e.g. gamma aminobutyric acid (GABA), glutamate, *N*-methyl-D-aspartate (NMDA), substance P) and brain-derived neurotrophic factor.

By contrast, mania is associated with monoamine overactivity. Bromocriptine (a dopamine agonist), L-dopa, amphetamine, and cocaine increase dopamine levels, and can induce manic symptoms, whereas antipsychotics (dopamine receptor antagonists) treat mania. Antidepressants increase monoamines and can trigger mania. Glutamate (the main excitatory neurotransmitter) overactivity is thought to play a role in BPAD and many mood stabilizers decrease glutamate activity.

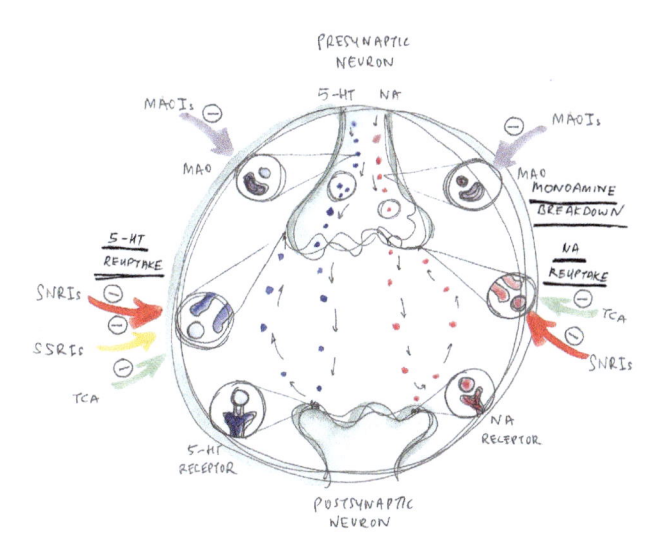

FIGURE 8.2 The mechanisms of antidepressant action. 5-HT, serotonin; MAO, monoamine oxidase; MAOIs, monoamine oxidase inhibitors; NA, noradrenaline; SSRIs, selective serotonin reuptake inhibitors; TCAs, tricyclic antidepressants; SNRIs, serotonin and noradrenaline reuptake inhibitors.

Neuroendocrine abnormalities

Cortisol, the main stress hormone, interacts with stressful experiences. In depression, abnormalities include higher baseline cortisol levels, disturbance of its normal diurnal secretion pattern, and loss of normal negative feedback. Excess cortisol causes hippocampal damage and affects neurotransmitters (e.g. serotonin): findings seen in depression. Hypercortisolaemia is also linked to cardiovascular disease and diabetes, which might explain the association between these chronic conditions and depression.

Neuroanatomical abnormalities

Depression is associated with neuroimaging abnormalities of the left anterior cingulate cortex, but it's unclear whether this is a cause or effect. Deep brain stimulation targets this area, and is a potential treatment for severe, treatment-resistant depression.

Depression

Clinical presentation

Depression may be *mild, moderate, severe,* or *severe with psychotic symptoms*, depending on the number and severity of symptoms and their impact on the person's day-to-day functioning (**Figure 8.3**). Biological symptoms tend to emerge as severity increases, with psychotic symptoms only seen in very severe cases (**Figure 8.4**).

Core symptoms

In ICD-11, a depressive episode is almost daily low mood or loss of interest in usual activities for at least two weeks, alongside other symptoms. (ICD-10 is similar, but requires two of: low mood, interest, or *energy*; ICD-11 places low energy under biological symptoms). Recurrent depressive disorder is when someone experiences at least two depressive episodes, separated by several months of wellness.

Low mood may include irritability, anxiety, or tearfulness and can show diurnal variation (typically, mornings feel worst). Lowered interest is closely associated with *anhedonia*—the inability to feel enjoyment or pleasure. Low energy (*anergia*) is often described as feeling 'tired all the time', 'worn out', or struggling to do everyday activities.

Cognitive symptoms

People may feel worthless, unconfident, or unworthy. They may feel disproportionately guilty, hopeless about the future, and helpless to improve their situation. They can struggle with concentration and memory and their thinking may feel slowed (slowed thoughts *and* movements are called psychomotor retardation). In older people, memory loss can resemble dementia, but resolves with treatment of depression ('pseudodementia').

Biological symptoms

People experiencing depression commonly report altered sleep patterns, typically initial insomnia (difficulty falling asleep) or early morning wakening (waking at least 2 hours earlier than usual). Reduced appetite can cause weight loss and low libido can place a further strain on relationships. Less commonly, people experience hypersomnia (oversleeping) and

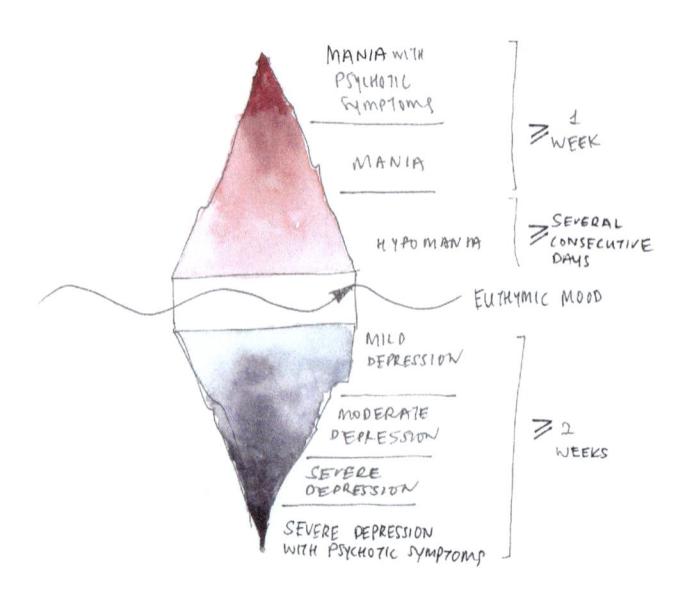

FIGURE 8.3 Diagnostic overview. Comparison of mania and depression severity and duration.

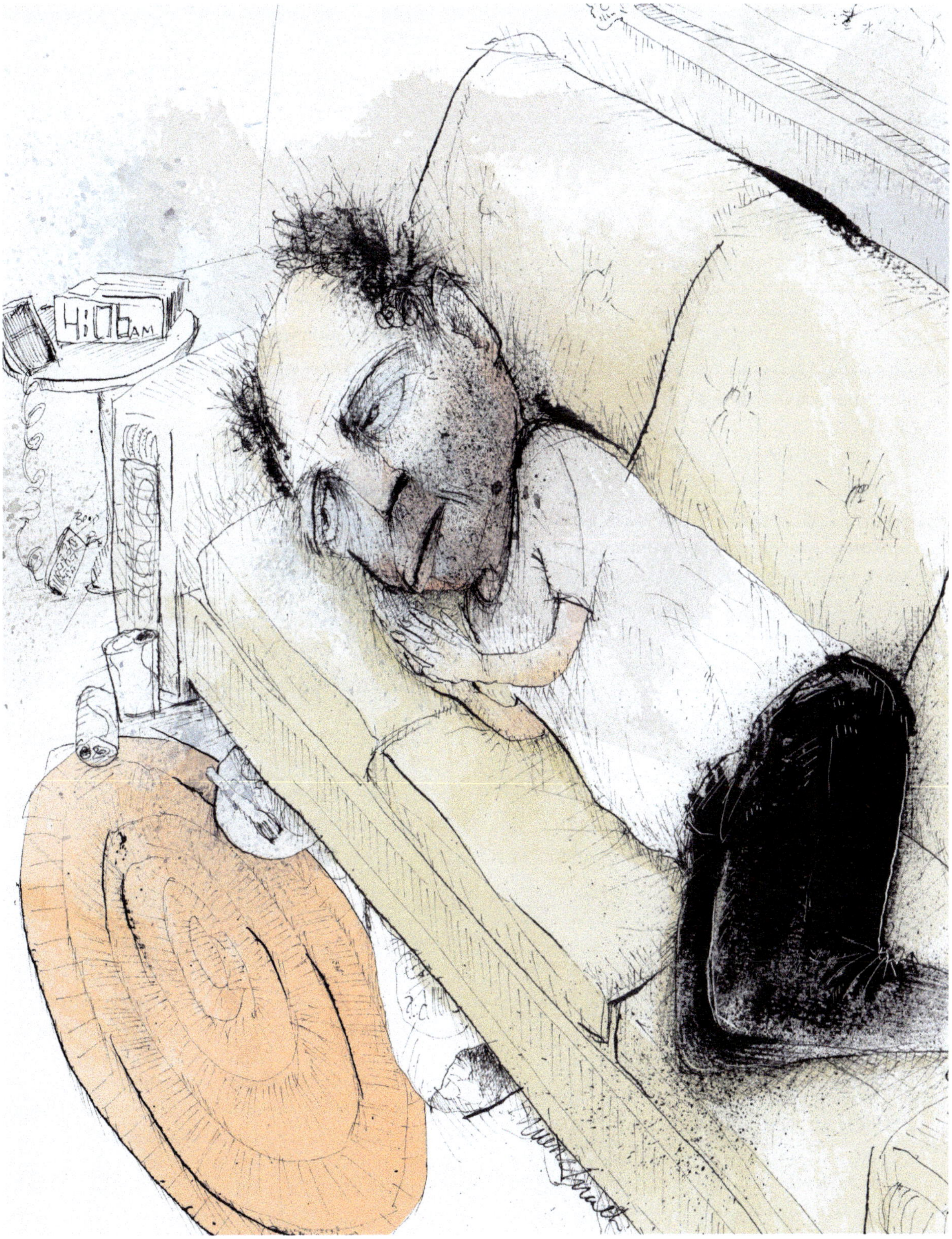

FIGURE 8.4 Clinical features of depression

hyperphagia (overeating) with weight gain. Associated physical symptoms may include constipation, aches, and pains.

Psychotic symptoms

People experiencing severe depression can have hallucinations and delusions (see p. 9) which are usually 'mood congruent'. For example, second-person, derogatory auditory hallucinations (e.g. 'You're worthless!') are typical; visual hallucinations (e.g. scenes of destruction) are uncommon. Delusions are often nihilistic (e.g. 'I'm losing my home', 'My blood has been removed', 'My organs are defective'), persecutory, or guilt related (e.g. 'I committed a crime').

Differential diagnosis

- **Organic causes**, e.g. hypothyroidism, hypoactive delirium, Addison disease. Dementia and other neurodegenerative disorders may cause low mood and apathy.
- **Sadness/bereavement:** *normal* responses to upsetting events or losses (**Box 8.2**).
- **Adjustment disorder:** mild affective symptoms after a stressful event, not severe enough to diagnose depression.
- **Dysthymia:** chronic low mood for more days than not, lasting years, but not continuous enough to diagnose depression.
- **BPAD:** recurrent mood episodes, with at least one hypomanic/manic episode.

BOX 8.2 Bereavement

Grief is a *normal* response to loss. Normal stages of grieving include:

- **Numbness.**
- **Pining.**
- **Depression.**
- **Recovery.**

People sometimes worry they're 'going mad' or will never recover. They may hear or see the deceased, experience anger, guilt, anxiety, sadness, or sudden 'pangs' of grief. It's important to listen and normalize experiences, rather than 'medicalizing'. In prolonged grief disorder, the response is:

- **Prolonged** (lasting >6 months *without any relief*).
- **Extremely intense** (longing for the deceased or persistent preoccupation, with intense emotional pain).
- **Exceeds expected social, cultural, or religious norms** for their context.
- **Significantly impairs functioning.**

The time-course of grief varies between people. Evidence that the person is moving *forwards* (albeit slowly), feeling slightly better than at first, is encouraging. If you lost your partner of 50 years, 6 months of intense grief would be normal.

- **Substance misuse:** substance misuse can cause or mask depression.
- **Postpartum depression** (see p. 226).
- **Burnout:** exhaustion, disengagement, and reduced productivity in response to chronic work stress. (Treatment focuses on addressing work problems. Committed, conscientious, compassionate people are at highest risk.)

Investigations

- **Collateral history.**
- **Physical examination.**
- **Blood tests** as suggested by history and examination, plus:
    - TFTs (exclude hypothyroidism).
    - FBC (anaemia causes fatigue).
    - Glucose/HbA1c (diabetes causes fatigue).
    - Vitamin D and B_{12} (low levels cause fatigue).
    - Calcium (hyperparathyroidism can cause depression).
- **Rating scales** measure severity or monitor treatment response, e.g. Beck Depression Inventory (BDI), Hospital Anxiety and Depression Scale (HADS), and Patient Health Questionnaire (PHQ-9), but are no substitute for history and MSE.
- **Cognitive assessment** where dementia/pseudodementia are differentials (p. 145).
- **CT/MRI head** are never routine but may exclude *suspected* cerebral pathology.

Management

Biological interventions

Medications

Antidepressants increase synaptic monoamines by decreasing their reuptake or breakdown (**Figure 8.2**). They're usually indicated for moderate to severe depression, ideally alongside psychological therapy. An antipsychotic is added in psychotic depression. All antidepressants are effective in treating depression, but selective serotonin reuptake inhibitors (SSRIs) are usually the first choice because of relatively mild side effects and being safer in overdose than older drugs (**Table 8.2**). Although several weeks' delay in effectiveness was previously reported, an effect is now expected within 1–2 weeks. Treatment should continue for 6–9 months *after* recovery, to prevent relapse. In recurrent depressive disorder, treatment should continue for longer (≥2 years).

Starting some antidepressants is associated with increased suicidal thoughts and acts, so people are warned and provided with information about accessing

Table 8.2 Comparison of antidepressants

Class	Examples	Common side effects	Good to know
Selective serotonin reuptake inhibitors (SSRIs)	Citalopram, Escitalopram, Fluoxetine, Fluvoxamine, Paroxetine, Sertraline	Nausea, vomiting; Dyspepsia, diarrhoea; Anxiety/agitation; Insomnia; Tremor; Headache; Sweating; Sexual dysfunction; GI bleeding; Hyponatraemia	• Enhance 5-HT neurotransmission by blocking 5-HT reuptake into the presynaptic neuron • Paroxetine has a very short half-life, so delaying a tablet can cause discontinuation symptoms
Serotonin and noradrenaline reuptake inhibitors (SNRIs)	Venlafaxine, Duloxetine	*As for SSRIs, plus*: Constipation; Hypertension; Raised cholesterol; Dry mouth; Dizziness; Drowsiness	• Avoid venlafaxine if risk of arrhythmia • Slowly withdraw venlafaxine; discontinuation symptoms are common, due to its short half-life
Tricyclic antidepressants (TCAs)	Amitriptyline, Clomipramine, Imipramine, Lofepramine	*Anticholinergic side effects*: Dry mouth; Blurred vision; Constipation; Urinary retention; Arrhythmia; Postural hypotension; Sedation; Sexual dysfunction	• Inhibit reuptake of NA and 5-HT • Infrequently used due to cardiotoxicity; even small overdoses can be fatal
Monoamine oxidase inhibitors (MAOIs)	Phenelzine, Tranylcypromine	Hypertensive crisis: the 'cheese reaction'; Drowsiness; Postural hypotension, dizziness; Insomnia; Nausea; Sexual dysfunction	• Inhibit monoamine oxidase, increasing 5-HT and NA • Rarely used as tyramine-rich foods (e.g. mature cheese, yeast extract) cause NA build-up and hypertensive crisis
Reversible inhibitors of monoamine oxidase A (RIMAs)	Moclobemide	Agitation/anxiety; Sleep disturbance; Nausea; Throbbing headache; Sexual dysfunction	• Reversible MAOI • Hypertensive crisis still possible: avoid tyramine-rich foods, report severe headache immediately
Noradrenergic and specific serotonin antidepressant (NASSAs)	Mirtazapine	Sedation; Appetite/weight gain; Oedema; Headache	• Sexual side effects relatively uncommon

(continued)

Table 8.2 Continued

Class	Examples	Common side effects	Good to know
Serotonin antagonist and reuptake inhibitor (SARI)	Trazodone	Sedation Dizziness, postural hypotension Headache Tachycardia Nausea/vomiting Tremor Priapism Sexual dysfunction	• Attend hospital if priapism (persistent and/or painful erection)
Melatonergic	Agomelatine	Nausea Dizziness Headache/migraine Insomnia Drowsiness Hepatotoxicity	• Melatonin receptor agonist and 5-HT receptor agonist • Monitor LFTs in early treatment • Can stop abruptly without discontinuation symptoms

services. Antidepressants are avoided in people with a history of hypomania/mania, due to the risk of 'switching' from depression into mania.

💡 People who respond 'too well' to antidepressants may be *switching* from depression to mania (undiagnosed BPAD).

💡 St John's wort is a herbal preparation for mild depression. It works like SSRIs but also induces enzymes, increasing metabolism of drugs (e.g. the contraceptive pill).

Stopping and swapping

Antidepressants are not addictive, but if suddenly stopped can cause unpleasant *discontinuation symptoms*. These vary with the drug, but include flu-like symptoms, 'electric shock' sensations, dizziness, headache, vivid dreams, and irritability. People should discuss stopping antidepressants with their doctor, so doses can be carefully reduced over a few weeks.

Antidepressants of different classes can interact dangerously. Some can be cross-tapered (reducing the old medication *while* increasing the new one); others need a drug-free 'washout' period, so this should always be checked before changing.

Serotonin syndrome is caused by excess serotonin (e.g. from giving two antidepressants at once). It's potentially fatal and symptoms include restlessness and sweating, myoclonus, confusion, and fits.

Treatment resistance

At least a third of people don't recover with a first antidepressant. Medication concordance and the diagnosis are reviewed, before considering a higher dose, different medication, or different class of antidepressant. Specialists can use *augmentation strategies* (adding something to the antidepressant), e.g.:

- Lithium.
- Second-generation antipsychotics (SGAs); lower doses than for psychosis.
- Tri-iodothyronine (T_3).
- Combining two antidepressants.

Electroconvulsive therapy (ECT)

ECT arose from the observation that people with epilepsy and depression felt better after a seizure. When first introduced, ECT was given without anaesthetic, making it painful and frightening. Today, psychiatrists and anaesthetists work together, using general anaesthetic and muscle relaxants to avoid these problems. People may still be understandably scared of trying modern ECT, but it can quickly and effectively treat life-threatening, treatment-resistant depression. It's usually given twice-weekly for 6–12 sessions, but the continuation is reviewed after each session.

A small electrical pulse is passed across the brain via electrodes, triggering a generalized tonic–clonic seizure. To observers, the fit is mild and brief, e.g. toe twitching and muscle tensing (no thrashing about). The person wakes up in a recovery room, and may feel briefly tired, achy, sick, or a little confused. Longer term, they may have residual memory loss of the time just *before* the ECT, though this can be minimized by placing electrodes unilaterally rather than bilaterally and keeping the dose of current as low as possible. *For some people, ECT is life-saving.*

Repetitive transcranial magnetic stimulation (rTMS)

In rTMS, a treatment coil is placed on the scalp, producing magnetic pulses which induce nerve cell firing in the dorsolateral prefrontal cortex. rTMS has similar efficacy to antidepressants, with few side effects and doesn't require anaesthetic. With expanding clinical use, larger studies including long-term follow-up are underway.

Light therapy

Seasonal depressive disorder (formally *seasonal affective disorder*, SAD) occurs in autumn/winter, often with reversed biological symptoms of hypersomnia and hyperphagia. A light box or dawn simulator can compensate for reduced daylight which is thought to be causative.

Exercise

Cardiovascular exercise can be very helpful in mild to moderate depression. 'Prescribing exercise' programmes, e.g. *Couch to 5K* and *parkrun*, or cycle commuting increase activity while connecting people with others through shared, achievable challenges.

Psychological interventions

'Talking treatments' are considered for mild depression which hasn't resolved spontaneously and for moderate or severe depression. The more severe the depression, the greater the benefit of combining psychological approaches with medication.

Cognitive behavioural therapy

CBT helps people think about their thoughts, feelings, and behaviours. It's delivered individually or in groups, usually weekly, for 8–24 weeks. It's goal orientated (sets and meets specific targets) and focuses on the *here and now*, rather than scrutinizing the past.

Behavioural activation (BA) is the first step in CBT for depression and can be a therapy in itself. Activity schedules are used to structure the person's day and encourage them to do things to raise energy levels, develop interests, and gain a sense of achievement.

CBT takes things a step further than BA, targeting thoughts *and* behaviours to raise mood. In depression, people's thoughts become distorted: the future feels hopeless; they feel worthless, guilty, and helpless; and the world seems overwhelming. Such symptoms mean everyday events are experienced as negative, creating a vicious circle: the person feels worse, so withdraws from activities and friends, further confirming beliefs that their life is pointless, empty, and lonely (**Figure 8.5**).

In CBT, the therapist helps the person notice *negative automatic thoughts* (NATs): the unhelpful ideas which pop into their head and trigger low mood and unhelpful behaviours. The therapist explains common thinking errors, e.g.:

- *Generalization*—'I *always* mess *everything* up'.
- *Minimization*—'I only passed that exam by *chance*. I'm not actually clever'.

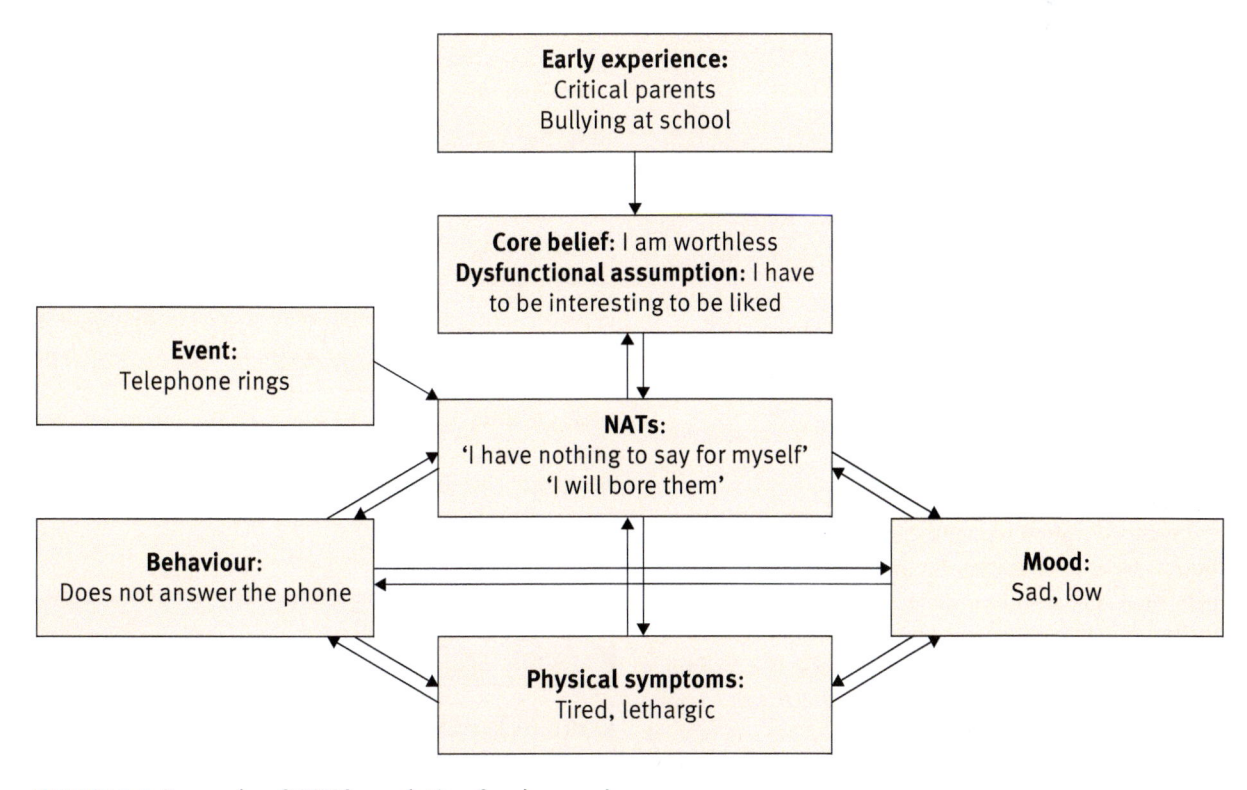

FIGURE 8.5 Example of CBT formulation for depression

The therapist and patient work together to challenge distorted beliefs through:

- *Discussion* during sessions, e.g. 'How can you be *sure* no one cares about you?'
- *Behavioural experiments* between sessions, e.g. inviting a friend to dinner to test the belief that nobody wants to spend time with them.

Through CBT, they build an alternative set of more realistic beliefs, e.g. 'I'm not perfect, but I'm OK'. Later, relapse prevention focuses on keeping away from old thinking and behavioural habits.

Psychodynamic psychotherapy

The developing relationship between the person and their therapist is the focus. The patient's *past experiences* of relationships cause them to behave (unconsciously) in certain ways, e.g. expecting the therapist to let them down. This distorted *transference* is picked up by the therapist, who can draw it to the person's conscious awareness through interpretations and comments, e.g. 'You're afraid I'll humiliate you', 'You expect me to dislike you'. Articulating these feelings allows the person to recognize and re-evaluate them, changing the way they see themselves and others, influencing their behaviour outside therapy. Although classical psychodynamic psychotherapy is provided over a year or more, a focused course can be delivered over 16–20 weeks.

Interpersonal therapy (IPT)

IPT focuses on unresolved loss, role transitions, relationship conflicts, and social skills deficits.

Mindfulness-based cognitive therapy (MBCT)

Individually or in groups, MBCT teaches *mindful awareness:* noticing what's happening externally and within the mind and body at any particular moment. It entails daily mindful meditation practice and reduces the risk of relapse in recurrent depressive disorder.

Social interventions

All grades of depression benefit from social interventions, and these are often all that's needed in mild depression, with active GP monitoring.

Psychoeducation is essential and may include self-help books, websites, or apps. Support groups may help by providing further information, peer support, and social inclusion activities. People should be supported to tell family and friends, rather than feeling ashamed of their struggles; this can mobilize their social network to offer practical and emotional support.

Exercise, a healthy diet, and sleep hygiene (**Box 8.3**) are important strategies. Problem-solving for social stressors is essential, e.g. brief sick leave if work is overwhelming, respite for carers, referral for debt or benefits advice, housing assistance, and signposting to support groups for substance misuse and other chronic problems.

Where depression is more severe, CMHTs provide support at home, e.g. home treatment/crisis teams can supervise medication and care coordinators can help with social stressors. Inpatient admission may be needed if someone is at risk of suicide or severe self-neglect.

> 💡 Depression is unlikely to lift if overwhelming social stressors remain, however good the treatment plan.

Prognosis

Approximately 50% of people have a second depressive episode. The risk of recurrence increases significantly with each subsequent episode. An average episode lasts 8–9 months, 2–3 months with treatment. Depression with psychotic symptoms has a worse prognosis but responds better to ECT. Up to 15% of people with depression die by suicide, with severe depression and depression with psychotic symptoms at highest risk.

Mania and bipolar affective disorder (BPAD)

Clinical presentation

A *manic* episode is an extreme mood state lasting at least a week (unless shortened by treatment; **Figure 8.6**,

---

BOX 8.3 Sleep hygiene: tips for a good night's sleep

- **Bed's only for sleep and sex:** not studying, eating, screen time, etc. *Being awake in bed teaches you to be awake in bed.*
- **Routine is essential:** get up and go to bed at specific times, even on weekends.
- **Daytime:** *don't* sleep; *do* exercise; avoid caffeine after lunch.
- **Evenings:** avoid alcohol/drugs (sedatives actually *disrupt* deep sleep).
  - Avoid heavy meals, nicotine, and excess fluids.
  - Avoid screens: blue light is stimulating.
  - Wind down for an hour before bed, e.g. soothing music, warm bath.
  - Ensure bedroom is quiet and dark, e.g. ear-plugs, sleep visors, mobile off.
- **Nights:** if awake after 30 minutes, *get up and be bored* for 20–30 minutes, e.g. read a dictionary. Then return to bed. Repeat until sleepy.

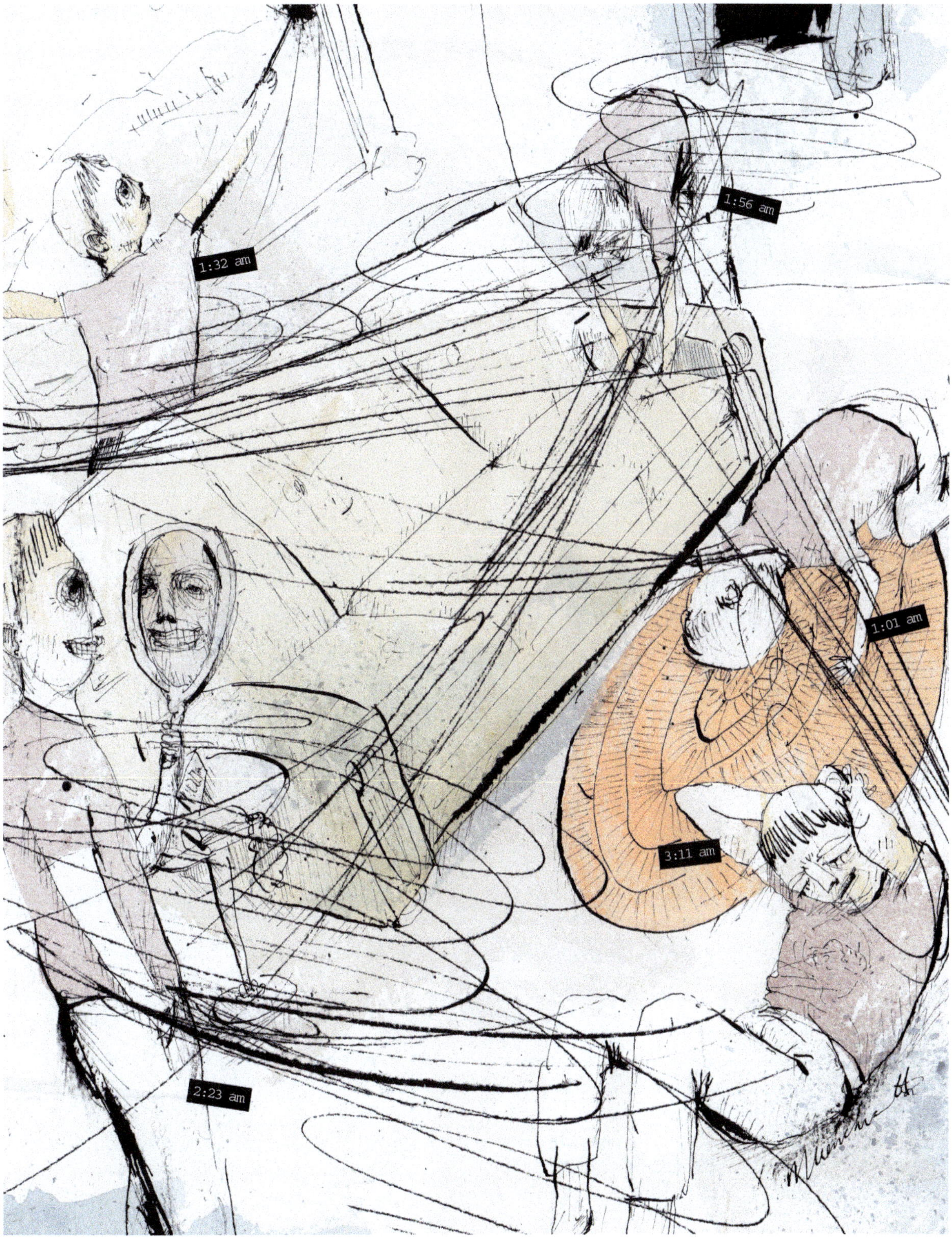

FIGURE 8.6 Clinical features of mania

Table 8.3). A *hypomanic* episode is a persistent mood state lasting at least several days, whose symptoms are less severe, and *don't* cause marked impairment in the person's work or social functioning. A *mixed* episode is a mixture or rapid alteration between manic and depressive symptoms on most days for at least 2 weeks. BPAD is diagnosed when someone has experienced at least one manic/mixed episode (type I) or a hypomanic episode and at least one depressive episode (type II). Episodes may alternate. BPAD may be 'rapid cycling' if

Mania and bipolar affective disorder (BPAD) **45**

Table 8.3 Overview: depression and mania

Factor		Depression	Mania
Duration		≥ 2 weeks	≥ 1 week
Core symptoms	Mood	↓ = Low	↑ = Elated/irritable
	Energy	↓ = Anergia	↑ = Energetic
	Interest/enjoyment	↓ = Anhedonia	↑ = New activities, contacts
Cognitive	Self	↓ = Worthless, guilty	↑ = Grandiose, talented
	World	↓ = Helpless: the world feels overwhelming	↑ = Capable: the world can be dominated
	Future	↓ = Hopeless, pessimistic	↑ = Hopeful, optimistic
	Concentration	↓	↓ = Distractible
	Memory	↓	↓
Biological	Sleep	↓ (Usually)	↓
	Appetite/weight	↓ (Usually)	↑
	Libido	↓	↑
Psychotic	Hallucinations	Auditory: often unpleasant, derogatory	Auditory: often positive/important
	Delusions	Nihilistic Persecutory Guilt	Grandiose Persecutory
Risk	Self	Suicide Self-harm Self-neglect Malnutrition Dehydration	Suicide Spending, gambling Reckless driving Self-neglect Exhaustion Dehydration Vulnerable to exploitation
	Others	Rarely	Aggression Sexual disinhibition

the person experiences four or more episodes within 1 year; this is commoner in women (**Box 8.4**).

Core symptoms

Mood, energy, and enjoyment, lowered in depression, are elevated in mania. The person is elated, excited, irritable, with rapidly changing (labile) mood, including brief tearfulness and distress. They're energetic, overactive, restless, and talkative, with rapid or pressured speech. They may take up new activities and make many acquaintances.

Cognitive symptoms

Self-esteem and confidence are elevated in mania: the person feels more capable than usual and thinks optimistically about the future, ignoring potential pitfalls of their many ideas. Their thoughts and concentration may

> **BOX 8.4** BPAD and related disorders
>
> - **Type I BPAD:**
>   – One or more manic/mixed episodes, often alternating with depressive episodes.
> - **Type II BPAD:**
>   – One or more hypomanic episodes and at least one depressive episode, *without* manic/mixed episodes.
> - **Cyclothymic disorder:**
>   – Persistent mood instability over at least 2 years.
>   – Numerous periods of hypomanic and depressive symptoms present during more of the time than not, causing significant distress and/or functional impairment.

feel clearer than ever before, but they're objectively distractible, with poor concentration and racing thoughts, which change topic rapidly ('flight of ideas').

Biological symptoms

Like depression, mania reduces the person's need for sleep. Unlike depression, libido and appetite are often elevated, although the person may be too 'busy' to eat.

Psychotic symptoms

In severe mania, the person can experience delusions and hallucinations, which are typically mood congruent. For example, auditory hallucinations of religious figures or celebrities instructing or praising them. Delusions are usually grandiose (e.g. of wealth, fame, a special purpose or talents) but sometimes persecutory (e.g. being hated because others envy them).

Risk

A person experiencing a manic episode may be impulsive and/or disinhibited, taking risks without considering the consequences, e.g. overspending, gambling, driving recklessly, drug and alcohol misuse. They may be sexually disinhibited, placing themselves and others at risk of unsafe sex, exploitation, or assault. Irritability can lead to verbal or physical aggression, inciting assault in retaliation. Self-harm and suicide attempts can occur in moments of sudden despair; illness or death from dehydration and physical exhaustion are possible if untreated.

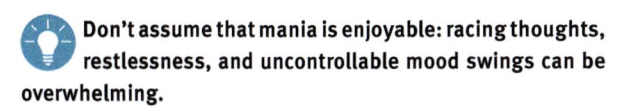

> 💡 **Don't assume that mania is enjoyable: racing thoughts, restlessness, and uncontrollable mood swings can be overwhelming.**

> 💡 **It's possible to 'mask' (hide) hypomania in a short assessment; collateral history is crucial.**

Differential diagnosis

- **Organic causes**, such as delirium, intoxication (e.g. amphetamines, cocaine), dementia, frontal lobe damage, cerebral infection (e.g. HIV), and 'myxoedema madness' (paradoxical state of hyperactivity in extreme hypothyroidism).
- **Schizoaffective disorder:** psychotic and affective symptoms evolve simultaneously (see p.85).
- **Emotionally unstable personality disorder:** labile mood and impulsivity can mimic mania, but will be persistent traits, not episodic symptoms.
- **Perinatal disorders** (see p. 227).
- **Attention deficit hyperactivity disorder:** can be hard to distinguish from emerging BPAD in young people, but ADHD is more persistent and develops earlier (by the age of 6).

Investigations

- **Collateral history**.
- **Physical examination**.
- **Blood tests**: FBC, TFTs, CRP, ESR for infection/autoimmune/thyroid problems; other tests as indicated by history, e.g. HIV.
- **Urinary drug screen**.
- **CT/MRI head** for intracerebral causes, if indicated (e.g. abrupt symptoms, change in consciousness, focal neurological signs).
- **Consider lumbar puncture** if encephalitis suspected.

Management

Priorities for acute mania/hypomania are containing risk and initiating mood stabilizing management (**Box 8.5**). Longer-term treatment is required after even a single manic episode, since likely future episodes are potentially devastating.

Biological interventions

Medications

Long term, BPAD is treated with mood stabilizers or mood-stabilizing antipsychotics. Other medications can be added during relapses or times of elevated relapse risk. People with BPAD and their loved ones may identify relapse indicators and initiate medication themselves.

BOX 8.5 Acute management of hypomania and mania

Hypomania may be managed in the community, but mania usually needs hospital admission, often under the Mental Health Act (see p. 29). For both, management entails:

- Stopping exacerbating medications, e.g. antidepressants, steroids, dopamine agonists.
- Limiting access to drugs and alcohol where possible.
- Monitoring food and fluid intake, to prevent dehydration.
- Considering a short course of benzodiazepines/hypnotics.
- Starting/optimizing mood stabilizing medication:
  - Second-generation antipsychotic (SGA) *or*
  - Mood stabilizer *or*
  - Mood stabilizer plus SGA for severe symptoms/poor response.
- Rarely, considering ECT (e.g. life-threatening overactivity and exhaustion despite medication).

Mood stabilizers 'even out' the extreme highs of mania and, to a lesser extent, the profound lows of depression (**Table 8.4**). Mechanisms of action aren't fully understood but the anticonvulsants may work through sodium channels and the inhibitory neurotransmitter, GABA.

Antipsychotics, e.g. olanzapine, can stabilize mood. They're initiated during a manic episode and may be continued for long-term prophylaxis. SGAs are preferred because of fewer side effects (see p. 87).

💡 **Switching between lithium citrate (usually liquid) and lithium carbonate (usually tablet) requires care: they can contain different amounts of lithium.**

💡 **Some people feel mood stabilizers curb creativity and hamper normal emotions so may discontinue medication. If *you* felt happier and more confident than ever (especially if you'd suffered depression), would *you* take a tablet to 'bring you down'?**

Table 8.4 Comparison of mood stabilizers

Drug	Adverse effects	Good to know
Lithium	Mild tremor GI upset Nausea/vomiting Fatigue Polyuria, polydipsia Hypothyroidism Hyperparathyroidism Weight gain Swollen ankles Metallic taste Teratogenicity	• Biologically similar to sodium, so difficult to prove mechanism of action • Therapeutic plasma range 0.6–1.0mmol/L • Levels taken 12 hours post dose • Narrow therapeutic index, with toxicity from 1.2mmol/L (**Box 8.6**) • Must check plasma level 1 week after starting/changing dose • Weekly monitoring until steady therapeutic level, then every 3 months • Monitor U&Es, calcium, and TFTs every 6 months (risk of renal impairment/hypothyroidism)
Valproate	GI upset, nausea Hair loss (with curly regrowth) Weight gain Fatigue Tremor Peripheral oedema Liver failure Pancreatitis Teratogenicity	• Anticonvulsant: treats acute mania and provides prophylaxis in BPAD • Active drug is valproic acid, but usually given as sodium or semi-sodium salt as fewer side effects • No need to monitor plasma levels (no agreed therapeutic range) • Not for women of child-bearing age (**Box 8.7**)
Carbamazepine	Nausea Headache Drowsiness Dizziness Diplopia, ataxia Leucopenia/rarely, agranulocytosis Rash (occasionally serious) Teratogenicity	• Anticonvulsant • Less effective than lithium or valproate, but can use for prophylaxis • Toxic at high doses • Induces liver enzymes that metabolize many drugs, including itself • Monitor levels closely • Check drug interactions before prescribing • Not for women of child-bearing age
Lamotrigine	Rashes (potentially life-threatening) Headache, tiredness Nausea Dizziness Insomnia	• Anticonvulsant • Good for depressive symptoms: often used in BPAD type II • Carefully titrate dose when starting/stopping to avoid Stevens–Johnson syndrome: flu-like symptoms, rash, blistering mucous membranes

> **BOX 8.6** Lithium toxicity
>
> - Levels greater than 1.2mmol/L.
> - Life-threatening.
> - Presents with diarrhoea, nausea/vomiting, drowsiness, ataxia, slurred speech, gross tremor, fits, and renal failure (Figure 8.7).
> - Triggers include:
>   - Electrolyte changes due to low-salt diets, dehydration, diarrhoea, and vomiting.
>   - Drugs interfering with lithium excretion, e.g. NSAIDs, thiazide diuretics, angiotensin-converting enzyme (ACE) inhibitors.
>   - Overdose.
> - Management: stop lithium and transfer for medical care (rehydration, dialysis).

> **BOX 8.7** Mood stabilizers and pregnancy
>
> - Mood stabilizers are *teratogenic*:
>   - Lithium risks Ebstein's anomaly (tricuspid valve defect).
>   - Valproate and carbamazepine risk spina bifida.
> - Mood-stabilizing antipsychotics are preferred in pregnancy and in women of child-bearing age; carbamazepine and valproate should not be started (if unavoidable, contraception and folic acid supplements are prescribed).
> - If medication *is* used in pregnancy, obstetricians monitor closely for complications.

Antidepressants

Depression in BPAD can be difficult to treat, since antidepressants can *switch* depression to mania. Antidepressants are only prescribed in BPAD *with* a mood stabilizer/antipsychotic; the person is monitored for signs of mania.

Withdrawing medication

Medication may be cautiously and slowly withdrawn if someone has been symptom-free for a sustained period. The risk of relapse and benefits of stopping medication are discussed in full, to support an informed decision, ideally with carer input.

> 💡 Suddenly stopping medication (particularly lithium) can trigger a manic episode.

Psychological interventions

Psychoeducation

The clinician (e.g. care coordinator, psychologist, psychiatrist) works with the person to identify *relapse indicators* (early warning signs), such as insomnia or increased energy. This helps to establish relapse prevention strategies, e.g.:

- Daily routine.
- Sleep hygiene (**Box 8.3**).
- Healthy lifestyle.
- Limiting excessive stimulation/stress.
- Addressing substance misuse.
- Medication changes.

Cognitive behavioural therapy

CBT reduces relapse frequency and the duration and number of inpatient admissions. It combines psychoeducation with opportunities to test and challenge grandiose thoughts, to regain perspective. CBT can inform a Wellness Recovery Action Plan (WRAP), which helps the person identify triggers and relapse indicators, agreeing a management plan for future episodes.

Social interventions

Family therapy works with the person, their family, and support network. It provides psychoeducation, builds trust, and encourages supportive communication to resolve conflicts and facilitate shared problem-solving. Family and friends play a vital role in managing BPAD, as a long-term condition.

Interpersonal and social rhythm therapy (IPSRT) incorporates aspects of IPT for depression, with attention to circadian rhythms. Stabilizing sleeping, waking, eating, and exercise times support the biological rhythms which regulate mood.

Supporting a person with BPAD to maintain their education or career is important. They may share their WRAP with occupational health staff, since stress levels, travel, and unsocial hours may affect recovery.

Support groups run by organizations such as Bipolar UK can facilitate self-monitoring, engagement with treatment, and psychoeducation.

Prognosis

Manic episodes often begin abruptly and are often shorter than depressive episodes, lasting 2 weeks to 5 months. Recovery is usually complete between episodes but remission becomes shorter with age and depressive episodes become more frequent. Up to 15% of people with BPAD die by suicide, although long-term treatment with lithium reduces prevalence to the general population level.

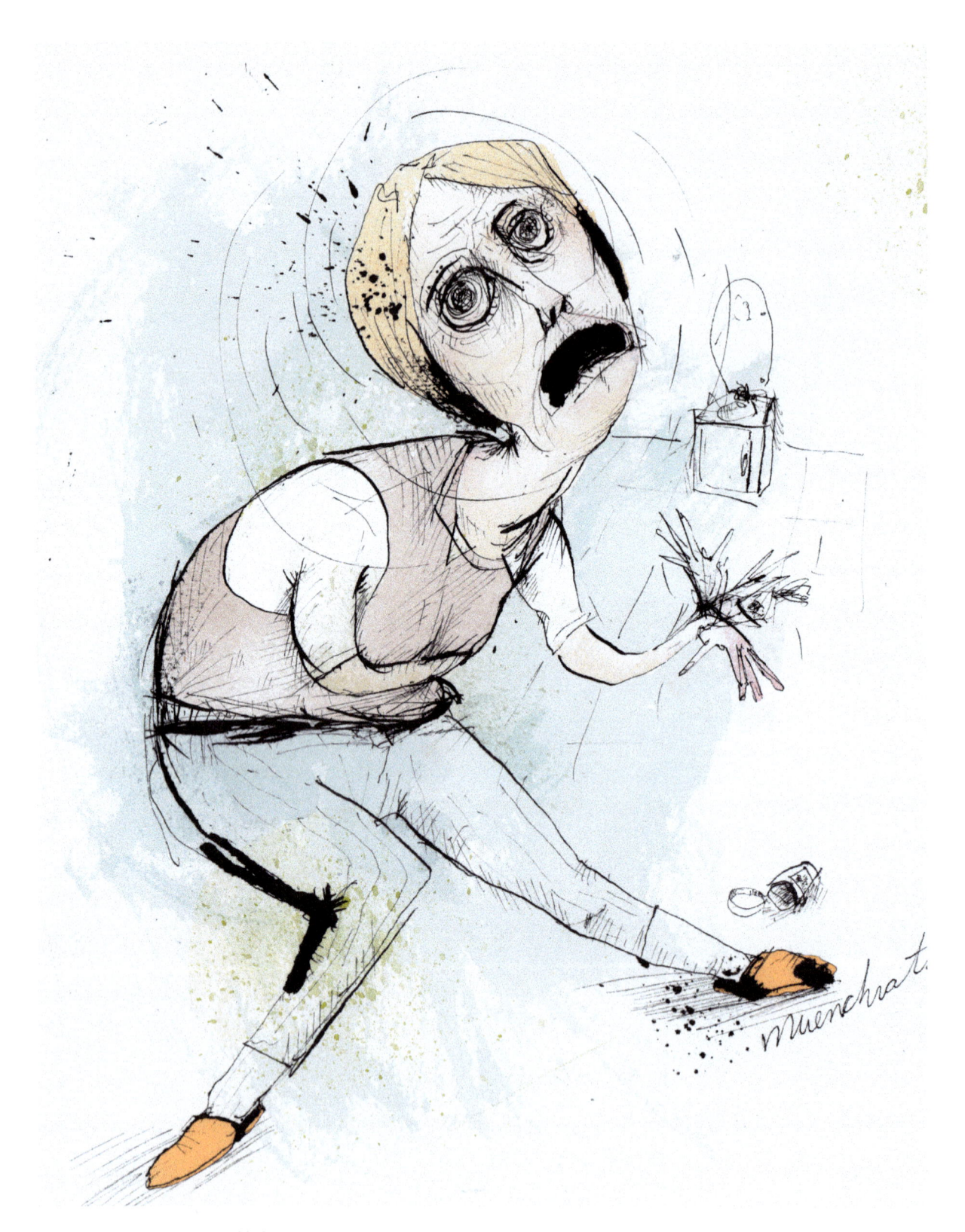

FIGURE 8.7 Symptoms of lithium toxicity

REALITY: DEPRESSION

General approach: tips, tricks, and cautionary tales

1. Don't say, 'I know how you feel'

Although this *seems* empathic, it usually comes across badly, causing despair or even anger that you could expect to know how awful someone else's experience feels. Paradoxically, it's often more empathic to say, 'I can't begin to imagine how that feels', since it recognizes the person's individual, profound experiences.

2. Avoid platitudes

We all grasp for something wise and comforting when we don't know what to say. 'Meaningful' phrases you've heard before are probably a bad idea. For example, if someone tells you their partner has died, *don't* say, 'Time's a great healer!' The inappropriate cheer will cause rapport to crash and burn.

3. It's not what you say, it's how you say it

What *should* you say? Apart from platitudes, almost anything works, if said compassionately. To find the right tone and make it meaningful, it's best to try and use phrases you'd use in everyday life. Note your response the next time a close friend tells you something difficult or painful. Your natural response is better than anything you can memorize from a book. Generally, the simpler the better, e.g. a heartfelt, 'I'm so sorry'/'How awful' often suffices.

4. Depression doesn't make people stupid

Suggesting 'quick fixes' can seem patronizing, e.g.:

> **Carrie:** *[sobbing]* He beats me 'til I do what he says. He says I'm a useless girlfriend and he wishes he'd never met me . . .
> **You:** You should leave him. Don't put up with that!

If it were that simple, she'd have done it by now. Rather than offering solutions, recognize the complexity of Carrie's situation—that she's justified in feeling upset.

5. Saying it's OK won't make it OK

People experiencing depression often make negative statements about themselves; it can be tempting to disagree, e.g.:

> **Beth:** I'm useless *[/fat/stupid/ugly/guilty, etc.]*
> **You:** No, you're not.
> **Beth:** How would you know?!

Beth isn't looking for a debate, just telling you how she feels. Contradicting her won't make Beth feel any better. Instead, try reflecting back the underlying message, e.g. 'You don't like yourself at the moment'. Let her realize that you understand and aren't dismissing her view. This can be difficult; a simpler response might be, 'It must be horrible, feeling like that'. You can also ask *why* she thinks she's useless.

6. Don't fear the tear

Don't panic if someone cries! Crying often shows you're doing everything *right*—that you've reached the most important bit of the interview: really close to the heart of the problem. You haven't done anything wrong, so don't apologize or try to stop someone crying. Let them cry—they'll often feel relieved, even grateful, afterwards. Simply recognize that they're upset and *be with them* as they cry; this may be the most therapeutic thing you can do. People are more likely to open up if you can cope with their sadness than if they think they're distressing you, so must protect you from the full force of their feelings.

Offering tissues *immediately* suggests you're uncomfortable and can't tolerate their emotions. On the other hand, don't leave someone gloopy, embarrassed, and struggling to wipe their face with their sleeve; tissues can be comforting and let people cry *more*, knowing they can mop up afterwards.

7. Slow down

Psychomotor retardation, shame, and sensitive topics make this unlikely to be a fast-paced conversation. Set aside plenty of time and *wait* for answers; accepting silence is essential. Open questions are still the rule, unless someone's very slowed: you might need to switch earlier to closed questions if simple *yes* or *no* answers, nodding, or head-shaking are all they can manage. Sometimes you can switch back to open questions once you've gained rapport.

8. Have hope

Depression can feel all-consuming and never-ending; people often think life will never improve (see **Figure 8.1**).

Gently offering hope—without dismissing their sense of hopelessness—is tricky but can be a lifeline. For example, 'It's really common to feel hopeless when you're depressed; as you recover that will change. There are lots of effective treatments to help you get better.'

The interview

• = Example question. ∗ = Question linking to other parts of the history.

Remember that symptoms must be present for at least 2 weeks for a diagnosis.

Core symptoms

Mood

- *How have you been feeling recently?*
- Have you felt very sad or tearful?
- Have you been more anxious or snappy than normal?
- Which bit of the day feels the worst/do you dread the most? *[Diurnal variation]*
- ∗ You've been low for a year. Did something happen a year ago?

Anergia

- *How are your energy levels at the moment?*
- Have you been feeling worn out or tired all the time?
- ∗ How's it affecting you? *[Screen: work/studies/childcare, etc.]*

Anhedonia

- *Can you enjoy things like you used to?*
- Have you lost interest in things you used to do?
- ∗ Do you still enjoy work/studies/hobbies?
- ∗ Can you still enjoy spending time with friends or family?

Cognitive symptoms

Worthlessness

- *How do you see yourself, as a person?*
- How would you compare yourself to other people?
- Can you think of something you're proud of? (Anything at all?)

Guilt

- *Why do you think you've had such a hard time recently?*
- Do you blame yourself for these problems?
- Do you worry you've let people down?

Helplessness

- *What do you think would help?*
- ∗ What about your family, friends, or the doctors...? Do you think they can help?

Hopelessness

- *How do you see the future?*
- Could things change for the better?
- ∗ Is it ever so bad you feel life isn't worth living?

Concentration/memory/thinking

- *How's your concentration been?*
- Can you focus enough to read a whole page (or watch a whole TV programme)?
- *How's your memory?*
- Can you remember details, say, after reading the news?
- Does your thinking feel more muddled or slowed down than usual?

Biological symptoms

Sleep

- *How's your sleep been lately?*
- Which part of the night is the problem? *[Screen: falling asleep/staying asleep/waking early]*
- ∗ How does that affect your energy levels?

Appetite

- *What's your appetite been like recently?*
- Has your weight changed? How much, roughly?
- Have you noticed your clothes getting baggy (or tight)?
- ∗ Can you be bothered (or find the energy) to cook for yourself?

Libido

- *When people feel low, they can lose their sex drive. Has that been a problem for you?*

💡 Both depression and antidepressants cause sexual dysfunction, but most people won't discuss this unless you've built rapport and asked directly.

Psychotic symptoms

See p. 92.

Hallucinations

- *Have you seen or heard anything recently that seemed strange or frightening?*
- Do people talk about you?

52   8 Affective Disorders

Delusions

- *Are you worried that people have turned against you?*
- Do you worry you've done anything unforgiveable?
- Is your body working properly? Is any part failing, dying, or rotting?

Risk

- *Have you felt so bad, you wanted to harm yourself in some way?*
- Are you eating and drinking enough?

- Are you looking after yourself? Washing, dressing, cleaning . . .?
- Have you had any thoughts of suicide?

💡 **If you believed you were worthless, what would make you question this more? A stranger saying you were worthwhile, *or* listening to everything you had to say?**

1. Depression history (15 minutes)

Candidate's instructions
Rahul Kapoor is a 19-year-old dental student presenting with tiredness. You are a medical student in general practice. Please interview Rahul to make a psychiatric diagnosis.

Patient's brief
Key characteristics
- I'm softly spoken and monotonous.
- I'm emotionally flat and feel sad.
- I'm uncomfortable, making poor eye contact, and crossing my arms as I speak.
- I want to 'get this fixed' but don't really want to admit that I'm depressed.

History
Though I've always been a hard-working student, I've been feeling drained for the past 3 months. Everything's an effort. My concentration's gone and I have to keep rereading the same paragraph to understand it. I feel like nothing's going in. My memory's terrible—I worry I just don't have the ability to learn the things I need to pass. I study late into the night (go to bed about 1am, though I couldn't sleep before then anyway) and wake up feeling exhausted when my alarm goes at 6am. I try to get 2 hours' reading in before lectures or clinics at 9am. I know I'm pushing myself hard, but since failing my exams last year I've lost a lot of confidence in my own ability. I'm in the bottom 5% of students, and I've got to compensate for my lower intelligence with hard work. I don't have time to cook and I'm not hungry often. I might have lost weight.

I used to enjoy dentistry. I wanted to go into maxillo-facial surgery and knew I needed top grades; I suppose this made everything challenging and interesting. Now, studies seem boring, I guess because I've done it all before. Right now, I can't even see myself graduating, let alone doing max-fax work. I was a member of the photography society, but I don't enjoy it enough to put the time aside, and I feel guilty when I'm doing things other than studying. I broke up with my girlfriend, Priya, a month ago—I'd lost interest in our relationship (including sex). I felt I was holding her back and making her miserable. Apart from the study group I attend every evening, I don't really socialize anymore. I deleted all the social apps on my phone to help me focus.

The final term was hard, last year. Dad was diagnosed with prostate cancer and I returned to India to support my family while he had treatment. He died just before my exams. He'd saved so much money for me to come to the UK and study; he was so proud of me and I've let him down and wasted his money. My family was so disappointed when they heard I'd have to re-sit, but they're certain I'll pass. It puts the pressure on. I'm not suicidal, but I just want this all to be over. Sometimes I daydream . . . It would be good to die heroically, save someone from being hit by a car or something. Everyone would remember me well, not see me as a failure.

Other history
- I have no medical problems and take no medication.
- I've never had mental health problems, though my mum had a breakdown, years ago.
- I've never smoked and don't drink or use drugs.

Question	Worry
Can you rule out anaemia, diabetes, and hypothyroidism? I know they cause tiredness.	You'll tell the university I'm depressed and it'll affect my future career—if I have one.

💡 This is a moderate to severe depressive episode. Exclude organic causes, psychoeducate, offer Rahul support to talk to his family and tutors, and refer for CBT. Keep checking his risk of suicide, especially if starting an antidepressant. *Many health professionals suffer from depression; this won't stop Rahul pursuing his career, as long as he seeks and accepts help.*

2. Depression with psychotic symptoms history (15 minutes)

Candidate's instructions
Annette Bristow is a 26-year-old accountant who underwent a termination of pregnancy 2 months ago, following the identification of severe abnormalities at her 12-week scan. Her boyfriend, Mark, has brought her to casualty. He is worried that Annette has stopped eating and drinking. You are a medical student working with the on-call psychiatrist. Please take a mood disorder history.

Patient's brief
Key characteristics
- My voice is quiet and monotonous but not slowed.
- I'm agitated and desperate to 'right my wrongdoing'.
- I make poor eye contact and am distracted at times by children's voices.

History
Mark and I were trying for a baby for 2 years. A good mother would have kept him and loved him . . . But I'm bad through and through; I'm a murderer. I told the doctors to kill my baby because he was disabled. When he died, he tore the cord between us and my life began to drain away. The doctors didn't take his corpse from my womb because they knew I should be punished for what I made them do. I know this because I can smell his corpse rotting inside me; it's so strong I don't know how Mark can't smell it. I'm becoming his grave . . . my organs are rotting and becoming earth over his corpse. I have no womb, just earth. I have no bowels, just earth. I'll soon be completely dead. *You* can't see it, because the death is from the inside, out.

I realized this was happening about 2 weeks ago. Before that (following the termination) I was sad and cried a lot. I cut my legs to punish myself. Then the tears stopped and I hardly needed the toilet because my body was dying. I haven't eaten in a week: there's no point. I last drank yesterday, but there's no point in that either: where would it go? I stay awake at night, praying for my baby's soul. I've no energy, but that's because I'm dying. I don't deserve to enjoy anything. My brain is dying too and everything is slowing to a standstill so I can't remember things or think clearly.

I came to hospital today because I need the doctors to open me up and exhume his corpse. They must hand him to the priests for a proper burial so that he can be blessed and properly buried. I won't need an anaesthetic; my nerves are already earth, so I won't feel it. If the doctors won't open me up, I'll do it myself . . . The skin barely holds back the soil so it won't take much to open me up; I could do it easily with a sharp knife. I hear children calling, 'You're too frightened to die! You'll never free the baby!' They're always with me like black whispers. They scare me, but all this will soon pass.

Other history
- My mother had postnatal depression.
- I was depressed and used to cut myself with scissors as a teenager, but never tried to kill myself.
- I smoked 20 cigarettes a day until 2 years ago. I don't drink and never used drugs.
- No medical problems.
- I don't have any friends now. I don't deserve them or their sympathy.

Question
When can you perform the operation?

Worry
I'll die before the baby can be freed and his soul will go to Hell.

> ⚠️ This is depression with psychotic symptoms, though a history of hypomania/mania would suggest BPAD or schizoaffective disorder. The risk of suicide (to exhume the baby) is high, and Annette will probably need hospital admission to keep her safe while starting an antidepressant and antipsychotic.

REALITY: MANIA

General approach: tips, tricks, and cautionary tales

1. Stay calm and slightly formal

The euphoria of a person experiencing a manic episode can be temporarily contagious. It's easy to be drawn into their excitement, causing the interview to spiral out of control. While gently mirroring people to enhance rapport is usually helpful, consciously *avoid* mirroring mania. Instead, sit still, speak calmly, and stay curious *without* becoming excited. The person may mirror *you* and become calmer but don't be lulled into a false sense of security. Lability means they may suddenly shift from relaxed to distraught or irritable. Again, staying calm is the best response.

To encourage a professional tone, it may help to be more reserved than usual, e.g. addressing the person formally, rather than using their first name.

2. The runaway conversation

Pressure of speech and flight of ideas can produce hefty monologues. Initially, let the person talk uninterrupted; if you cut them off early, you risk a power struggle. As they speak, glean as much information as possible, looking for themes and making a mental note to refer back to them. Then:

- Take control of the conversation, firmly but politely steering back to something you'd like to explore.
- To hold their attention, use short questions, closed questions, and echoes.
- Comment on what you see (e.g. energy/elation).
- Summarize or clarify to show understanding, then refocus the conversation.

> **Dan:** ... by that time, I'd healed all diseases and holy powers were oozing out of me. People were drawn to me and my beautiful, *sexy* body!
> **You:** You could heal? *[Redirection]*
> **Dan:** Yes! Anything at all!
> **You:** When did that start? *[Short question]*
> **Dan:** About 3 weeks ago. It was so exciting! I didn't realize I had anything like this going on until God told me I could heal.
> **You:** God told you? *[Echo]*
> **Dan:** Yes!
> **You:** Did anyone else hear Him? *[Closed question]*
> **Dan:** No! Just me!
> **You:** So, 3 weeks ago, God said you could heal and that's when you got these healing powers. Right? *[Summary]*
> **Dan:** Right! *[Doing a little dance]*
> **You:** Did you always have this much energy? *[Redirection, comment on behaviour]*

3. Be safe, not brave

Disinhibition and irritability can cause rude, sexualized, or aggressive behaviour; you don't want to be on the receiving end. Your safety is the priority (see p. 17). Remember that insults may precede aggression, so view verbal abuse rather like haematemesis: an unpleasant but important sign that you need experienced staff present.

No history or learning opportunity is more important than your well-being—don't 'bravely' stay, if feeling unsafe. Even experienced psychiatrists may only gain the mental state examination of a very unwell person from a distance; they then piece together the story from collateral historians and previous notes.

4. Know your boundaries, spot breaches

Boundaries can feel unclear or irrelevant during a manic episode, causing people to do things they'd never do when well. By protecting your boundaries, you're also protecting *them* from later embarrassment or guilt.

In *clinical* relationships, you wouldn't expect any:

- Intrusive personal questions.
- Flirting.
- Touching (unless clinical).
- Threatening or abusive behaviour.

If *you* know these rules beforehand, you'll spot them being bent or broken. Signs are often *subtle at first*, e.g. a vigorous, prolonged handshake; compliments about your clothing or hair; a brief touch of your shoulder. Context is everything—a euthymic, elderly male patient may simply feel paternal towards you, but someone experiencing a manic episode could be testing your boundaries. If you think it's a boundary push, don't reinforce the behaviour, e.g. by copying, laughing, returning compliments. Set your chair a little further back than usual, keep your own body language and speech formal, and stay alert for further signs.

5. Set boundaries, match defences

Don't run from the room if somebody cheekily winks at you; match the level of your defence to that of the 'breach': a small infringement should result in a small defence; bigger threats need bigger defences. For example:

- Ignore the behaviour/change the topic.
- Increase personal space.
- Verbally set boundaries.
  - Explain 'OK' behaviour (e.g. just talking).
  - Point out inappropriate behaviour, saying why.
  - Warn them you'll have to end the interview if the behaviour continues.
- Leave.

Telling the person that their behaviour is inappropriate feels awkward, but it's really important, e.g.:

> **Dan Davis:** *[Touching your knee]* Sexy legs!
>
> **You:** *[Moving out of reach]* Don't touch me, Mr Davis—that's not OK. I'm here to *talk* to you.
>
> **Dan:** I just wanted to see what it felt like.
>
> **You:** I don't want to be touched. If you do it again, we'll stop the interview. OK?
>
> **Dan:** Fine. So, as you were saying . . . *[Touches your knee again]*
>
> **You:** *[Getting up to leave]* I asked you not to touch me, but you're making me uncomfortable.
>
> **Dan:** I'll be good! Please?
>
> **You:** We can talk another time. Thank you. *[Leaves]*

It's firm, but fair. Always tell experienced staff if you are feeling uncomfortable or threatened—your experience may affect management plans, including whether medical students should see this person alone.

6. Focus on them

Innocent personal questions can pave the way to inappropriate ones—so if you answer initial questions (e.g. whether you can drive), it's harder to avoid later ones without looking awkward (e.g. if you're single). Cut questions off early and turn the focus back on the person, e.g.:

> **Dan:** What are you doing this evening?
>
> **You:** I'm more interested in hearing about your healing powers. Which illnesses did you heal?
>
> **Dan:** Polio, TB, AIDS, dementia . . .

During a manic episode, the person is distractible, with elevated self-esteem, which is why this often works. If not, politely explain that you're there in a professional capacity: you want to talk about them and *can't* talk about yourself.

7. Humility and irritability

However intelligent you are, a manic patient may find your relative 'slowness' and attention to 'meaningless details' rather tiresome. By recognizing this and being humble, you can make the conversation easier. For example:

> **Dan:** I could cure HIV with my eyes, no chemicals needed! I do exactly what it says on the tin! It was obvious to everyone why they'd want my songs!
>
> **You:** I know I sound a bit slow, but why would they want your songs?

💡 **People experiencing a manic episode have an incredible ability to spot your flaws. Don't be surprised, outraged, or upset if they mention that spot on the end of your nose, your coffee breath, or that haircut you wish you'd never had. It's a superpower, of sorts.**

The interview

You're unlikely to see someone experiencing a manic episode in an OSCE, as they'd disrupt the exam (collateral histories are commoner). Get experience interviewing people with mania during your ward placements or shadowing on-call shifts.

Core symptoms

Mood

- *How have you been feeling recently?*
- Are you happier or more cheerful than usual?
- * Do people irritate you more easily these days?
- * When did you start feeling like this? What was happening in your life around then?

Energy

- *How are your energy levels?*
- Have you always had this much energy?
- * How do you spend your energy?

56 8 Affective Disorders

Interests/enjoyment

- **You seem interested in so many things. Are these new interests?**
- You must have a lot of energy to do so much . . .
- You're so busy. When do you manage to sleep/eat/work?

Cognitive symptoms

Self-worth

- **How do you see yourself, as a person?**
- How do you compare to other people?
- What are you most proud of/best at? *[Grandiosity]*
- Are you more daring than other people? *[Risks]*

Optimism/hope

- **You seem such a positive person. Where do you see yourself in a month/year?**

Concentration/thoughts

- **How's your concentration?**
- Can you focus enough to read/watch a whole TV programme?
- Do you find your thoughts jump around a lot?
- Are your thoughts racing?
- You have so many ideas. Where do they come from?

Biological symptoms

Sleep

- **How's your sleep been lately?**
- How does that affect your energy levels?
- You haven't slept in a week? You must be exhausted!

Libido

- **Have you noticed a change in your sex drive?**
- How's that affected you?

Psychotic symptoms

See p. 93.

Hallucinations

- You seem a very sensitive person. **Do you pick up on things other people can't see or hear?**
- Do people gossip or talk about you?
- Is anyone important or famous speaking to you?

Delusions

- **Do you have any special talents (or powers)?**
- Does your life have a mission or special purpose?
- Have you noticed anything in the news that had a special meaning for you?
- Are people jealous of you?

Risk/impulsivity

- **Have you done anything you wouldn't usually do?** *[Screen: drugs/sex/gambling]*
- Have you spent more than usual?
- Have you been in any trouble recently?
- What happens when people irritate you?
- Do you find time to eat and drink?
- Although you're feeling good now, **have you had moments of wanting to harm or kill yourself?**

Manic episode history (15 minutes)

Candidate's instructions

Sally Bateman is a 22-year-old secretary who was admitted to a psychiatric ward 5 days ago under Section 2 of the Mental Health Act. The ward psychiatrist has asked you to take a mood disorder history.

Patient's brief

Key characteristics

- I speak very quickly and jump between subjects, sometimes bursting into song.
- I'm distractible and restless, pacing and moving about.
- I'm over-familiar, asking personal questions and trying to touch or flirt with the student.
- I can abruptly become irritable, giggly, or tearful.
- I'm wearing sunglasses and colourful clothing.
- At times, I hear the producers talking and may answer them.

The interview

History

About 2 weeks ago I felt something amazing was going to happen! I hadn't slept properly for a few days but still had loads of energy. I was so efficient at work, I had time to paint my office purple! My manager was amazed and gave me the week off as a reward. It was a nice change, what with my boyfriend leaving me the week before. Bastard cheated on me. Well, we'll see who's laughing now!

On the way home, I noticed an ad for *Love Island*, looking for contestants with beauty, brains, personality, and heaps of talent. It was *me*! I bought new outfits, saw a plastic surgeon and personal trainer. I used my savings . . . It's only a few thousand but an important investment! People started staring at me in the street, and the paparazzi were everywhere on mopeds; cameras were put up in the shops to film me . . . I love the attention; I kiss my fans and give them cash handouts. I even had (unprotected) sex with a fan who recognized me in the street! I show off my moves and sing the songs I'm writing, for my career outside the villa! I've got more ideas than ever before, coming out so fast I can barely keep up with them! I sometimes hear the producers, you know? 'Sally, darling! You're why we make this show!' I'm not sure how I hear them, but it's got to be a microchip or a widget or a digit or a fidget or something.

A week ago I was strip teasing for fans in Sainsbury's when the TV company staged a police pick-up! (It's all actors, of course, but what a treat!) Anyway, I've ended up in the villa (yes, yes, 'hospital', of course it's a hospital) and it's just amazing! The cameras are everywhere and I've already given them plenty to watch! There's a cute guy here, Juan. He's the *Juan* for me! *Juan*, two, three, four, five . . . I pulled him into the shower and was about to give him *Juan* when the staff stopped us. I put up a good fight for the cameras and had a cry afterwards (got to keep the general public on side). I don't need to sleep! I think it's something the producers put in the water, to keep me awake so I don't bore the viewers. I practise my singing and dance routines throughout the night. I feel great! The best I've ever felt! After I win *Love Island* I'll be bigger than Adele! I'm designing my own line of clothing to complement my new perfume, which I'm calling *Sex*. Would you like my autograph?

Other history

- Depression 2 years ago, treated with antidepressants.
- No medical problems.
- They've started me on olanzapine but it's for show: just a sugar pill.
- I was drinking quite a bit before I came in, champagne mostly! No drugs.
- No one in my family has psychiatric problems.

Question

Do you have a boyfriend/girlfriend? I'm pansexual . . .

Worry

The other contestants are jealous and want me out of the villa.

! This is a manic episode with psychotic symptoms. The history of a previous depressive episode confirms BPAD; schizoaffective disorder is a differential diagnosis. Sally's risk-taking behaviour makes her very vulnerable, and she shouldn't currently have unescorted ward leave. Benzodiazepines would be a useful short-term sedative, and a mood stabilizer or antipsychotic will be needed. Once better, offer sexual health screening, sleep hygiene, and CBT.

NEXT STEPS

Poor recovery post myocardial infarction (MI)

You're a cardiology FY2. Mr Jacobs is a 74-year-old man admitted 2 weeks ago in a dishevelled state, post-MI. He has a history of congestive cardiac failure and stroke. The cardiology team is frustrated because he isn't making progress with his rehabilitation programme and appears withdrawn and unmotivated. You note that his wife died 3 months ago. At the multidisciplinary team meeting, someone proposes that he should be sent to a nursing home.

- What could be wrong with Mr Jacobs?
- How would you manage this situation *before* discharge planning?

Differential diagnosis

Includes bereavement, depression, adjustment disorder, dementia, and delirium.

Preparation

Review Mr Jacobs' notes and gain team members' views. Contact his GP for background, including psychiatric history and how he'd been coping prior to admission. Check for causes of delirium: investigation results, stool chart (constipation?), and drug chart (recent changes, anticholinergic medications).

Assessment

Explore Mr Jacobs' bereavement in more detail, including risk factors for pathological grief, e.g. marital harmony/*discord*, the circumstances of his wife's death, and how he's been since. Elicit depressive symptoms. Check substance misuse, past psychiatric history, and family history. Explore his personal history, including how he coped with previous losses and adversity. Your social history will explore activities of daily living (ADLs) and identify key social contacts for practical and emotional support.

Focus your mental state examination on mood, psychotic symptoms, and cognition. Formally assess Mr Jacobs' cognition using a recognized scale, e.g. the Mini-Addenbrooke's Cognitive Examination (M-ACE). Inattention, disorganized thinking, or clouded consciousness suggests delirium. Ask Mr Jacobs what he understands about the current situation and what he wants in the short and longer term.

Perform a risk assessment, especially considering suicide, self-harm, and accidental injury or self-neglect if he were discharged home imminently. Seek Mr Jacobs' consent to speak with relatives or friends for collateral information, including how he's coped since he lost his wife and whether any cognitive impairment predates his bereavement.

Management

Transfer to a nursing home is a major decision, which should be delayed if Mr Jacobs could regain lost function; a premature move could mean losing his independence and his home. Treat any physical or mental health problems that might prevent rehabilitation; only then can you consider his level of functioning and need for placement.

Bereavement may simply require empathy, normalization, and recruitment of family, friends, or faith leaders for support; if they don't know he's in hospital, *call them*! Normal and pathological bereavement benefits from social support and counselling, e.g. through Cruse Bereavement Care.

If delirium is present, investigate fully and treat the underlying medical cause(s) (see p. 129). Dementia can only be diagnosed after delirium is treated, and with a clear history of decline. Contact liaison psychiatry (the mental health team in a general hospital): they can help further assess dementia and advise on ongoing management.

If Mr Jacobs is experiencing a mild/moderate depressive episode, ensure appropriate blood tests (see p. 40) and consider using a depression rating scale to grade severity and track progress, e.g. Hospital Anxiety and Depression Scale (HADS). Psychological therapy (e.g. CBT) might be possible through liaison psychiatry or upon discharge via the GP. Consider cardiac safety before starting an antidepressant, and check options with liaison psychiatry; an SSRI or mirtazapine are probably safest but discuss choices with Mr Jacobs beforehand. Organize an occupational therapy assessment of his functional ability, both in hospital and at home; this will inform your risk assessment and need for a home-care package. He'll need follow-up by his GP or an older adult CMHT, depending on his response to treatment. More severe depression needs specialist review and management by liaison psychiatry; they may recommend admission to a psychiatric ward.

💡 **In the 6 months after spousal bereavement, mortality rates increase from various sources, including heart disease, cancer, suicide, and accidents. Depression affects as many as 35% of people in Mr Jacobs' position.**

> **Movie buff**
>
> *Homeland* (2011 onwards): this political drama follows Nicholas (Damian Lewis), an American soldier returning home from an Iraq prisoner of war camp. Suspecting his recruitment by Al Qaeda, CIA agent Carrie (Claire Danes) monitors his potential threat to national security. Carrie is a strong female character whose BPAD was praised for its accuracy by people with lived experience. Look out for its sensitive depiction of mania and depression, treatment with lithium and clozapine, and issues of concordance.
>
> *Melancholia* (2011): with a blue planet hurtling towards Earth and the population grappling with imminent mortality, Justine (Kirsten Dunst) finds peace in the knowledge that her world is ending. This beautiful, painful film captures how a person struggling with depression can seem to be functioning, cut off from everyone else.
>
> *Silver Linings Playbook* (2012): Pat (Bradley Cooper) meets Tiffany (Jennifer Lawrence), who suffers from depression, soon after discharge from hospital, where he was treated for BPAD. This Oscar-winning comedy tells their story of recovery through friendship and dance routines.

Book shelf

Gale, P. (2007) *Notes from an Exhibition*: Gale's acclaimed novel accurately portrays the difficulty of living with BPAD through the story of artist Rachel Kelly. Manic and hypomanic episodes allow Rachel to paint; depressive episodes provide darker inspiration but impinge on her marriage and parenthood. Gallery-style postcards link Rachel's mental state directly to her work and the tension between dampening creativity and staying well on medication are sensitively handled.

Jamison, K.R. (1995) *An Unquiet Mind: A Memoir of Moods and Madness*: an autobiographical account of BPAD by an eminent psychologist. Jamison explores the agony of living with BPAD and attempting to maintain her clinical reputation amid her colleagues' stigmatizing views.

Plath, S. (1963) *The Bell Jar*: Plath's semi-autobiographical account of depression demonstrates the waxing and waning nature of the disease with tense clarity.

Styron, W. (1990) *Darkness Visible*: one of the best written accounts of depression, *Darkness Visible* is beautifully written and brutally honest. Styron conveys the horror of depression and its experience as loss: of self-confidence, motivation, and belief that life is worth living. By capturing his descent into the 'despair beyond despair', and his subsequent recovery, Styron shines a light of hope, into the darkest corners of human experience.

Notes

1. Rowling, J.K. (1999). *Harry Potter and the Prisoner of Azkaban*. London: Bloomsbury. Copyright © J.K. Rowling 1999.
2. Jamison, K.R. (1995). *An Unquiet Mind: A Memoir of Moods and Madness*. Toronto: Random House.

Journal club

Beck, A.T., Rush, A.J., Shaw, B.F., et al. (1979) *Cognitive Therapy of Depression*. New York: Wiley.

Cipriani A., Furukawa T.A., Salanti G., et al. (2018) Comparative efficacy and acceptability of 21 antidepressant drugs for the acute treatment of adults with major depressive disorder: a systematic review and network meta-analysis. *The Lancet*, **391**, 1357–66.

Hawton, K., Salkovskis, P., Kirk, J., et al. (1996) *Cognitive Behaviour Therapy for Psychiatric Problems: A Practical Guide*. Oxford: Oxford Medical Publications.

Maier, S.F., Seligman, M.E.P. (1976) Learned helplessness: theory and evidence. *Journal of Experimental Psychology: General*, **105**, 3–46.

McGuffin, P., Rijsdijk, F., Andrew, M., et al. (2003) The heritability of bipolar affective disorder and the genetic relationship to unipolar depression. *Archives of General Psychiatry*, **60**, 497–502.

Rush, A.J., Trivedi, M.H., Wisniewski, S.R., et al. (2006) Acute and longer-term outcomes in depressed outpatients requiring one or several treatment steps: a STAR*D Report American. *Journal of Psychiatry*, **163**, 1905–17.

Sartorius, N. (2001) The economic and social burden of depression. *Journal of Clinical Psychiatry*, **62**(Suppl 15), 8–11.

Go to www.oup.com/uk/stringer2e for a wealth of additional resources, including an OCSE mark scheme, filmed scenarios, and self-assessment questions.

9 Self-Harm and Suicide

True or false?

Answers on p. 277

1. Suicide rates are highest in social classes IV and V.
2. People attending hospital following self-harm are 50 times more likely to die by suicide in the next 12 months.
3. About 60% of people dying by suicide have self-harmed in the past.
4. Limiting paracetamol pack size and installing catalytic converters had little impact on suicide rates.
5. Most people who die by suicide have a psychiatric disorder.
6. If paracetamol levels are significantly elevated, overdose is treated with activated charcoal.
7. Most people who self-harm are admitted to hospital to minimize the risk of suicide.
8. SSRIs are the safest antidepressants where there is a risk of overdose.
9. Gastric lavage deters people from attempting another overdose.
10. Treating the physical complications of self-harm against a person's will requires use of the Mental Health Act.

Contents

Principles
Introduction
Epidemiology
Aetiology
- Genetics
- Childhood and life experiences
- Social isolation
- Occupation
- Physical illness
- History of self-harm
- Psychiatric illness

Theories
- Mentalization
- Self-preservation

Clinical presentation
- Presentation
- Method
- Function and lethality
- Discovery
- Self-cutting
- Overdose

Management
- Immediate interventions
- Follow-up
- After suicide

Prognosis

Reality
General approach: tips, tricks, and cautionary tales

The interview
- Risk assessment following self-cutting
- Risk assessment following overdose

Next steps
Self-harm treatment refusal
- Immediate management
- Ongoing management

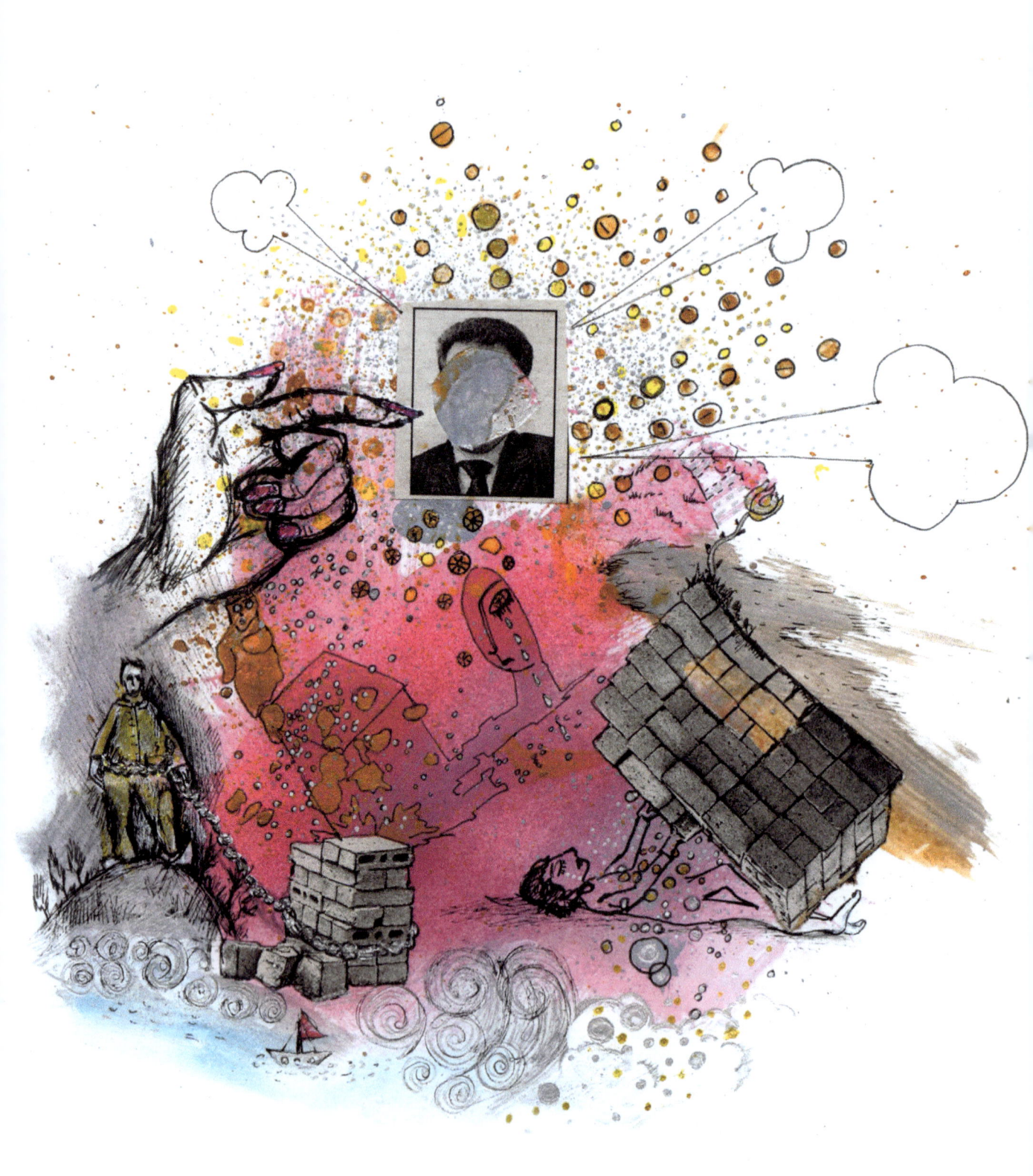

PRINCIPLES

Dearest, I feel certain that I am going mad again. I feel we can't go through another of those terrible times. And I shan't recover this time. I begin to hear voices, and I can't concentrate. So I am doing what seems the best thing to do [. . .] What I want to say is I owe all the happiness of my life to you. You have been entirely patient with me and incredibly good. I want to say that—everybody knows it. If anybody could have saved me it would have been you. Everything has gone from me but the certainty of your goodness. I can't go on spoiling your life any longer. I don't think two people could have been happier than we have been.

Virginia Woolf's suicide note[1]

Introduction

Self-harm and suicide can be highly emotive areas of medicine, for the person concerned, carers, and staff. Self-harm is any intentional act of self-injury, *irrespective* of the motive. It ranges from milder harm (e.g. self-scratching) to attempted suicide (e.g. near-fatal hanging). Older terms include non-suicidal self-injury and parasuicide. Suicide is when someone ends their life. This chapter explains self-harm, helping you to navigate your own and other people's emotions, to compassionately help those affected by self-harm or suicide.

> The term *deliberate self-harm* is now avoided as it carries a sense of blame. Likewise, saying someone *committed suicide* implies it's a crime, like committing murder (in the UK, suicide was legalized under the Suicide Act 1961).

Epidemiology

The lifetime risk of self-harm is 7–13%; it accounts for 10% of medical admissions. It's under-reported, but commonest in adolescents and young adults. Women are more likely than men to be treated for self-harm but male prevalence may be similar. People in social classes IV and V are at highest risk.

Up to 2% of all deaths are suicides, representing nearly a million worldwide each year. Globally, suicide prevalence increased from 10 to 16 per 100,000 in the past 50 years but declined in the UK (10–11 per 100,000), where suicide is highest among people who are:

- Male: they're three to four times more likely than women to die by suicide, partly due to more violent methods, e.g. hanging, shooting.
- In social class I (professional occupations) and V (unskilled occupations).
- Middle aged (40–54 years).
- Over 80 years old.

However, suicide rates are increasing fastest in young people (15–30 years). It's the leading cause of death in young people and new mothers. Suicide *attempts* are up to 20 times more frequent than suicide (**Box 9.1**).

> Worldwide, suicide is the second leading cause of death in 15–29-year olds and the leading cause of death among adolescent girls.

Aetiology

Genetics

A family history of self-harm is common in people who self-harm, while a family history of suicide is common in people who self-harm with suicidal intent. The risk of completed suicide is elevated in people with a family history of mental illness *or* suicide. Twin and adoption studies suggest the heritability of suicide is 43%. Low levels of serotonin metabolites have been detected in the cerebrospinal fluid (CSF) of people who've attempted or completed suicide.

Childhood and life experiences

Many people who self-harm have a history of childhood abuse (including sexual abuse), neglect, or bullying; these may also predispose to suicide, years later. Self-harm is commoner among certain adolescent subcultures, e.g. LGBTQ (lesbian, gay, bisexual, transgender, queer) and 'goth' young people.

Self-harm is associated with stressful life events in adulthood, including current domestic violence. Completed suicide is particularly associated with loss events, especially bereavement.

Social isolation

People who die by suicide are more likely to be isolated: *living alone, unemployed, divorced, widowed,* or *single*. Connectedness (family/community support) is a protective factor.

Occupation

Access to lethal means is associated with higher risk of suicide, e.g. vets, farmers, military personnel. Suicide rates in highly skilled professionals (e.g. doctors) have reduced recently; the highest risk occupations are now manual, male-dominated trades, e.g. building, metalwork, construction.

Physical illness

Chronic, painful, and terminal illnesses increase the risk of suicide. Risks are particularly high in neurological (e.g. epilepsy) and stigmatized conditions (e.g. HIV).

History of self-harm

Any history of self-harm increases the risk of future self-harm. Up to 60% of people who die by suicide have previously self-harmed. The lifetime risk of suicide in people who have self-harmed is 3–5%, increasing to 10–15% if there was clear suicidal ideation. *Self-harm with suicidal intent is the strongest predictor of eventual suicide.*

Psychiatric illness

The risk of self-harm is increased in people with depression, anxiety disorders, and BPAD. It's associated with personality disorders (especially borderline and dissocial types), conduct/dissocial disorder (CDD), autism spectrum disorders (ASDs), and substance use disorders. Impulsivity may mediate this relationship. Nine out of 10 people dying by suicide have a psychiatric disorder at the time of death.

BOX 9.1 Suicide prevention strategies

Government interventions at a national level can lower suicide rates. UK strategies include:

- Limiting paracetamol pack sizes and pack numbers purchased.
- Installing barriers, free telephones, and helpline posters at suicide 'hotspots'.
- Mandatory catalytic converters to cut carbon monoxide in car exhaust fumes.
- Media guidance for reporting: limited detail to prevent copying.

- *Depression*: 15% lifetime risk of suicide; up to 80% of suicides are associated with depression. High-risk symptoms include recurrent suicidal thoughts, insomnia, weight change, extreme hopelessness, worthlessness, or guilt. Risk may *increase* as severe depression lifts, providing the energy and motivation to act on suicidal thoughts.
- *Bipolar affective disorder*: 15% die by suicide and 30% attempt suicide.
- *Personality disorders*: present in up to 50% of people dying by suicide. Dissocial, disinhibited, and borderline traits are particularly associated.
- *Schizophrenia*: 10% lifetime risk of suicide. People experiencing command hallucinations to self-harm; and young, high-functioning, recently diagnosed people, with insight into the severity of their illness, are at highest risk.
- *Anxiety disorders*: suicide risk is elevated in people with all anxiety disorders.
- *Substance use disorders*: increase the risk of suicide, as intoxication can exacerbate distress and impulsivity. Fifty per cent of suicide attempts are associated with alcohol use within 6 hours. Alcohol dependence carries a lifetime suicide risk of 7%.

Theories

Mentalization

Childhood should provide a validating environment, where supportive parental figures take the child's emotional experiences seriously and reflect them back, e.g. 'That looks sore! Does it hurt? Poor you.' This encourages *mentalizing*: the ability to reflect on, process, and manage emotions. It allows the child to understand their emotional experiences and gain insight into other people's feelings. When childhood is traumatic, abusive, or neglectful, there's little opportunity for reflection. Rather than learning to tolerate and understand uncomfortable emotions, they may learn *behaviours* to manage their mood or ventilate their emotions, e.g. shopping, punching walls. When mentalization skills are underdeveloped, self-harm may be used to deal with difficult emotions like anger, sadness, or anxiety.

Self-preservation

Although it looks destructive, self-harm may represent a coping strategy: attacking only a *part* of the body (representing the condemned self), to secure the survival of the whole person. For some people, painful, non-lethal self-harm *protects* them from suicide.

Clinical presentation

Although self-harm is an umbrella term for all self-injury, it's clinically important to identify people at high risk of suicide. Don't make assumptions about risk—explore all presentations thoroughly for risk factors associated with completed suicide (**Table 9.1**).

Preparation

Self-harm may be impulsive or planned in detail, over days, weeks, or months. In-depth preparation poses a higher risk of completed suicide. Preparation includes research on methods, obtaining equipment, visiting potential locations, and rehearsal. Someone putting their affairs in order ('last acts') suggests expected fatality and is particularly worrying, e.g. writing a will, rehoming pets, seeing friends, apologizing to enemies.

Method

Explore what the person did in detail (see p. 71), including location, timing, precautions taken against discovery (e.g. locking doors, turning off phones), suicide notes (or 'signing off' online), and drug and alcohol use. Methods include:

- Scratching, punching, head-banging.
- Cutting, burning, interfering with wounds.
- Self-poisoning, e.g. overdoses, ingesting bleach, pesticides.
- Inhaling toxic fumes (e.g. car exhausts) or inert gases (e.g. helium).
- Swallowing or inserting items, e.g. razor blades.
- Self-stabbing.
- Jumping from a height (e.g. bridges, car parks) or in front of trains/vehicles.
- Hanging, asphyxiation.
- Shooting.
- Drowning.
- Self-immolation (setting yourself on fire).

Violent or medically dangerous methods elevate the risk of completed suicide but do not always reflect the extent of the person's distress.

Function and lethality

The *function* (purpose) of self-harm may or may not be suicide (**Box 9.2**), although dangerous methods more often represent a suicide attempt; this needs to be clarified with the person.

Explore the person's view of the act's *lethality* (whether they thought it could kill them). This can be surprising: someone may believe a medically insignificant overdose would be lethal or expect to survive a large overdose.

> 💡 **It's not always a good sign when an agitated person suddenly appears calm: they may feel peaceful, having decided to die.**

Discovery

The person coming to hospital after calling an ambulance or messaging a friend (and accepting help when it arrived) is less concerning than if they were accidentally discovered (and resisted assistance).

Self-cutting

Self-cutting is the commonest form of self-harm, often with a knife or razorblade on concealed parts of the arms or thighs. Although cuts are usually superficial, people may sever blood vessels, nerves, and tendons or even amputate body parts. They may describe superficial cutting relieving emotional tension and replacing it with calmness or mild elation. Using safety measures to prevent serious harm suggests a lower risk of suicide, e.g. cleaning blades, cutting 'safer' fleshy areas, bandaging wounds. When someone has a long history of cutting, a changed cutting pattern is worrying, e.g. superficial cuts becoming deep gashes, cutting the throat instead of thighs.

> 💡 **Many people self-harm secretly, hiding their scars: the opposite of 'attention-seeking'!**

Overdose

Overdose is the self-harm most commonly treated in hospital. The agent and quantity ingested affects symptoms, risk, and treatment. Overdose is a differential diagnosis for unexplained sedation, confusion/coma, arrhythmia, bradycardia/tachycardia, hypotension/hypertension, or respiratory depression. 'Accidental' overdoses, including of recreational drugs, may have been deliberate. Over-the-counter analgesia is often used in overdose; people may visit multiple shops to overcome sales restrictions and avoid arousing suspicion. Prescriptions for people at risk of suicide are limited and monitored by their GP.

- *Paracetamol*: usually causes nausea, vomiting, or no symptoms initially. Untreated, it causes fulminant liver failure, with jaundice, abdominal pain, confusion, coma, and death. Staggered overdoses (excess tablets taken over more than 1 hour) are particularly dangerous: blood paracetamol levels are misleadingly low, and damage is cumulative.
- *Non-steroidal anti-inflammatory drugs (NSAIDs)*, e.g. ibuprofen. Symptoms include headache, nausea,

Table 9.1 Self-harm: risk factors for completed suicide

Risk factor	Higher risk	Lower risk/*Protective
Demographic		
Sex	Male	Female
Age	Middle aged / elderly (over 80)	Under 18 years
Marital status	Widowed > divorced > single	*Married/supportive partner
Social network	Isolated/living alone	*Supported
Employment	Unemployed/job with access to means	*In work/education
Accommodation	Homeless	Stable
Personal history		
Self-harm	Especially with suicidal intent	✗
Mental illness	Any	None
Physical illness	Painful, neurological, terminal, stigmatizing	Healthy
Family history	Suicide, mental illness	None
Substance use	Harmful use, dependence	No misuse
Personality traits	Dissocial, disinhibited, borderline	None
Self-harm		
Triggers	Insoluble/ongoing	Resolved
Preparation	Extensive	Limited
Last acts	✓	✗
Suicide note	✓	✗
Method	Violent/medically risky	Less harmful
Access to means	Access to firearms or pesticides	✗
Function	Suicide	Not suicide
Lethality	Believed lethal	Believed non-lethal
Alone at time	✓	✗
Precautions against discovery	✓	✗
Substance use involved	✓	✗
Discovery	Found accidentally	Sought help
Help-seeking	Refusing/resisting	Engaging
Hope	Hopeless	*Hopeful
Ongoing suicidal plans	✓	✗

> **BOX 9.2 Self-harm functions**
>
> - Coping strategy: to survive stressful situations/avoid suicide.
> - Relieving or regulating strong emotions, e.g. anger, despair.
> - Feeling *something* instead of numbness.
> - Exchanging emotional pain for physical pain.
> - Escaping consciousness, e.g. overdose to sleep.
> - Self-punishment.
> - Communicating distress.
> - Changing intolerable situations, e.g. relationship issues.
> - Suicide.

vomiting, drowsiness, dizziness, blurred vision, and sometimes tinnitus. Large overdoses cause acute kidney injury, seizures, hepatic dysfunction, cardiovascular collapse, and coma.

Management

Any self-harm must be taken seriously, as it communicates distress and is a risk factor for suicide.

Immediate interventions

Biological

The initial priority is assessing and treating physical consequences, e.g. fractures, burns, blood loss. The mental capacity of people trying to leave hospital before treatment is assessed, due to the risk of active suicidal intent. If they lack capacity to decline treatment (e.g. acute intoxication), treatment in their best interests may be required (see p. 29).

Lacerations

Superficial cuts are sutured under local anaesthetic and closed with butterfly sutures or skin glue. Deep cuts causing functional (nerve/tendon) or cosmetic damage (e.g. facial cuts) require surgical closure.

Overdoses

Depending on the substance, physical observations, blood tests, and ECGs are needed, sometimes over several hours. ToxBase (www.toxbase.org) provides management guidance for rarer overdoses without established protocols. Treatments include:

- *Antidotes*—available for some poisons, e.g.:
  - Paracetamol: *N*-acetylcysteine (NAC; **Box 9.3** and **Figure 9.1**).
  - Benzodiazepines: flumazenil.
  - Insulin: glucagon.
  - Opiates: naloxone.
  - Digoxin: digoxin-specific antibody fragments (Digibind®).
  - Iron salts: desferrioxamine mesylate.
- *Activated charcoal*—binds many poisons, preventing absorption from the gut into the blood, e.g. antidepressants. Useful only within 1 hour.
- *Active elimination*—some poisons can be eliminated more quickly with haemodialysis (e.g. lithium, salicylates, valproate), urine alkalinization (e.g. salicylates), or repeated activated charcoal (e.g. carbamazepine).
- *Gastric lavage* ('stomach pumping')—washing out stomach contents within 1 hour of overdose. Rarely used and never for corrosive substances.

Supportive management is sometimes all that can be offered immediately, and may require transfer to intensive care, especially for respiratory depression.

Psychosocial

See also p. 69.

Risk assessment

Once physical consequences are treated or stabilized, a psychiatrist or psychiatric liaison nurse conducts a thorough psychosocial assessment. Assessment can be therapeutic, by validating distress and identifying the person's support needs. It includes:

- Details of current and previous self-harm.
- Social circumstances and stressors, and triggers for self-harm.
- Diagnosis of underlying mental illness and its relationship to self-harm.
- Evaluation of hopelessness, suicidal intent, and persistent plans to self-harm.
- Strengths and coping strategies.
- Risk and protective factors for future self-harm/completed suicide.

This evaluates immediate and longer-term risks of self-harm and suicide. Labelling risk as *low, medium,* or *high* is less helpful than elaboration of the person's risk (e.g. presence of continuing stressors versus resolution of relationship conflict following hospital admission).

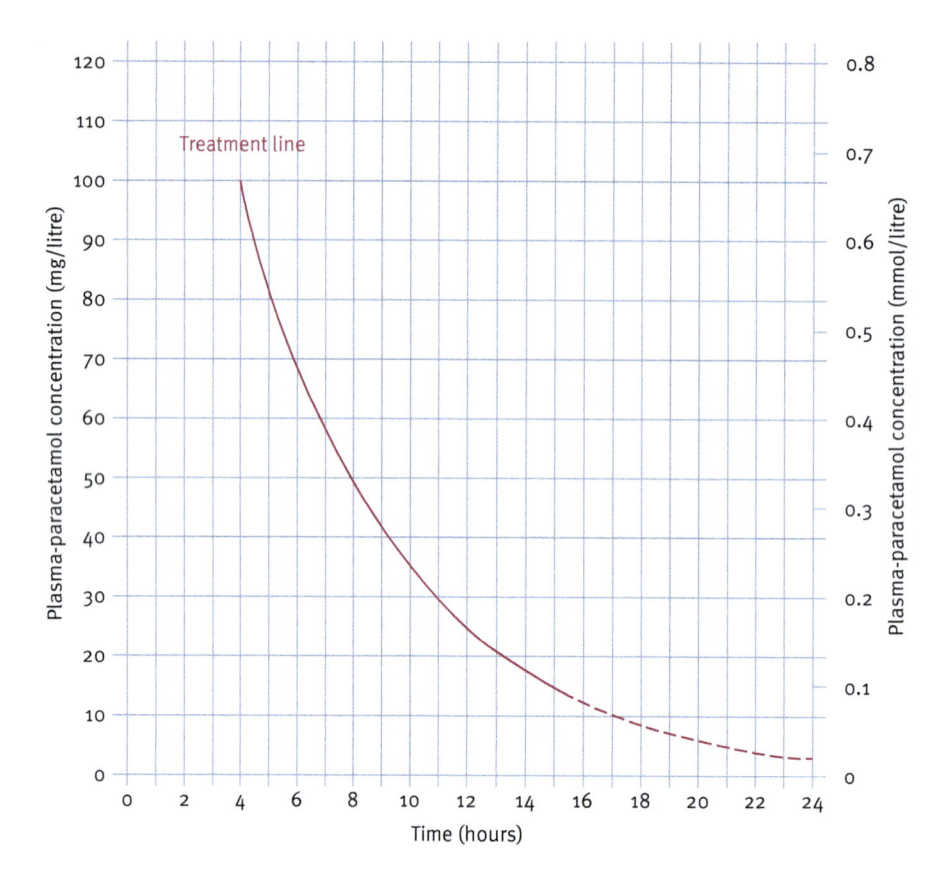

FIGURE 9.1 Treatment nomogram.

Reproduced from Medicines and Healthcare products Regulatory Agency (2014). Treating paracetamol overdose with intravenous acetylcysteine: new guidance. *Drug Safety Update*. Contains public sector information licensed under the Open Government Licence v3.0. https://www.gov.uk/

BOX 9.3 NAC and paracetamol overdose

- Paracetamol metabolism produces a toxic by-product, N-acetyl-p-benzoquinone imine (NAPQI). Glutathione usually immediately conjugates NAPQI, but paracetamol overdose depletes glutathione stores.
- NAPQI starts causing hepatotoxicity around 8 hours post overdose.
- Within 8 hours of overdose, IV NAC is almost 100% effective in preventing liver damage by replenishing glutathione stores.
- Three infusions over 21 hours are dosed according to the person's weight.
- NAC is administered for:
  - Plasma paracetamol levels on or above the treatment line, 4–15 hours post overdose.
  - Staggered overdoses.
  - Overdoses with unclear timing.
- See Figure 9.1.

Risk management

A problem-solving approach addresses stressors and risk factors (e.g. accessing emergency accommodation if homeless). People at immediate risk of suicide can be admitted to psychiatric hospital for further assessment and treatment in a safe, supportive environment. This may include close observation (e.g. 1:1 nursing), restricted leave, treatment of underlying problems (e.g. depression, psychosis). The Mental Health Act (MHA) may enforce admission if the person refuses or lacks capacity to consent because of a mental health problem.

Before discharge, a care plan is agreed with the person, including how they'll handle future thoughts of self-harm, and access crisis support (e.g. calling a support line, attending hospital). With the person's consent, this plan should involve family or friends.

Follow-up

Most people can be safely managed at home, especially if they have a supportive network, aren't actively suicidal, and will seek help if feeling worse. Follow-up should be arranged *within a week*, e.g. with a CMHT, outpatient clinic, GP, or therapist. The crisis/home treatment team can visit daily to monitor the person's mental state and risk and supervise medication, limiting impulsive overdoses.

Biological

Disorders underlying self-harm require treatment. If needed, medications with the lowest risk of toxicity in overdose are prescribed, for short periods (e.g. 1–2 weeks), reviewed regularly to prevent stockpiling. Treatment of physical illnesses and chronic pain (risk factors for suicide) is optimized.

> ❗ **Tricyclic antidepressants (TCAs) caused many suicides until the advent of selective serotonin reuptake inhibitors (SSRIs), which are safest in overdose.**

Psychological

Brief psychological interventions (3–12 sessions) effectively reduce self-harm. CBT has the strongest evidence, but therapists may also introduce problem-solving and psychodynamic techniques. Coping strategies include distraction techniques and uplifting activities (e.g. exercise, socializing). Some people find particular strategies helpful (**Box 9.4**), while others find them patronizing.

Borderline/emotionally unstable personality disorder is strongly associated with self-harm. Longer-term psychological therapies reduce repeated self-harm, e.g. dialectical behaviour therapy (DBT; see p. 262) and mentalization-based treatment (MBT).

Social

Stressors triggering self-harm or depression are tackled (see p. 44). Recruiting friends and family to a support network for times of crisis shows the person that they're loved, important to others, and not alone in coping with problems.

If the person isn't ready to stop self-harming, psychoeducation and harm reduction can make them safer, e.g. never sharing blades, basic first aid.

After suicide

Death isn't the end of the story; on average, six people suffer intense grief reactions following every suicide. When qualified, you may need to speak to friends or family after a suicide. Beforehand, obtain all available facts about the death, including names of key staff, the method, injuries sustained, and treatments given. Be clear and compassionate in your explanation, using 'chunking' to provide small pieces of information one at a time. Keep to the facts, remembering that providing all details initially may not be helpful.

Bereaved people often feel responsible or think they should have prevented the death; allowing them to express these feelings can help. Encourage them to seek support from friends or family, including when identifying the body; it's a difficult time to be alone. Don't avoid the topic of organ donation (if relevant); this may salvage a sense of purpose for the person's life. Signpost potential supports, e.g. chaplains/counsellors, the Survivors of Bereavement by Suicide charity. All suspected suicides have a coroner's inquest (often delaying funeral arrangements). It may comfort the family that the healthcare trust will investigate the suicide (if in hospital), to learn from it. Depending on your role and time commitments, you may offer to meet again at a later point.

Prognosis

In the year after an episode of self-harm, one in six people self-harms again and the risk of completed suicide is over 50 times that of the general population. Although risk factors can be managed, suicide isn't 100% preventable. For some people, surviving a suicide attempt becomes a turning point in their life, when their recovery begins.

> 💡 **The semicolon (;) has become a symbol (often a tattoo) of people reaching the point of suicide but choosing to continue; just as a semi-colon continues a sentence, rather than ending it with a full stop.**

> ❗ **One-third of suicides by people accessing mental health services occurs within 3 months of discharge from a psychiatric ward; the first week is particularly high risk.**

BOX 9.4 Strategies to reduce or prevent self-harm

Prevention

- Avoid things that 'trigger' self-harm, e.g. websites.
- Store tablets/sharp objects out of sight and easy reach.
- Contact friends when tempted to self-harm.
- Carry friends' and helpline telephone numbers.
- Avoid drugs and alcohol (increase likelihood and severity of self-harm).

Alternatives to painful, damaging self-harm

- Snap a rubber band around the wrist.
- Squeeze ice cubes/plunge fingers into ice cream.
- Bite something strongly flavoured, e.g. chilli, lemon.

REALITY

General approach: tips, tricks, and cautionary tales

1. Stigma and assumptions

People who self-harm can face a lot of stigma, even from healthcare professionals, who may struggle to understand and judge them as attention-seeking or selfish. These assumptions are ignorant and unprofessional. Worse, they may increase the person's level of risk by causing conflict, escalating distress, and alienating them from services.

If making assumptions, let it be: *self-harm was the best or only option this person had at the time*. This encourages an attitude of compassion and respectful curiosity, lowering risks by building rapport and allowing comprehensive assessment.

2. Bear the unbearable

Self-harm is often a way of communicating that emotions, thoughts, memories, or events feel unbearable or overwhelming. It suggests that the person struggles to talk about these issues or doesn't have someone to listen.

Don't accidentally minimize their problems (e.g. 'It'll be OK')—they won't feel you're taking them seriously. Instead, *bear to hear* them. By listening and bearing witness to their problems, you're communicating that they're not alone. This raises hope that others might also bear to listen and that they don't have to deal with problems alone, through self-harm. You're also modelling a calm response, which 'contains' their distress and might differ from how those closest to them usually react.

Strong emotions may follow, including frustration, guilt, shame, fear, and despair. Stay calm: these show that you're exploring essential issues.

3. Find the function

Self-harm serves many functions. A person may feel annoyed if you assume the function, e.g. that they attempted suicide when they were actually punishing themselves, or vice versa.

Asking 'Why did you do this?' can feel intrusive or overwhelming, and some people struggle to put their reasons into words. Instead, draw out the story of what happened *and* (if possible) how they were feeling. Then explore how the self-harm fitted in, e.g.:

Helen: Look! *[Showing cuts]* I cut down to the bone and needed surgery!

You: That looks painful. Things must have been awful for you to cut so deep.

Helen: Yeah. Everything was shit!

You: What was happening?

Helen: Well . . . *[Explains]*

You: *[Summarizes]* . . . then Ryan cheated on you and left, and you couldn't pay the rent. Is that right?

Helen: Yes.

You: How did you feel when all that happened?

Helen: *[Sarcastically]* How do you *think* I felt?

You: Pretty awful . . . Maybe . . . Lonely? Rejected? Angry?

Helen: Yeah.

You: Which?

Helen: Rejected and angry . . . And let down. Gutted.

You: That makes sense. So how does cutting help when you feel like that?

Helen: It sort of lets it out. Makes me feel a bit calmer.

It would have been easy to be distracted by Helen's cuts or frustration, missing the opportunity to draw out the function (coping with distress). By eliciting the function, you'll help her feel understood and identify situations where she'll be vulnerable to future self-harm.

4. Brains and guts

Your brain makes sense of the story, waves red flags when you discover risk factors, and creates management plans. Your *gut feeling* is a less nuanced instinct telling you 'everything's OK' or 'something's wrong. Usually, brain and gut agree: you spot concerning risk factors and feel worried for the person's safety *or* decide they're safe and feel untroubled as they go home. Brain–gut *mismatches* are important, e.g.:

- *You're worried about the person, despite an intellectually 'low-risk' presentation.* Your gut may say something doesn't add up: the person hasn't been completely honest, or you've missed something important.

- *You feel calm, despite a multitude of risk factors.* You *should* worry that they planned to die for months, changed their will, stabbed themselves, and were found by accident. The person may have hoodwinked your gut feeling, by reassuring you. Are they *really* safe, given the risk factors your brain's noticed?

> **BOX 9.5** Screening for self-harm/suicide
>
> If someone *hasn't* presented with self-harm, assessing suicidal thoughts can feel awkward. Don't be too blunt. Try:
>
> A sequence, e.g.:
> - How do you see the future?
> - Do you ever feel hopeless/life isn't worth living?
> - Do you ever want to harm yourself? Or end your life?
>   – Tell me about those thoughts.
>
> Or
>
> Empathic reasoning, e.g.:
> - I'd imagine that many people in your situation might feel life wasn't worth living. Do you ever feel that way?
> - It wouldn't surprise me if this made you feel desperate sometimes—even suicidal. Do you ever feel like that?

Listen to your brain *and* gut in every interview; check in with both *before* considering risk and explore mismatches thoroughly, especially once you're qualified to discharge people home after self-harm.

💡 **Psychodynamically, the person may subconsciously *want* you to feel worried, for some reason.**

5. Address ambivalence

Following a suicide attempt, people can feel they've crossed a 'point of no return,' making it hard to think or talk about living or hope. Recognizing ambivalence gives the person permission to change their mind, e.g. 'Part of you wanted to die and maybe a part didn't?' The self-harm may have temporarily 'cured' a problem by changing the person's circumstances (e.g. activating their social network), offering a way forward.

6. Self-care

Discussing self-harm can be upsetting, especially if you've self-harmed in the past, or lost someone to suicide. When someone takes their own life, those left behind can blame themselves or feel they should have done something to prevent it. Whether you're a relative, friend, student, or doctor, there's no shame in looking after yourself: find people you trust and talk about it.

The interview

- • = Example question. ✱ = Question linking to other parts of the history.

Encourage the person to tell their story chronologically, from the first thought of self-harm until now. Summarize and fill gaps with questions—a seamless story ensures you don't forget important details. Then turn to the future, covering risk and protective factors.

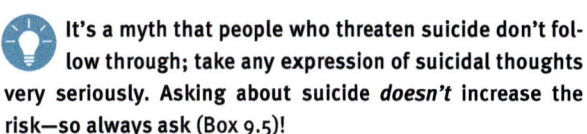

💡 **It's a myth that people who threaten suicide don't follow through; take any expression of suicidal thoughts very seriously. Asking about suicide *doesn't* increase the risk—so always ask (Box 9.5)!**

Beforehand

- (You've been through a lot today.) *It may be hard to talk about, but could you tell me what happened?*
- ✱ What first made you think of harming (or killing) yourself?
- ✱ Was there a final straw?
- ✱ Did you have any problems or worries? *[Screen: work/studies, relationships, money, health]*

Planning

- *Was this planned? Tell me about that . . .*
- How long were you planning this?
- How did you prepare yourself?
  – How did you choose this method? *[Screen: online research, peers]*
  – Where did you get the [tablets/equipment]?
  – Did you practise beforehand?
- Did you put your affairs in order?
  – Did you write/change your will?
  – Did you say goodbye to anyone?
- Did you do anything else because you wouldn't get another chance?
- ✱ Did you tell anyone what you were planning/how desperate you felt?

During

Method

- *Talk me through exactly what you did . . .*
- *Overdose*:
  – Which tablets did you take? *[Type, number]*
  ✱ What did you know about them? *[Lethality]*
- *Cutting*:
  – What did you use to cut yourself?
  – Where did you cut? How deeply?
  – Did you clean the [blade] beforehand?
  – Did you care for yourself afterwards? *[Clean wounds, bandage]*
  – How were you feeling . . . ? *[Check: before, during, after]*

- Did you write a note or leave a message online?
  - What did it say?
- *Did you take any drugs or alcohol?*

Precautions against discovery

- *Did you do anything to make sure you couldn't be interrupted?* [Screen: locking doors, saying they were elsewhere, turning off phones]
- Were you alone?

View at the time

- *What did you hope would happen?* [Function]
  - ... To die? Something else?
- *Did you think this would kill you?* [Lethality]
  - [If yes] How confident were you that you'd die?
  - [If no] How confident were you that you'd survive?
  - Did you think anyone could save you if they found you?

Discovery

- (It sounds as though you planned things very carefully.) **How did you come to hospital?**
- Were you found? Did you call for help?
  - How do you feel about that?

Afterwards

View now

- Looking back, how do you feel about trying to harm/kill yourself?
  - Do you regret it?
  - What do you regret? [Screen: trying/'failing' to die]
  - [If this was a suicide attempt] Do you wish you'd died?

Current problems

- **Has anything changed?** (Are things as bad as before?)
  - How?
- *How do you feel now?* [Screen: active symptoms, especially depression, psychosis]
- *Do [family/friends/partner] know you self-harmed? How did they react?*

❗ If someone's made a suicide attempt and nothing has changed (or it worsened their situation), be very suspicious of a sudden, miraculous wish to live. People may pretend (and even lie) that they're feeling better, to avoid admission and make another attempt.

Future

General

- *How do you see the future?*
- *Are you looking forward to anything over the next week or so?*
- What will you do if you leave hospital today?
- What will you do if [stressor] happens (again)?
  - Do you have other ways to cope?
- *Could anything make life easier for you?*
- *Would you like any help?*

Plans to self-harm

- *Do you still want to harm yourself? Tell me about that.*
- *Do you (still) want to end your life?*
- What plans do you have?
  - How will you do it? When?
  - Have you taken any steps towards this?
- Is anything stopping you?
- Is there anything that could push you to do it sooner?

Risk and protective factors

Risk factors

- *Have you tried to harm or kill yourself before?*
- *Have you had any mental health problems in the past?*
- *Do you think you're suffering from any mental health problems now?*
- *How's your physical health? Are you in pain?*
- *Do you drink alcohol? Do you take drugs?*

Protective factors

- *Who can you talk to about your worries?*
  - *Is there anyone you'd like me to contact now?*
- Are there things you still want to live for? Tell me about them.

❗ As a medical student, you'll never discharge people (although you can add a valuable perspective). When qualified, always request a psychiatric opinion before discharging someone who's self-harmed.

1. Risk assessment following self-cutting (15 minutes)

Candidate's instructions

Anthony Fowler is a 19-year-old pet shop worker. His father brought him to hospital after discovering Anthony cutting himself. You're a medical student in the emergency department (ED). The psychiatric liaison nurse has asked you to assess Anthony's risk.

Patient's brief

Key characteristics
- I'm sarcastic and irritable.
- This is pointless. I want to go home.

History

I cut myself today. So? I've been cutting for years. Today, my manager had a go at me in front of *everyone* for not cleaning out the rabbits properly. Not my fault—I was doing someone a favour; it wasn't even my job! I was so angry I just walked out. All I could think about was cutting myself. It took 20 minutes to walk home, and I went straight upstairs and got my kit out. I cut my arm (I allowed myself five cuts) and was about to start taping up when Dad walked in. He went ballistic when he saw the blood and started yelling, calling me a freak. He *literally* dragged me to the car, screaming all the way to hospital. He doesn't *care*—it's just another excuse to have a go at me.

I wasn't *trying* to kill myself, but if I *did* die, nobody would care. I'll keep cutting; it's my right to do what I want with my body. I use a fresh razorblade and always disinfect it. I get excited building up to it, but I'm patient and don't rush; it feels best that way. I focus on the blood bulging along the edges of skin—it calms me down when I'm angry or stressed. I know the safe places to cut (I've done this since I was 15), and always clean and bandage up afterwards.

I've been depressed for years—nothing helps. My girlfriend, Anna, understands. We met in an online cutting forum and we're going to live together when we've saved enough. *Pets at Home* is looking for staff, so I need to get to the library to print off a CV. I'm hardworking and good with animals, so I reckon they'll employ me. I'll stay with a friend this week—that'll teach Dad not to do this again—he only wants me for my rent.

Other history
- I tried to kill myself at 14: I overdosed when mum walked out.
- I saw the children's mental health team for counselling from age 14 to 18. They said I was depressed. Nothing helped.
- Dad beat me, so I was in foster care from 16 to 18. I've been living with him again this year. He needs my rent, so doesn't hit me so much.
- Dad drinks himself to sleep every night. Mum died of breast cancer just after leaving us.
- I had asthma as a kid but grew out of it—I'm fit and well.
- I smoke 20 cigarettes a day. I don't drink, but smoke weed (cannabis) most evenings. No other drugs.
- My mood's up and down. Energy's good. I enjoy seeing Anna and working with animals.

Questions
When can I go home?

Worries
If I didn't cut, how would I handle my stress?

💡 Anthony's cut for many years to cope with stress, and his story *suggests* a diagnosis of emotionally unstable personality disorder (EUPD). Unless today's cutting is a change from his usual pattern, an admission will probably exacerbate distress. His immediate risk of suicide seems low, but he's likely to continue self-harming, and is at increased risk of suicide (deliberately or accidentally) in future. A therapeutic assessment now could help him accept CMHT support and psychotherapy, e.g. DBT or MBT, providing other ways to manage emotions, reduce or stop self-harm, and improve his relationships.

2. Risk assessment following overdose (15 minutes)

Candidate's instructions
Scarlet Gillespie is a 25-year-old single mother and freelance DJ. She was admitted after an overdose yesterday and is medically cleared for discharge. You're a medical student in ED. The liaison psychiatrist asked you to assess risk.

Patient's brief

Key characteristics
- I'm putting on a brave face but feel miserable and hopeless.
- I lie about my future plans.

History
Two months ago I got stranded in town, about 3am, so rang my best friend, Dee. She came to get me but never turned up: she died in an accident on the way. It wouldn't have happened if I hadn't called her out. I've been depressed since. I lie awake every night thinking about her. It leaves me drained and I can't work; I just sit around the house. Mum moved in to look after my 4-year-old daughter, Erica; I wasn't coping. Erica shouldn't have to see me in that state.

About 3 weeks ago, I started thinking about killing myself. I wanted everything to stop and not have to think anymore. I got the tablets 2 weeks ago. My GP's nice: he gave me antidepressants and sleeping pills. I bought four packets of paracetamol from different shops. I knew I needed to provide for Erica, so I made Mum her legal guardian.

Last week I told Mum I'd start DJing again. I organized some trips out together and made sure they knew I loved them. Yesterday I took the train into town like I was going to a gig and booked into a hotel. I locked the door and wrote a letter explaining I was sorry but couldn't go on. I took the tablets with a bottle of wine: fluoxetine (28×20mg), zopiclone (14×7.5mg), and paracetamol (4 packs: 64×500mg). I was sure I'd taken enough to kill myself but woke up in hospital. Some maintenance man got his rooms mixed up and found me unconscious. He called an ambulance 'just in time'.

I'm glad I was found and regret everything that happened; it was so stupid. I'd never do it again. I just want to go home to look after Erica—I've realized she needs me.

What I'm really thinking
- My heart sank when I woke up—I'm still here. There's nothing to live for.
- Erica doesn't need me—Mum's much better than me.
- I'll jump in front of a train tonight.

Other history
- I have rheumatoid arthritis; the flare-ups are very painful.
- I'm prescribed fluoxetine 20mg, zopiclone 7.5mg.
- I got depressed and took an overdose when Dad killed himself 10 years ago.
- I don't drink/smoke/take drugs.
- I've got friends but none I can talk to, not like Dee.

Questions
Can I go home?

Worries
The doctors might put me in a mental hospital.

Scarlet is at immediate risk of suicide. She has many risk factors for completed suicide and nothing has changed—she needs inpatient admission. If Scarlet refuses, she may require admission under Section 2 of the MHA. In hospital, she'll need visits from her mum and Erica, escorted leave (to prevent impulsive suicide attempts), treatment of depression, review of her arthritis, and exploration of guilt around Dee's death. A ward social worker can organize benefits while off work or organize childcare. As her depression lifts, she'll benefit from bereavement counselling or CBT. She'll probably receive home treatment team support on discharge before CMHT follow-up.

NEXT STEPS

Self-harm treatment refusal

You're an ED FY2, about to assess 22-year-old Duncan Moore. He was admitted after jumping from a car park (second floor) with bilateral femoral fractures. The paramedic reported no evidence of head injury or abdominal trauma but Duncan was muttering to himself. After basic observations, he's refused X-rays because 'the government will read my mind'.

- What is your immediate management?
- What's his likely ongoing management plan?

Immediate management

Ensure that Duncan is physically stable with no urgent medical needs. Check his records for previous ED presentations, which may include psychiatric and self-harm history. Offer analgesia (even if he's refused it)—it's hard to think while in pain. Assess his injuries as far as possible.

Perform a focused psychiatric history and MSE. Find out what Duncan was doing in the car park and why he jumped/fell. Look for symptoms of psychosis, depression, and mania, asking whether he:

- Was *trying* to harm or kill himself?
- Heard someone tell him to jump? (*Auditory hallucinations*)
- Was escaping something? (*Persecutory delusions*)
- Believed he wouldn't be harmed? (*Grandiose delusions*)
- Tried to harm himself before?
- Had contact with mental health services?
- Uses drugs?
- Plans to harm/kill himself or jump from a height again?

Assess his risk of self-neglect, harming others, and—given his unpredictability—accidents or retaliation from others. If he hasn't previously seen psychiatric services, an acute and transient psychotic episode triggered by substance use is most likely. In first-episode psychosis, organic causes (e.g. encephalitis) must be ruled out.

Assess Duncan's capacity to refuse medical treatment: can he *understand*, *retain*, and *weigh* pertinent information and *communicate* his decision? If he's refusing X-rays due to persecutory delusions, these may prevent him understanding the nature of the investigations or fully weighing the pros and cons. If so, he lacks capacity as defined by the MCA (see p. 29). Explain his options and check whether he might accept scans if accompanied by someone he trusts. If still refusing, discuss with seniors. They'll probably suggest performing investigations under the MCA in Duncan's best interests, to identify and treat fractures. If he becomes acutely agitated or aggressive, sedation may help, e.g. lorazepam 1–2mg PO/IM.

Ongoing management

The MCA can be used to treat Duncan's fractures but it's logistically difficult if he's actively resisting or refusing interventions. Discuss with liaison psychiatry, who may conduct a MHA assessment with a view to detain Duncan on the orthopaedic ward for further *psychiatric* assessment and treatment. Medical treatment would still usually happen under the MCA but the MHA will prevent him leaving and is occasionally used to treat the *consequences* of mental disorder, e.g. self-harm injuries.

Liaison psychiatry will monitor Duncan and may suggest one-to-one nursing to support him and monitor his mental state. They may start antipsychotic medication, review him regularly, and consider whether he needs inpatient admission once medically fit for discharge.

Risk assessment is a continuous process. Medication should improve Duncan's psychotic symptoms, reducing his risk of self-harm. However, as insight improves, the risk of suicide can increase following recovery from first episode psychosis, requiring close monitoring. He'll be reviewed regularly post discharge by an early intervention CMHT.

> 💡 **Did you miss a head injury?** Although the paramedic reported no evidence of head injury, a full medical examination is vital, especially after falling from a height. Head injuries cause confusion but can be masked by psychosis or intoxication. Never assume that 'strange behaviour' is psychiatric!

> **Movie buff**
> *The Bridge* (2006): the Golden Gate bridge is the second most popular site in the world for attempting suicide. Eric Steel's documentary captured some of these attempts, and showed the impact on friends and family.
> *The Hours* (2002): suicide and Virginia Woolf connect the narratives of three women in 1923, 1951, and 2001.

The Virgin Suicides (1999): based on Jeffrey Eugenides' novel, Sofia Coppola's film tells the story of five sisters confined to their home after the youngest attempts suicide.

Thirteen (2003): Tracy (Evan Rachel Wood) grapples with adolescence after befriending the school 'queen bee' (Nikki Reed).

Book shelf

Coelho, P. (1998) *Veronika Decides to Die*: this philosophically informed novel begins with Veronika's suicide attempt and admission to a psychiatric unit, during which she meditates on life and death.

Honeyman, G. (2017) *Eleanor Oliphant is Completely Fine*: a lighter read than some, this page-turner sensitively explores risk and protective factors for self-harm, starting with loneliness.

Kettlewell, C. (1999) *Skin Game: A Memoir*: an autobiographical narrative on cutting.

Ray, R. (1998) *A Certain Age*: a 13-year-old girl becomes enmeshed in an exploitative relationship with a much older man and begins to self-harm. Essential reading on the relationship between childhood abuse, self-harm, suicidality, and risk factors in young people.

Yanagihara, H. (2015) *A Little Life*: this tale of the intersecting lives of four university friends takes in addiction, self-harm, suicide, severe abuse, resilience, hope, and love in all its guises.

Note

1. Virginia Woolf (1882–1941): Woolf wrote this note to her husband, Leonard, before drowning herself in the River Ouse.

Journal club

Bateman, A., Fonagy, P. (2016) *Mentalization-Based Treatment for Personality Disorders: A Practical Guide*. Oxford: Oxford University Press.

Clark, S.E., Goldney, R.D. (2000) The impact of suicide on relatives and friends. In: *The International Handbook of Suicide and Attempted Suicide* (eds. K. Hawton, K. van Heeringen), pp. 467–84. Chichester: John Wiley.

Department of Health (2017) *Preventing Suicide in England: Third Progress Report of the Cross-Government Outcomes Strategy to Save Lives*. London: Department of Health.

Main, T. (1989) *The Ailment and Other Psychoanalytic Essays*. London: Free Association.

National Institute for Health and Care Excellence (NICE) (2013) *Self-Harm* (QS34). London: NICE. www.nice.org.uk/guidance/qs34/chapter/Introduction-and-overview

Go to www.oup.com/uk/stringer2e for a wealth of additional resources, including an OCSE mark scheme, filmed scenarios, and self-assessment questions.

10 Psychotic Disorders

True or false?

Answers on p. 277

1. A hallucination is the misperception of a stimulus.
2. People with schizophrenia are more likely to be born in January than June.
3. The incidence of schizophrenia is twice as high in urban than rural areas.
4. Depression is a core negative symptom of schizophrenia.
5. Haloperidol has fewer extrapyramidal side effects than clozapine.
6. Neuroleptic malignant syndrome is an antipsychotic side effect characterized by hyperkinesia and clonus.
7. 5% of people with at-risk mental state (ARMS) will go on to develop psychosis.
8. Late onset predicts poor prognosis in schizophrenia.
9. It's important to strongly challenge delusions when first interviewing a person with psychosis.
10. When assessing the risk of violence, past behaviour is an important factor in predicting future behaviour.

Contents

Principles
Introduction
Epidemiology
Aetiology
- Genetics
- Obstetric complications
- Childhood adversity
- Social disadvantage
- Urbanicity
- Migration and ethnicity
- Associated conditions
- Substance use disorders

Main theories
- Neurodevelopmental theories
- Neurotransmitter theories
- Psychological theories

Clinical picture
- ARMS
- Acute phase
- Chronic phase

Diagnosis
Differential diagnosis
- Organic
- Non-organic
- Other differentials

Investigations
- Risk assessment

Management
- Biological interventions
- Psychological interventions
- Social approaches

Prognosis

Reality
General approach: tips, tricks, and cautionary tales
The interview
- Psychosis histories

Next steps
Early adverse complications of clozapine
- Differential diagnosis
- Essential investigations
- Immediate management
- Longer-term management

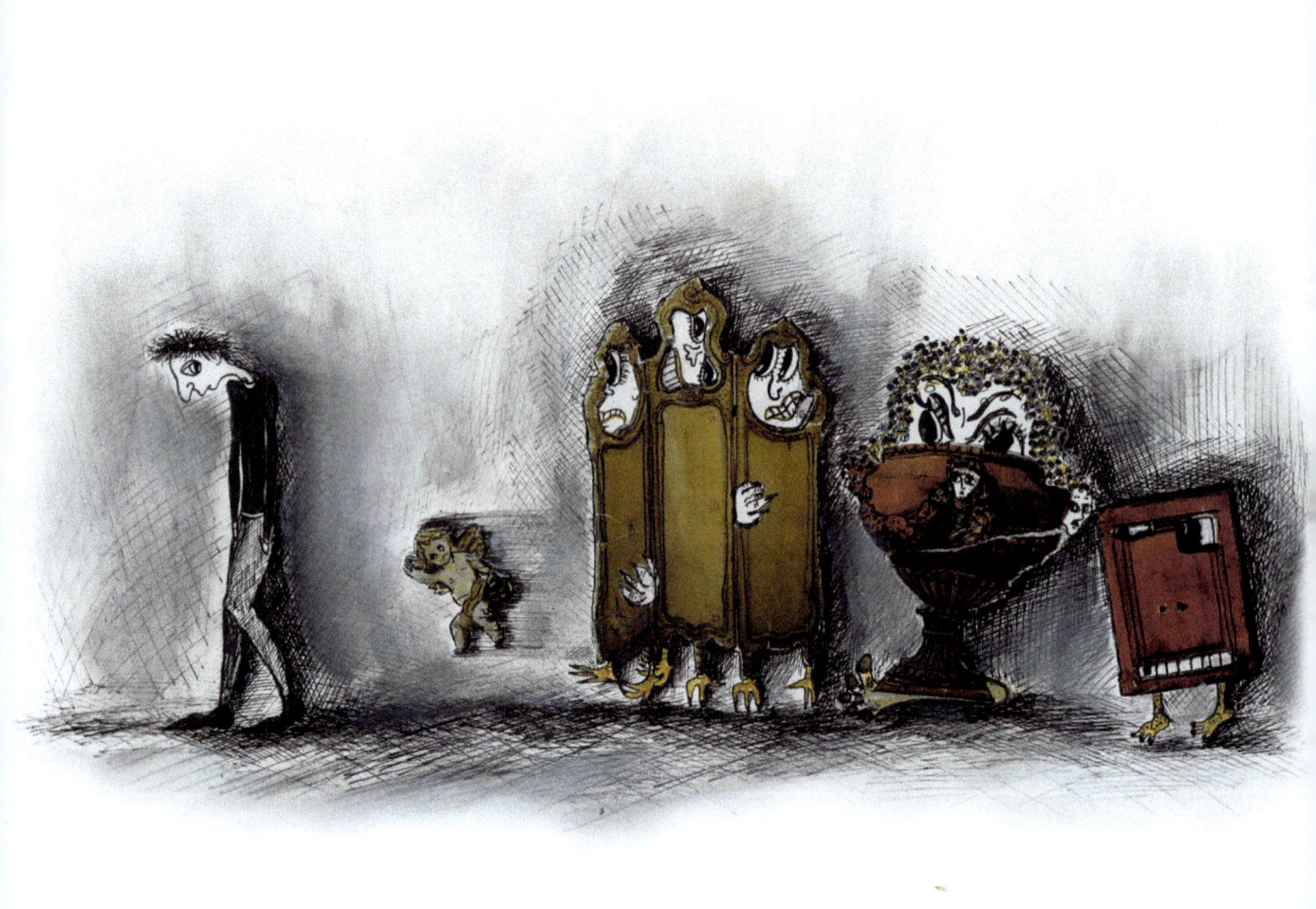

PRINCIPLES

Was it there? Again that awful uncertainty—I would seem to have it, then it was gone. I sat hunched on the bed, clutching myself around the shins, my forehead on my knees. Did I have it? Was there gas? Was it seeping from my groin? I lifted my head and turned it helplessly from side to side. Gas from my groin? It was at that moment that I became aware of the noise in the attic overhead, quiet laughter followed by a sort of bump—then there was silence again.

Patrick McGrath, *Spider*[1]

Introduction

Psychosis refers to experiences where someone loses touch with reality. Key psychotic symptoms are:

- **Hallucinations:** perceptions without an external stimulus, i.e. hearing, seeing, smelling, touching, or tasting something that isn't actually there.
- **Delusions:** fixed, false beliefs, held despite rational argument or evidence to the contrary. These can't be explained by the patient's cultural, religious, or educational background.
- **Formal thought disorder:** illogical or muddled thinking; people may experience this as struggling to think clearly.

People with psychotic illnesses have always suffered stigma. Historically, they were thought to be 'demon possessed' or afflicted with 'madness' as a divine punishment for their sins. Nowadays, they're often portrayed as dangerous criminals by the media, and recurrently rejected by employers, relatives, and friends (see **Box 10.1** on *schizophrenia*). This stigma also results from the unsettling experience of encountering psychosis without understanding it. As a medical student and future doctor, your knowledge and explanations are powerful antidotes to stigma against all mental disorders, but particularly psychosis.

Epidemiology

The lifetime risk of developing schizophrenia is ~0.7% and of *any* psychotic disorder 3%. Onset is typically from late adolescence to the early twenties; though it can occur at any age. The male:female ratio is 3:2; and men are usually affected earlier and more severely than women.

> **BOX 10.1** Schizophrenia: what's in a name?
>
> Schizophrenia is a *type* of psychotic illness. In 1908, the psychiatrist Eugene Bleuler coined the term from the Greek *schizein* ('to split') and *phren* ('mind'), trying to describe the fragmentation of thought, memory, perception, and personality he saw in people with the illness.
>
> Schizophrenia is a controversial label, not least because it's misunderstood and often *wrongly* thought to mean violent, 'split personality', or incurable. Understandably, many patients and carers reject the label, and increasingly clinicians and researchers are thinking more broadly about people who have psychosis, not just those meeting the specific criteria for schizophrenia. In this chapter, we'll talk generally about psychotic illnesses, but use the term schizophrenia when appropriate, e.g. when defining the diagnostic criteria or when quoted research uses this specific term.

Aetiology

Schizophrenia has a complex, multifactorial aetiology, in which genetic and environmental factors interact.

Genetics

The genetic basis is supported by twin concordance and adoption studies. Lifetime risk increases around 10-fold for first-degree relatives of people with schizophrenia, and 40-fold for someone whose parents are both affected. Overall, heritability (see p. 35) is estimated at 85%.

Multiple *susceptibility genes* of small effect are thought to interact, each making someone slightly more likely to develop schizophrenia. Genes of interest include those coding for proteins involved in neurodevelopment, receptor function, and synaptic pruning (the elimination of weaker brain synaptic links, occurring from childhood until the twenties). These susceptibility genes are probably not specific to schizophrenia, but increase the risk for a range of disorders including bipolar disorder, schizoaffective disorder, and autism. Increased paternal age is a risk factor for schizophrenia, probably due to increased genetic mutations.

Obstetric complications

Maternal prenatal malnutrition, viral infections, stress, and analgesic use increase the risk of schizophrenia; as do obstetric complications causing hypoxia (e.g. pre-eclampsia, emergency Caesarean section), and foetal growth retardation. These factors may be causal, or associations due to shared genetic/neurodevelopmental abnormalities.

> 💡 Rates of schizophrenia are higher in people born in the winter (December–March in the northern hemisphere), when viral infections are rife.

Childhood adversity

Childhood abuse, neglect, and bullying increase the risk of schizophrenia. Though this may be due to confounding factors such as genetics, it's possible that adversity has a direct impact on neurodevelopment.

Social disadvantage

The higher prevalence of schizophrenia among adults of lower socioeconomic status isn't reflected in their status at birth, suggesting a downward 'drift' due to the damaging effects of psychosis on social function, education, and employment.

Urbanicity

Schizophrenia is twice as prevalent in urban as in rural areas. This may be due to those affected gravitating to cities, or to stress specific to living in cities.

Migration and ethnicity

First- and second-generation migrants have an average threefold increase in the risk of schizophrenia compared with indigenous populations. Rates vary with ethnicity, with black Caribbean and black African people showing the highest rates (a four- to sixfold increase compared to white British people). This isn't fully understood: it isn't explained by preferential migration, diagnostic bias, higher rates of schizophrenia in country of origin, or socioeconomic status. Possible factors include childhood separation from parents and adult stresses, e.g. social exclusion and experience of racism.

Associated conditions

Schizoid personality (see p. 258) precedes schizophrenia in up to a quarter of people affected. Schizotypal disorder (see p. 85) is more commonly associated with schizophrenia, possibly due to a shared genetic basis.

Substance use disorders

Some drugs produce psychotic symptoms which subside as the drug wears off ('drug-induced psychosis'), e.g. cannabis, amphetamines, cocaine, and novel psychoactive substances (NPS). Drug use can also trigger a relapse in people with a history of psychosis.

Additionally, there's a dose-dependent association between cannabis use (particularly as a teenager) and the risk of later developing schizophrenia. The risk is heightened for *skunk*, a form of cannabis with higher concentrations of *tetrahydrocannabinol* (THC), the chemical particularly associated with psychosis. Some of this association might be explained by 'self-medication' of subtle prodromal symptoms of psychosis (see p. 81), or by confounding factors such as urbanicity. However, there's an increasing consensus that cannabis is a causal factor, probably in those already genetically susceptible to schizophrenia.

> 💡 In south-east London, it's estimated that skunk use is responsible for nearly a quarter of new psychosis presentations. Compared with people who've *never* smoked skunk, those who smoke skunk are roughly three times more likely to experience psychosis (and five times more likely if daily users).

Main theories

Neurodevelopmental theories

Studies show brain changes in some people with schizophrenia, including enlarged ventricles, reduced cortical, amygdala, or hippocampal volume, and disorganization of white matter tracts in frontal/temporal regions. Children who will later develop schizophrenia may show subtle neurological signs, lower premorbid IQ, and particular deficits in learning, executive function, and social function.

These findings suggest that schizophrenia can be viewed as a neurodevelopmental disorder. Initial, possibly imperceptible, brain abnormalities (from genetic origin or early brain damage) progress as the brain matures through ongoing myelination and synaptic pruning. Maturation, together with other risk factors (e.g. cannabis), may allow abnormalities to evolve until overt psychotic symptoms emerge.

Neurotransmitter theories

The dopamine hypothesis explains psychosis as a result of dopamine dysregulation in the brain. *Positive symptoms* (hallucinations and delusions) are thought to result from excess dopamine in the mesolimbic tracts (**Box 10.2**). By contrast, *negative symptoms* (e.g. apathy, social withdrawal) may result from dopamine underactivity in the mesocortical tracts. Evidence for the dopamine hypothesis includes:

- All known effective antipsychotics are dopamine antagonists (dopamine receptor blockers).
- Antipsychotics work better against positive, rather than negative, symptoms.
- Dopaminergic agents like amphetamine, cocaine, L-dopa, and bromocriptine can all induce psychotic symptoms.

Dysfunction of glutamate (the main excitatory neurotransmitter in the brain) may be fundamental:

- Glutamate transmission affects dopamine transmission.
- The street drugs phencyclidine (PCP) and ketamine cause a schizophrenia-like psychosis by blocking glutamate transmission at NMDA receptors.

Serotonin overactivity may also be important, e.g. atypical antipsychotics are effective serotonin antagonists.

Psychological theories

Cognitive models suggest that *thinking errors* lead to delusions, e.g. the tendency to *jump to conclusions* without properly looking at evidence to the contrary.

From a psychodynamic perspective, fear of 'going mad' may prompt the defences of denial and rationalization, resulting in a delusional system to explain persecutory voices.

Clinical picture

This can be divided into three stages: *at-risk mental state* (ARMS), *acute phase*, and *chronic phase*.

BOX 10.2 The salience hypothesis

Dopamine has a role in attributing meaning or 'salience' to potentially rewarding stimuli. The *salience hypothesis* suggests that excess dopamine in the mesolimbic system leads to over-attribution of meaning to irrelevant environmental or internal events. This, it proposes, might lead to the formation of delusions or—when salience is given to innocuous internal experiences—to auditory hallucinations.

ARMS

About 20–30% of people who develop the ARMS go on to develop psychosis, half of whom meet criteria for schizophrenia. The term *prodrome* has lost popularity since it wrongly suggested that psychosis was inevitable.

The ARMS may include a period of very mild or brief psychotic symptoms, a change in function such as social withdrawal or loss of interest in activities, or mood symptoms in those with a genetic risk of psychosis. The picture might be of someone in their late teens or early twenties who's dropped out of work or education after a period of increasing absence. They might seem distant, isolating themselves in their bedroom without giving reasons. They may deny emerging psychotic symptoms for fear of their significance. Psychosocial treatment with CBT and family intervention is recommended.

💡 **The ARMS can be hard to distinguish from depression, substance misuse, or 'normal' teenage behaviour!**

Acute phase

This has the most striking and florid 'positive symptoms' (the things that are 'added' in psychosis):

- Delusions—of any kind, but often persecutory.
- Hallucinations—most commonly auditory, especially hearing voices.

These may count as 'first-rank' symptoms (**Box 10.3** and **Figure 10.1**)—worth knowing about as they pop up surprisingly commonly in exams!

Formal thought disorder is common: thoughts become muddled, making speech disorganized. Vagueness may progress to very disjointed speech that's hard to follow and apparently senseless. Thought blocking (a sudden stop in the flow of thoughts, leading to silence) may also occur.

Behaviour may be withdrawn, overactive, or bizarre. People may have a number of acute psychotic episodes over the years, with full or partial recovery between relapses.

💡 **Imagine your skull is permeable. How would you feel if, while sitting on a bus, other passengers dipped into your mind, removing your ideas, forcing you to think things against your will, or knowing your *every* thought (however personal or embarrassing)?**

Chronic phase

Over time, people may develop disabling 'negative symptoms' (the things that are *lost* in schizophrenia). These include:

- Apathy—the opposite of enthusiasm; loss of motivation.

> **BOX 10.3** Schneider's first-rank symptoms
>
> Schneider described symptoms that he felt suggested schizophrenia in the absence of an organic disorder. However, they're neither necessary nor sufficient to make the diagnosis: they can occur in other states (e.g. mania, delirium) and may be absent in schizophrenia.
>
> **Delusional perception**
>
> A two-stage process where a *real* perception is then interpreted with delusional meaning, e.g.:
>
> - 'The traffic lights changed to green: I knew I was Jesus.'
>
> **Thought interference**
>
> The person believes that their thoughts are controlled by someone/something else. These delusions all share the subjective sense that something abnormal is happening in the usually private confines of someone's head.
>
> - *Thought insertion*—believing that thoughts are placed directly into the person's mind (these thoughts *feel* alien), e.g.:
>   - 'She uses black magic to make thoughts suddenly pop up in my mind. They're not my thoughts—they *feel* completely different to mine . . .'
> - *Thought withdrawal*—believing that thoughts are taken from the person's mind (there is a sudden *feeling* of loss), e.g.:
>   - 'Spies use a neodymium magnet to pluck the thoughts from my head!'
> - *Thought broadcasting*—believing that thoughts are withdrawn, then publicly disseminated, so that others know what the person is thinking, e.g.:
>   - 'As I think, my thoughts flash up as words on a website. Anyone logged on can read my thoughts.'
>
> **Passivity phenomena (delusions of control)**
>
> The belief that a movement, emotion, or impulse is made or controlled by someone else, e.g.:
>
> - 'He makes my eyes go round and round and I can't keep them still.'
>
> These share the experience that the movement, emotion, or impulse is somehow *alien*, and not originating from the person.
>
> **Auditory hallucinations**
>
> - 'Third person' voices discussing or arguing about the person, e.g.:
>   - First voice: 'Nobody likes him.'
>   - Second voice: 'Yeah . . . It's because he's ugly.'
> - *Voices giving a running commentary* on the person's actions, e.g.:
>   - 'He's going into the bedroom now. He's taking off his shoes . . .'
> - *Thought echo*—a voice says the person's thoughts aloud, e.g.:
>   - Person thinks: I'm hungry.
>   - Voice: 'I'm hungry.'

- Blunted affect—decreased reactivity of mood (not to be confused with low mood).
- Anhedonia—the inability to enjoy interests/activities.
- Social withdrawal.
- Poverty of thought and speech.

These may manifest as self-neglect, social isolation, inactivity, or withdrawal. There may also be residual and less prominent 'positive symptoms', e.g. the person may still hold persecutory delusions but seem less distressed and affected by them. See **Box 10.4** for an early example of acute and chronic phase untreated symptoms.

> Depression and antipsychotic side effects can resemble negative symptoms, but are often much easier to treat. Don't overlook them, since treatment can give someone a new lease of life.

Differential diagnosis

When people first experience psychotic symptoms, clinicians often avoid using specific labels like schizophrenia or schizoaffective disorder—keeping to the more general term of 'psychosis' or 'first-episode psychosis' (FEP). The more specific labels may become appropriate if the illness continues or recurs.

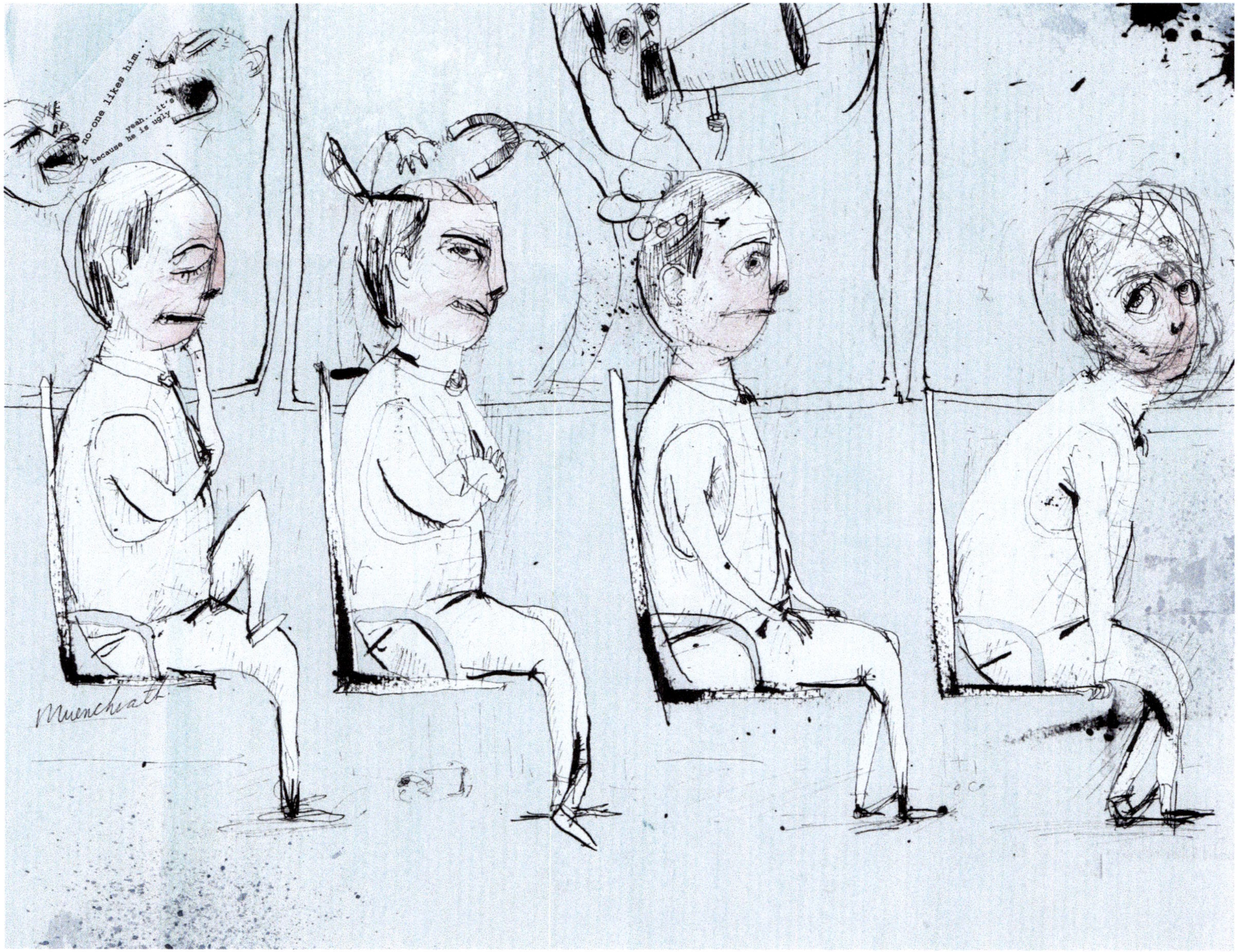

FIGURE 10.1 Some first-rank symptoms of schizophrenia

> **BOX 10.4** Schizophrenia in Britain: the first clear description
>
> James Tilly Matthews was a London tea merchant. He travelled to France in the 1790s to dispel the threat of war between England and revolutionary France with his *own* set of peace terms. James gained the French government's trust, but was later arrested, suspected of spying. Upon his release, he returned to England, consumed by conspiracy theories; he was committed to the Bethlem Hospital in 1797, after shouting, 'Treason!' in the House of Commons.
>
> James believed he was persecuted by a gang of 'active worriers,' who operated the *Air Loom* (which he drew: Figure 10.2). He thought it ran on a mixture of 'male and female seminal fluid' and 'gaz (sic) from the anus of the horse'. James experienced first-rank symptoms, for example, 'Laugh Making' (Passivity of Affect) and 'Kiteing' (Thought Insertion), e.g.:
>
>> As boys raise a kite in the air, so these wretches, by means of the Air Loom and magnetic impregnations, contrive to lift into the brain some particular idea, which floats and undulates in the intellect for hours together. [The victim] is, during the whole time, conscious that the kited idea is extraneous, and does not belong to the train of his own cogitations.
>> (J. Haslam, *Illustrations of Madness*)
>
> Although James was decreed both 'insane' and dangerous, he helped to design the new Bethlem Hospital, and spent his final year in a private asylum, bookkeeping and gardening for a doctor who regarded him as entirely sane. His case illustrates the controversy regarding illness and dangerousness—issues still relevant today.

Organic causes ('organic psychosis')

- **Dementia** (see p. 152) *or* **delirium** (see p. 129)—especially in elderly patients.
- **Medication side effects**, e.g. steroids, dopamine agonists, levetiracetam.
- **Cerebral pathology**, e.g. stroke, space-occupying lesion, encephalitis (including autoimmune encephalitis), epilepsy (especially temporal lobe), multiple sclerosis, cerebral lupus, HIV, neurosyphilis.
- **Systemic illnesses**, e.g. Wilson disease, porphyria, Cushing syndrome, hypo-/hyperthyroidism.
- **Drug use**. Drugs causing psychosis through intoxication include amphetamine, cocaine/crack cocaine, LSD, ecstasy, ketamine, GHB (gamma-hydroxybutrate)/GBL (gamma-butyrolactone), phencyclidine (PCP) and many NPS. GHB and GBL can cause psychotic symptoms during withdrawal.
- **Alcohol.** Heavy use can cause:
  - *Alcoholic hallucinosis*—hearing voices in clear consciousness.
  - *Delirium tremens* (see p. 106)—a life-threatening alcohol withdrawal state; symptoms include hallucinations (visual, auditory, tactile) and delusions (often persecutory).

Non-organic causes ('functional psychosis')

These can be considered *once* organic causes have been excluded.

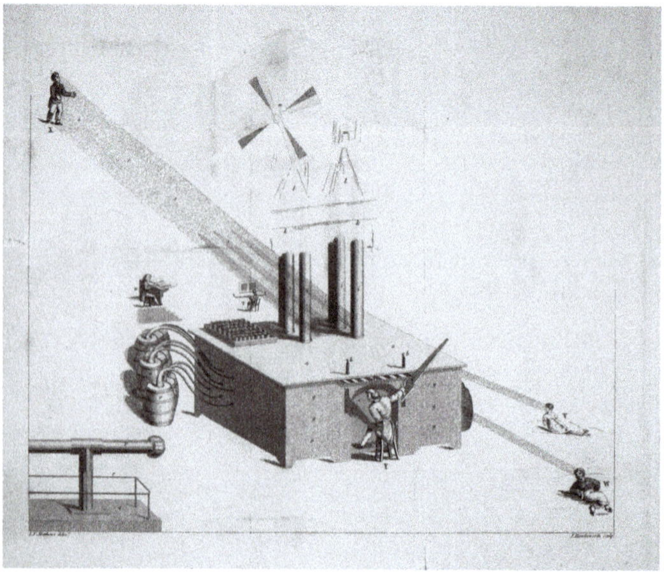

FIGURE 10.2 The Air Loom.

Reproduced from James Tilly Matthews, Air-loom machine. Credit: Wellcome Collection. Distributed under the terms of the Creative Commons Attribution 4.0 International (CC BY 4.0). https://creativecommons.org/licenses/by/4.0

- **Schizophrenia:** symptoms should be present for at least 1 month, and affect multiple areas of the mental state, e.g. hallucinations, delusions, thought disorder, affective blunting, apathy, impaired attention/memory, and experiences of being controlled by others. There may be psychomotor disturbances such as catatonic symptoms (**Table 10.1**). Schizophrenia shouldn't be diagnosed in the presence of striking mood disturbance.
- **Acute and transient psychotic disorder:** psychotic symptoms occur suddenly and relatively briefly. They peak within 2 weeks and usually resolve within a month (the maximum duration is 3 months). Symptoms can fluctuate rapidly, and may be acutely disabling. It's not diagnosed if there's a history of another psychotic illness, e.g. schizophrenia.
- **Schizoaffective disorder** is diagnosed when there's a picture of schizophrenia, but with a mood disorder (moderate/severe depressive or mania) developing *simultaneously*. This is in contrast to primary mood disorders, such as bipolar affective disorder, where psychotic symptoms emerge only as mood becomes more extreme, e.g. psychotic depression, mania with psychotic symptoms.
- **Delusional disorder** describes delusions lasting more than 3 months, without a clear mood disturbance, and lacking other schizophrenia symptoms such as thought disorder, persistent hallucinations, or negative symptoms.
- **Schizotypal disorder** is an enduring state lasting several years or more (it's actually classed under personality disorders in the DSM-5). Eccentricity is central to the diagnosis: people may dress, behave, think, and speak oddly. They may be suspicious, aloof, and struggle to make close relationships. They have unusual ideas, and may experience low-level or fleeting delusions or hallucinations (not sufficient to diagnose another psychotic illness). The risk of developing schizophrenia is increased.
- **Puerperal (postpartum) psychosis:** psychosis triggered by childbirth; it usually occurs within a few weeks of delivery (see p. 227).

Other differentials

- **Personality disorder** (PD, see p. 258) should be considered when there's a *lifelong* pattern of interpersonal difficulties.
    - *Paranoid PD (prominent detachment and negative affectivity traits)*: suspiciousness and paranoia.
    - *Schizoid PD (prominent detachment traits)*: lack of interest in others or social norms (can resemble ARMS or negative symptoms).

Table 10.1 Subtypes of schizophrenia. Schizophrenia was traditionally divided into subtypes based on the most prominent symptoms. Don't get too tied up in this though, since patterns may overlap or change over time—the ICD-11 describes the main symptom profiles, e.g. positive, negative, cognitive, psychomotor symptoms

Subtype	Features
Paranoid	Most common type: prominent hallucinations and (usually persecutory) delusions
Catatonic	Dominated by psychomotor disturbance, e.g.: • *Stupor*—immobility, mutism, and unresponsiveness, despite being conscious (eyes are open and can track movement) • *Excitement*—periods of extreme, purposeless motor activity (may alternate with stupor) • *Posturing*—assuming and holding inappropriate or bizarre positions • *Rigidity*—holding a rigid posture against efforts to be moved • *Waxy flexibility*—the person's limbs offer minimal resistance to being placed in seemingly uncomfortable positions, which are maintained for unusually lengthy periods • *Automatic obedience*—to any instructions • *Perseveration*—inappropriate repetition of words or movements (see p. 139) NB: catatonia can kill—people can stop eating and drinking; this is an indication for ECT
Hebephrenic	• Predominantly disorganized and chaotic mood, behaviour, and speech • Shallow or inappropriate affect • Aimless behaviour • Delusions and hallucinations are less prominent
Simple	Negative features only, having never shown positive psychotic symptoms
Residual	Prominent negative symptoms that remain after delusions and hallucinations subside

- *Borderline personality pattern*: brief psychotic or psychotic-like symptoms can occur at times of stress, e.g. hearing voices, paranoia.

💡 **Catatonia can be seen in a range of illnesses, including organic conditions, e.g. encephalitis.**

Investigations

A full physical workup is required, not only to exclude organic causes, but also to pick up comorbid physical health problems, and ensure baseline tests have been done before starting an antipsychotic.

- **Full physical examination and vital signs**.
- **Blood tests:** FBC, U&Es, LFTs, TFTs, ESR, CRP, CBG, lipid profile. Routine HIV testing is advisable; consider syphilis serology.
- **Urinary drug screen** (UDS) can identify common illicit substances (e.g. cannabis, amphetamine) but many drugs, especially NPS, can't yet be detected.
- **Baseline ECG:** ideal, before starting an antipsychotic.

Additional tests are indicated if the clinical presentation suggests organic pathology, e.g.:

- **CT/MRI brain** in older patients, those with a history of head injury, or focal neurological signs. Routine neuroimaging isn't indicated.
- **EEG**—if epilepsy or another organic cause is suspected, e.g. prominent confusion.
- **Anti-NMDA and voltage-gated potassium channel (VGKC) antibodies**—if autoimmune encephalitis is suspected (see p. 141).
- **Lumbar puncture** for suspected encephalitis.

A **collateral history** is an essential social investigation; loved ones' perspectives add crucial context to the assessment.

💡 **A medication-free period of inpatient observation may clarify the diagnosis if someone develops psychosis while using drugs.**

Risk assessment

Contrary to popular belief, people who have psychosis pose a greater risk to themselves than to others. Only a small subgroup of people with psychotic illnesses are violent; they commit fewer than 10% of all violent crimes in the UK.

- **Risk to self** includes suicide, self-neglect, social decline, and victimization by others.
- **Risk from others:** people with psychosis are more than ten times more likely to be victims than perpetrators of violent crimes.
- **Risk to others:** aggression may be a direct response to persecutory delusions or command hallucinations.

Factors increasing the risk of violence include substance misuse, medication non-concordance, specific threats of violence, or a history of aggression.

Management

See **Box 10.5**.

> **BOX 10.5 Early intervention services**
>
> The duration of untreated psychosis (DUP) is the time from the first clear-cut psychotic symptom until the start of effective treatment. Psychosis itself seems to be 'toxic'—the longer the DUP, the greater the damage to someone's cognitive abilities, insight, and social situation (e.g. dropping out of school, work, relationships). The sooner effective treatment is started, the better the prognosis. Early intervention services were set up to engage people with very early symptoms and offer antipsychotic medication and psychosocial interventions, aiming to keep the DUP below 3 months.

Biological interventions

Physical healthcare

People with psychosis have higher rates of smoking and *metabolic syndrome* (a cluster of vascular risk factors including obesity, hypertension, pre-diabetes/diabetes, and dyslipidaemias) than the general population. Antipsychotic side effects worsen this risk, contributing to an average 20-year reduction in life expectancy. It's therefore critical to support people to access physical healthcare. Psychiatrists build close links with people's GPs and proactively offer advice and support on smoking cessation, diet, exercise, and substance misuse. Anyone with a severe mental illness such as psychosis should receive a yearly GP health check; if prescribed an antipsychotic, they need additional monitoring (**Box 10.6**).

> **BOX 10.6 Antipsychotic monitoring**
>
> Everyone should have the following measured regularly:
> - BMI and waist circumference.
> - Blood pressure.
> - FBC, LFTs, U&Es, lipid profile, CBG (followed by a glucose tolerance test and HbA1c if abnormal).
>
> Some people need:
> - Prolactin levels—if hyperprolactinaemia is suspected or likely (e.g. risperidone).
> - ECGs—important in older people and those on high-dose antipsychotics or clozapine—to monitor the QTc interval.

Antipsychotics

Antipsychotics are *dopamine antagonists*; they block postsynaptic D_2 receptors. In general, the greater the affinity, the more effective they are in treating positive symptoms, caused by dopamine excess. Where possible, medications should be chosen *with* the person (see **Box 10.5** on early intervention), using the lowest dose that controls symptoms without causing unpleasant side effects. Lower doses may be possible during remission, but the general advice is to continue medication for up to 3 years after a first episode of psychosis; longer periods are often needed with recurrent psychosis. Routine use of more than one antipsychotic is avoided, as combinations widen the side effect profile and can increase the risk of serious cardiac events. See **Table 10.2** for side effects of antipsychotics.

First-generation (or 'typical') antipsychotics (FGAs)

These are the older drugs, e.g. chlorpromazine, haloperidol, sulpiride, trifluoperazine, zuclopenthixol. They're effective and cheap, but more likely to cause distressing extrapyramidal side effects (EPSEs) and/or hyperprolactinaemia at normal treatment doses. Some are available as long-acting injections ('depots')—useful when people have difficulties taking daily tablets consistently, e.g. flupentixol decanoate, fluphenazine decanoate, haloperidol decanoate, zuclopenthixol acetate.

Second-generation (or 'atypical') antipsychotics (SGAs)

These are later-developed drugs, e.g. olanzapine, risperidone, quetiapine, aripiprazole, amisulpride, lurasidone, clozapine. They block dopamine receptors *and* serotonin $5\text{-}HT_2$ receptors, giving them a different side effect profile to FGAs. They cause fewer EPSEs and generally don't increase prolactin levels, but are more likely to cause *metabolic side effects*: hypertension, central obesity, raised fasting plasma glucose, hypertriglyceridaemia, low high-density lipoprotein cholesterol. These increase the risk of cardiovascular disease and type 2 diabetes, so physical health monitoring is essential.

Atypicals are often used when:

- Choosing first-line treatment in newly diagnosed psychosis.
- There are unacceptable side effects from typical antipsychotics.
- Relapse occurs on a typical antipsychotic.

Several SGAs are available as depots, e.g. aripiprazole, risperidone, paliperidone, olanzapine.

Clozapine

Treatment resistance is when psychotic symptoms fail to reduce following treatment with two or more antipsychotics, at least one of which is atypical, each at a therapeutic dose for at least 6 weeks. Clozapine is the first-line drug for *treatment-resistant schizophrenia*. It can work when everything else has failed, but causes the potentially fatal complication of agranulocytosis in 0.7% of patients. People starting it need a weekly blood test for FBC to detect early signs of neutropenia; this occurs in 3% of patients and means that clozapine must be stopped since it may herald agranulocytosis. In the absence of problems, blood tests are gradually reduced to monthly.

The sooner an effective treatment is started, the better the person's prognosis. Hence, if other treatments fail, a trial of clozapine should follow promptly. This can improve quality of life through symptom reduction, and reduce admissions and the risk of suicide. Some people with schizophrenia don't respond well to clozapine either, and require augmented treatment with other medications.

> When admitting someone taking clozapine to a medical ward, seek advice regarding doses and blood monitoring from a psychiatrist or pharmacist as soon as possible.

Psychological interventions

A number of psychological approaches are used to treat psychosis as part of a biopsychosocial management plan (see **Box 10.3**).

Cognitive behavioural therapy

CBT is offered to anyone experiencing psychosis *or* at increased risk of developing psychosis (i.e. ARMS, especially if there are transient psychotic symptoms, experiences or behaviours suggesting possible psychosis, or they have a first-degree relative with psychosis).

General principles of CBT apply (see p. 43), and emphasis is placed on reality testing. During a psychotic episode, *aberrant salience* places excessive importance on neutral events and delusions result from jumping to conclusions to explain these events. In CBT, the therapist aims to gently challenge the person's beliefs, helping them to spot illogical thinking, e.g. 'I'm a bit confused by that. If the Prime Minister's stalking you all day, how do they find the time to run the country and appear on TV?' The person is encouraged to think about the evidence for and against a belief and to consider alternative explanations. As well as improving self-esteem and problem-solving, CBT may help people live their lives productively, even if still experiencing some hallucinations and delusions.

Table 10.2 Side effects of antipsychotics

Side effect	Description	Treatment	Worst offenders
EPSE	**Dystonia** • Onset: early, sometimes within hours • Sustained, painful muscle spasm • E.g. torticollis; oculogyric crisis (eyes twist upwards)	Anticholinergic, e.g. procyclidine Consider decrease or change antipsychotic	FGAs Risperidone
	Akathisia • Onset: hours–days • Unpleasant subjective feeling of restlessness • Causes pacing/leg jiggling	Decrease dose/change to SGA (avoid aripiprazole) Add propranolol	FGAs Aripiprazole
	Parkinsonism • Onset: days–weeks • Resting tremor, bradykinesia + rigidity (experienced as stiffness) • ± Reduced facial expressivity, shuffling gait	Decrease dose/change to SGA Try anticholinergic (e.g. procyclidine), but review for effect	FGAs
	Tardive dyskinesia • Onset: months–years • Rhythmic, involuntary movements (mouth, face, limbs, trunk) • Grimacing, chewing/sucking movements of mouth and tongue common • Socially stigmatizing • Can be irreversible	*Stop any anticholinergic* Decrease antipsychotic/switch to SGA (quetiapine or clozapine best) Consider tetrabenazine	FGAs
Metabolic side effects	• Weight gain • Hypertension • Dyslipidaemia • Raised fasting glucose	Decrease or change drug Diet, exercise Antihypertensives, statins, hypoglycaemics Add metformin or aripiprazole to help weight loss	SGAs (clozapine > olanzapine > risperidone > quetiapine)
Hyper-prolactinaemia	• Galactorrhoea, amenorrhoea, gynaecomastia, hypogonadism • Sexual dysfunction • Increased risk of osteoporosis	Decrease or change drug Add aripiprazole	FGAs Amisulpride Risperidone

Sedation	• Hard to wake up • May be drowsy, clumsy and/or feel muddled throughout the day	Decrease or change drug Nocte dosing ± take earlier in the evening	Chlorpromazine Clozapine Olanzapine Quetiapine
Anticholinergic	• Dry mouth • Blurred vision • Constipation • Urinary retention • Confusion • Tachycardia	Decrease or change drug Symptomatic treatment	Trifluoperazine Clozapine (NB: clozapine more often causes hypersalivation than dry mouth; this risks aspiration penumonia)
Increased QTc interval on ECG	• Increased risk of arrhythmias and cardiac arrest	Decrease or change drug ECG monitoring	Haloperidol Quetiapine
Decreased seizure threshold	• Seizures	Decrease/change drug Add valproate or lamotrigine	Clozapine
Neuroleptic malignant syndrome	• Rare but life-threatening (rhabdomyolysis causes acute kidney injury) • Usually triggered by new antipsychotic/increased dose • Hyperthermia • Autonomic instability • Rigidity (muscle stiffness) • Drowsy/delirious (fever, tachycardia, labile BP)	• Bloods: ↑CK, ↑WCC • Stop antipsychotic • Supportive care (may need ICU): cooling, fluid resuscitation • Dantrolene/amantadine/bromocriptine • Once well, cautiously try different SGA if antipsychotic needed	FGAs

Cognitive remediation therapy (CRT) is particularly helpful in negative symptoms: it aims to improve neurocognitive skills such as concentration, memory, and problem-solving—often using computer-based programmes.

Family intervention

It can be extremely stressful living with somebody who has a psychotic illness, since they see the world very differently to others, and may behave in ways that are worrying, upsetting, or frustrating. Unfortunately, stressed relatives may not communicate their concerns in a helpful way. The term *high expressed emotion* (high EE) describes unhelpful communication styles, measured as *hostility, critical comments*, or *emotional over-involvement*. High EE is a recipe for further family tension, and although it doesn't cause psychosis, it increases the risk of relapse after an acute episode.

Family intervention is a type of therapy that works with the patient and their family or cohabitees. It can reduce the effects of high EE through communication skills training, education about psychosis, and problem-solving techniques. Improving understanding and empathy on both sides can help reduce conflict, as can encouragement to take time out from each other, and expand respective social networks.

Arts therapies

Arts therapies can help people to discover new forms of expression and communication with others. They are often provided as group therapies, and can be effective during an acute episode, or for the negative symptoms in chronic illness.

Social approaches

Multidisciplinary approach

Practical needs should be addressed, e.g. benefits, housing, training, and education. Social workers, benefits advisors, and occupational therapists are all involved in good management planning. Some teams have specialist vocational workers, who are skilled in getting people back into education, training, voluntary work, or paid work. Befriending and peer support may help develop social confidence. Mental health organizations such as Rethink and Mind provide a wealth of patient resources, as well as carrying out important work in promoting social inclusion and helping tackle stigma at a personal and societal level (see 'The recovery model' in **Box 10.8**).

People are encouraged to develop skills to care for themselves in the least restrictive environment possible. Those with the greatest needs may require fully supported accommodation (with specialist staff on site, 24 hours a day), but many people manage with much lower levels of support, e.g. an independent flat with visits from their care coordinator or a housing keyworker.

Social skills training

This is primarily aimed at improving interpersonal skills. Using methods such as role-play, people develop improved confidence and skills in their day-to-day functioning.

Psychoeducation

This a collaborative approach where people are encouraged to ask and find out more about their illness. An important part of the therapeutic alliance is encouraging people to consider the pros and cons of their treatment, improving insight into their needs (**Box 10.7**).

Carer support

All carers should have their needs assessed. They may require more formal support from social services, or may benefit from carers' groups.

Admission

Hospital admission may be needed for further assessment or treatment when this isn't possible at home, e.g. due to risks, difficulties engaging the person, or particularly complex physical, mental health, or social circumstances.

BOX 10.7 'Open Dialogue'

'Open Dialogue' has been Finland's approach to psychosis since the 1980s. On evidence gathered so far, it claims dramatically improved outcomes for people experiencing psychosis, e.g. within 2 years, 75% of people have returned to work or education, and only 20% still require an antipsychotic. Regular *network meetings*—involving the patient, their family, extended social network, and their care team—develop a therapeutic conversation, *listening and responding* to each member, while placing the person with psychosis at the centre of all discussions. There's reduced hierarchy, with respect for non-medical viewpoints and recognition that *we all* suffer mental distress at times (health professionals included). Clinical decisions are *only* made *openly* in front of the patient, decreasing the feeling that treatments are 'done to' them. It's an exciting approach, but still in the early stages of research in the UK.

Rehabilitation

Rehabilitation psychiatry focuses on quality of life, overcoming disability where possible, and accepting limitations where not. It's a long-term approach, addressing varied needs, including:

- Accessing education, training, or employment (supervised or in the open job market).
- Skills, e.g. budgeting, cooking.
- Housing, e.g. supported accommodation, independent flats.
- Accessing social activities.
- Developing personal skills and pursuing interests, e.g. music.

Summary

See **Table 10.3** for a management summary.

Prognosis

A quarter of people recover and experience no further difficulties after a single psychotic episode. Two-thirds develop schizophrenia, which can relapse when medication is stopped. One in ten will be seriously and continuously disabled, and up to a third will develop a treatment-resistant illness. However, the prognosis of schizophrenia varies between people (**Box 10.8**), depending on numerous factors (**Table 10.4**).

BOX 10.8 The recovery model

Not everyone will be completely free of symptoms forever, but that doesn't mean you should give up on them! *Recovery* isn't necessarily about getting back to life exactly as it was before, but about getting the most out of life, *despite* experiencing mental health problems. The *recovery model* encourages professionals to be optimistic and holistic: to see the person and believe in their potential, to help build their resilience, and not simply concentrate on their symptoms. It encourages people with mental health problems to see their recovery as a process or a journey, rather than a specific destination. There may be challenges and tricky times, but rather than just surviving these, there is opportunity for learning, building relationships, setting goals, and choosing activities that give life meaning. Hope, creativity, empowerment, and holism are essential components.

Life expectancy for people with schizophrenia is reduced by up to 20 years, with the greatest impact among men due to increased rates of accidents, substance use disorders, and suicide. Poor physical health, lifestyle, smoking, and medication side effects contribute greatly to reduced life expectancy, so need proactive management. The lifetime risk of suicide is 10%, ten times that of the general population. Intelligent young men with good premorbid functioning are especially vulnerable. Risk is highest in the early years after diagnosis, following first admission, or if the person becomes depressed.

Table 10.3 Management summary

	Biological	Psychological	Social
Immediate	Exclude organic cause Medication-free assessment if possible Start (atypical) antipsychotic	Reassurance Psychoeducation	Carer support Psychoeducation
Medium term	Continue medication Monitor side effects and concordance Optimize physical health	CBT Family intervention Arts therapies	Housing and financial support Vocational support Carer assessment and support
Long term	Treatment resistance: try clozapine Adherence problems: consider depot Optimize physical health Support and psychoeducation if trying to reduce/stop medication	Family intervention Arts therapies	Rehabilitation: housing, education, work, recreation, etc. Recovery: fostering hope, meaning, and resilience Helping to tackle stigma

Table 10.4 Prognostic indicators in schizophrenia

Factor	Prognosis Good	Prognosis Poor
Sex	Female	Male
Onset	Later, acute	Earlier, insidious
DUP	<3 months	>3 months
Premorbid IQ	High	Low
Prominent symptoms	Mood	Negative
Social support	Good	Poor/social withdrawal
Medication adherence	Good	Poor
Family history	No	Yes
Clear stressor	Yes	No
Substance use disorder	No	Yes (especially cannabis)

REALITY

General approach: tips, tricks, and cautionary tales

1. Suspend your disbelief

When you read a novel or watch a film, you become absorbed in the story and forget to question whether there really *is* (for example) a school for wizards, or an evidence base for kryptonite causing fatigue. Without suspending disbelief, you'd miss the point of the story. The same is true when talking to people who have psychosis. Rather than questioning their story, try to relax and be absorbed in it. *Listen as though everything you hear is true* and you'll find people open up to you.

2. Avoid the language of disbelief

People who suffer with psychosis have often been ridiculed or criticized for their beliefs, so may be sensitive to words that suggest you don't believe them, e.g.:

> You: *[Trying to summarize]* So you think you're the Messiah . . .
> Johan: I don't *think—I know!* You're not taking me seriously!
> You: Um . . . Sorry. And you've been hearing voices saying . . .
> Johan: I'm not *hearing voices*! I'm not mad!

Avoid the word 'think' when describing the *certainty* of a delusional belief. Unless *they* describe hallucinations as 'voices', simply talk about the people they hear, e.g.:

> You: You realized you were the Messiah when God said you were the Chosen One, last week.
> Johan: Right.

💡 How would you feel if someone said 'You *think* you're a medical student' or asked 'Do you hear voices?' What would you think they thought about you?

3. Respond!

Listen as a human being, rather than a doctor who's spotting pathology. Don't do this:

> Ola: I realized they were gassing me to take my organs for experiments! I woke last night and heard them say, 'You take her head and I'll have the eyes!'
> You: Oh dear. Do you have any allergies?

Step into Ola's shoes for a moment: her *experience* is absolutely real to her (even though the threat is imagined). She *absolutely believes* her organs will be harvested; empathize with *that*. Under those circumstances, any response less than 'That's terrifying!' seems heartless and disbelieving.

4. The balancing act

People may ask if you believe them. You can't lie and say you do—colluding is unethical and creates confusion. Neither should you rudely say, 'Of course not—that's delusional.'

Deflection may work, e.g.:

- I don't know. Can you tell me a bit more so I understand it better?
- I haven't been through anything like this, but I can see it's really scaring you.
- I know you're not lying. What do your family think about it?

Otherwise, you might try to explore the possibility of mental health problems, e.g.:

- I come from a medical background—I think stress has a lot to do with what you're experiencing. What do you think about that?
- I wonder if this might be understood as a mental health crisis. What do you think?

Avoid arguments—you'll seem arrogant and won't 'cure' anyone. Sometimes you'll need to *agree to disagree* with people, in order to move forward.

5. State the obvious

If someone's doing something unusual (e.g. wearing tinfoil, recording you with their mobile, or giggling incongruously), gently *ask why*—don't ignore it. You may unearth important issues you'd otherwise miss.

When people hear voices, they may openly talk or whisper back in response—if so, ask who it is they're speaking to. Often, it'll be subtler, e.g. distracted pauses, or needing questions repeated, as they couldn't concentrate on you *and* the voices. Try these questions:

Ola: They always wanted . . . *[surreptitiously glances away]*

You: Ola? What's happening at the moment?

Ola: Sorry? What?

You: You seem distracted by something. What's distracting you?

Ola: I heard them.

You: If we go really quiet for a moment, can you listen and tell me what they're saying?

Ola: OK . . . *[Listens intently]* They say they'll kill me for talking to you . . .

You: *[After further exploration]* I'm a bit confused—I know you can hear them, but I can't. What do you make of that?

---

6. Gain trust

If someone's suspicious of you, don't become defensive—you'll look dodgy! Calmly explain who you are, offer to show ID, and explain confidentiality. You may be able to turn their mistrust into a talking point by asking why they're concerned, whether they're specifically worried about *you*, or have had bad experiences with other people.

7. Logical, curious questions

If a friend said they'd been followed home, you'd automatically ask logical, curious questions (LCQs). Do the same in a history: curiously ask the next logical question. Questions often start with: *Who?/Why?/What?/How?/Where?/When?*

The 'L' in LCQs is important—you must have listened to their last answer in order to make your next question connect *logically* and smoothly (otherwise, you're just asking *random* curious questions).

The interview

• = Example question. ✱ = Question linking to other parts of the history.

Don't *start* by awkwardly screening for psychotic symptoms. Instead, start with any information you already have (e.g. stress over bullying at work), and explore it as you would any problem, looking out for things which sound unusual, or for evidence that the person's family, friends, or colleagues see things differently. This approach normalizes the search for psychotic symptoms, and will tend to help people open up.

The areas to cover are:

- Delusions.
- Passivity and thought interference.
- Hallucinations.
- Formal thought disorder.
- Strength of conviction.
- Risk.

Delusions

General

- *Have you had any strange experiences lately that are hard to explain?*

Persecutory

- *How have you been getting on with other people recently?*
- Is anyone trying to make life difficult for you?
  - E.g. follow/spy on/hurt/watch/trick/poison . . . you?

- Are you worried that people have turned against you?
- Has anyone been acting suspiciously?
* Have you got people around you who you can trust?

Grandiose

- *How do you see the future?*
- Do you have any special talents (or abilities)?
- Does your life have a special purpose?

Nihilistic

- *Is there anything important missing from your life?*
- Does your body work properly? Is any part failing, dying, or rotting?

Guilt

- *Do you worry you've done anything unforgiveable?*

Religious

- (Are you a religious or spiritual person?) *Have you had any important religious (spiritual) experiences recently?*

Delusions of reference

- *Have people said or done things with a special meaning, just for you?*
- Have you noticed anything in the news that had a special meaning for you?
- Have you noticed any signs or messages in everyday things?

Delusional perception

- *Did something happen which alerted you to what was going on?*

Passivity and thought interference

Passivity

- *Do you ever feel like you're not fully in control of yourself?*
* Have you ever felt that someone else can control your movements or feelings? (Almost as if they have a remote control for you?)

Thought interference

- *Can anyone interfere with your thoughts? Tell me about that...*
- Do you ever feel like...
  - ...there are thoughts in your mind that don't belong to you? [Insertion]
  - ...people can put *their* thoughts into your mind without talking to you? [Insertion]
  - ...people can steal thoughts from your mind? [Withdrawal]
  - ...everyone knows what you're thinking? [Broadcast]
  - ...your thoughts aren't private anymore? [Broadcast]

NB: *if yes, always ask for an example and explore how this might work.*

💡 Ask for *examples* of thought interference. Someone may then say 'Mum puts thoughts in my head. She'll say we're having chips for dinner, then I really want chips'. This isn't thought insertion, just a great dinner suggestion.

💡 If you've fully explored delusions, but not discovered any hallucinations, ask if the people in the delusion have spoken. For example, if the story focuses on spies, simply ask, 'Have you heard the spies talking?'

Hallucinations

General

- (You seem a very sensitive person.) *Do you pick up on things other people don't seem to see or hear?*

Auditory

- *Have you ever heard people talking when you thought you were alone?*
- Do people gossip or talk about you?
- Do people say these things to your face or behind your back?
- Voices:
  - Who do you hear?
  - What do they say?
  - Do they talk to you or about you?
  - Do they ever describe everything you do, just as you do it?
  - Do they ever say your thoughts aloud?
  - Do they ever tell you to do things? What? Can you resist?
  - Can you hear them now?
- Have you heard strange noises and not been able to work out where they were coming from?

Visual

- *Have you seen anything recently that was frightening or hard to explain?*

- Have you seen things that other people said they couldn't see?
- Have you ever had visions?
- Have you ever seen ghosts or spirits?

Somatic/tactile

- *Have you had any unusual feelings in your body?*
- Any strange feelings on or just under your skin?
- Do you ever get strange feelings in your insides/organs?

Gustatory/olfactory

- *Have you noticed any strange tastes or smells recently?*
- Does food taste normal?

💡 If someone's said they hear people talking, the key questions to cross over to delusions would be, 'How can you hear them when other people don't seem to?' or 'Why is this happening to you?'

Formal thought disorder

If you feel increasingly confused as the conversation goes on, this may signal formal thought disorder.

- (I'm finding it hard to follow what you're saying at times.) *Do you ever find it's hard to think clearly?*
- Have your thoughts felt a bit muddled up?

Strength of conviction

Politely test how strongly they hold their beliefs (this isn't about trying to prove them wrong).

- *Why is this happening to you?*
- Do you have a theory about what's going on here?
- How can you be sure this is definitely happening?

- Have you been able to gather any evidence or proof (e.g. for the police)?
- ∗ What do your family/friends think?
  - Why do you think they don't agree with you?
- Sometimes people's minds can play tricks on them (under stress). Is that possible in your case?

💡 Be aware that someone might share your patient's delusional view! In folie à deux, two people with a close relationship develop a shared delusion.

Risk

Think about the risks pertinent to the person's story, but always check suicide and aggression.

General

- *You've put up with a lot so far. Have you done anything about it?*
- What will you do if this goes on?
- Would it ever get so bad that you'd . . .
  - . . . have to kill yourself?
  - . . . need to defend yourself? How?
  - . . . have to take the law into your own hands? How?
  - . . . lose your temper or get aggressive with them?

If command hallucinations/passivity/thought insertion

- *What do they want you to do?*
  - Can you resist? How?
  - What do you think will happen if you don't do as they want?
  - How likely is it that someone could get hurt?

1. Psychosis history (15 minutes)

Candidate's instructions

Samuel Winstanley is a 60-year-old grandfather. His GP referred him to the CMHT, following concerns from his family that he's become strangely worried about his grandson, Jake (aged 6). You're a medical student at the CMHT. The consultant has asked you to see Mr Winstanley, while she talks to his daughter. Take a psychiatric history with a view to suggesting differential diagnoses.

Patient's brief

Key characteristics
- I'm annoyed at being told to attend a 'mental health facility'.
- I'm initially suspicious, and may think the student is part of the 'paedophile plot'. If they laugh, I'm *sure* they're involved.
- If the student is kind and empathic, I talk earnestly about my fears.

History

I'm only here because the Devonshire Paedophile Society (DPS) want me committed to silence me! It began 6 months ago when I read some articles about paedophiles; I couldn't stop worrying about them. It became clear there are powerful people in Devon who are DPS members or being paid to turn a blind eye.

There's *plenty* of evidence! A middle-aged man always uses the computer nearest the crèche at the library (allows the webcam to film the children). Local newsagents only let one child in the shop at a time (lone children are more vulnerable; newsagents are part of the DPS network). The school caretaker replaced after-school club posters with recycling posters (if children don't know about the clubs, they'll play on the estates where he can molest them more easily). My MP wrote back to my letters about the paedophiles and included the line 'Direct Policing Strategy' (DPS! I realized he and the police were members).

Apart from my family, I trust nobody. I've been trying to keep Jake off school, but my daughter (Jenny) thinks I'm over-reacting and makes him go. I need to walk him to and from school, to protect him. I'm gathering evidence to take the DPS to court, and don't go anywhere without my notepad and camera.

Other history
- I've never heard the paedophiles talking (I keep my distance) and don't hear other voices or noises. No visions, strange smells, tastes, or bodily feelings.
- People can't control my movements/thoughts. They can't read my thoughts.
- My family and I haven't had any mental health problems.
- I'm not depressed, just annoyed and worried. My energy levels are good and I enjoy playing with Jake. My memory is excellent. I'm not suicidal.
- My wife, Maria, died 10 years ago. I miss her, but I've learned to cope alone.
- I don't smoke, drink, or use drugs.
- I'm prescribed steroid creams for eczema.
- I'd like to castrate the caretaker, but *won't*. He needs to go to prison!

Questions
You *do* believe me, don't you?/Are you DPS?

Worries
What's happening to Jake while I'm here?

💡 In the absence of hallucinations, thought disorder, or first-rank symptoms, a psychosis lasting longer than 3 months is likely to be delusional disorder. However, a first-episode psychosis in a man of this age should trigger thorough physical investigation to exclude organic causes, including early-onset dementia. Treatment should be possible in the community, given the low immediate risks. Inpatient admission might be needed if he began to endanger himself (e.g. by accusing strangers of paedophilia) or decided to take the law into his own hands.

2. Psychosis history (15 minutes)

Candidate's instructions
Bilal Ali is 38 years old and works at the postal sorting office. He's been off work for 2 weeks and was told he needs the GP to provide a 'sick note'. You're a medical student at the practice. Please take a history with a view to making a diagnosis.

Patient's brief

Key characteristics
- I'm scruffy, perplexed, and reluctant to talk as I don't think I'll be understood.
- I just want a sick note and to leave (before the jinn settles on me).
- When rapport is gained, I explain about the jinn.

History
My manager's angry I haven't been in work for 2 weeks. She wrote to say I needed a sick note and should have called her . . . I'm a good worker but it's been stressful since I was promoted to supervisor (6 months ago). My colleagues are jealous, and started treating me differently around 3 months ago, excluding me from conversations and staring at me. Then I noticed strange things in the sorting office . . . Objects were moved when I wasn't there: first, stationery, then letters and parcels. I realized it was black magic—from jealous colleagues, so threw these things away, even though I know I shouldn't. I haven't been to work since I found soil under my desk (a brown lump—someone wanted everyone to think I was *dirty*).

Things still move around at home, but now I'm getting *prickly feelings* up and down my body . . . it's a *jinn* (supernatural creature). I can feel it in the air and sometimes it gives me electric shocks and my arms move when I don't want them to. It whispers to me: says my name, tells me to touch the sockets or electrical appliances. It wants to electrocute me! My parents visited last week and got worried when they saw my flat: I'd taped over sockets and thrown all the electrical appliances in the garden. I told them about the jinn and they called a Mullah. He gave me verses of the Qur'an to recite but I think it's made the jinn angry and things are worse: it's spending more time with me, and trying harder to possess me.

I spend as much time out of the flat as possible, walking the streets. I only go back at night, but I barely sleep because the jinn might possess me while I'm sleeping and can't actively resist. I just need a sick note while I work out what to do . . .

Other history
- I was diagnosed with schizophrenia 5 years ago, but the diagnosis was wrong. I went to hospital twice, and they made me take olanzapine. I was discharged to my GP last year, and haven't taken olanzapine since.
- An uncle had some kind of mental illness but we don't talk about it.
- I don't drink, smoke, or use drugs.
- I'm single and live alone in my flat.
- I sometimes take sumatriptan for migraines.
- Not depressed or tired, but the jinn won't let me enjoy things.
- Not suicidal, but worried I'll touch the electric sockets and die.
- I don't want to hurt anyone (I'm peaceful).

Questions
Are you a Muslim? (How can you understand if not?)

Worries
The jinn will possess me and make me touch the sockets.

💡 Bilal has a history of schizophrenia, and it's most likely he's relapsed secondary to stopping medication. Due to the risks of electrocution or rough sleeping, admission is probably sensible at first. Bilal may have good reasons for non-adherence, e.g. side effects, a poor understanding of his illness, or social stigma. Interventions would address these issues to help him get and stay well, such as finding a more acceptable medication, psychoeducation for him and his family, and vocational input to help managers support him at work. The medical model is only one way of making sense of mental illness—religious (and other) beliefs offer a different framework. It can help to include faith leaders, as they may be able to legitimize the use of both medical treatments *and* prayer.

NEXT STEPS

Early adverse complications of clozapine

You're an FY2 psychiatrist, clerking a new admission, under Section 2 of the MHA, to your ward: 24-year-old Emmanuel Ochieng has treatment-resistant paranoid schizophrenia, and started clozapine 7 weeks ago. He was under the HTT, due to increased distress that a 'microchip' was implanted in his heart, causing him to say he'll dig it out with a knife if his team doesn't remove it. Emmanuel is thought disordered and hard to follow, but says that the government is making his heart 'flip' and 'twist' with the microchip, and some 'technology' is 'stealing' his breath. You repeat his physical observations: temperature 38.7°C, HR 122, BP 118/70mmHg, RR 21, SaO$_2$ 98%.

- What are your key differentials?
- Which investigations are essential?
- What is your immediate management if his FBC is normal?
- What is the longer-term management?

BOX 10.9 Neutropenia and clozapine

Regular FBC testing is used to monitor potential neutropenia/agranulocytosis in people prescribed clozapine. A 'traffic light system' is used to indicate the safety of continuing the medication.

	Green	Amber	Red
WCC (×10^9/L)	≥3.5	<3.5/≥3.0	<3.0
Neutrophil count (×10^9/L)	≥2.0	<2.0/≥1.5	<1.5

BEN refers to baseline lower neutrophil counts (non-pathological) seen in a proportion of people of African ethnicity. Ranges for the traffic light system are adjusted for those with established BEN.

Reproduced from Royal College of Psychiatry online CPD module 'Managing the adverse effects of Clozapine' by Dr James MacCabe and Dr Jennifer Brook, last updated in 2019. www.psychiatrycpd.co.uk/learningmodules/managingtheadverseeffectso.aspx. Data from Semple, D, Smyth R (2009) *Oxford Handbook of Psychiatry*. Oxford University Press.

Differential diagnosis

Although Emmanuel has delusions and possibly somatic hallucinations (heart 'flipping' and 'twisting'), you mustn't fall into the trap of assuming his physical complaints are due to psychiatric illness. Emmanuel may be trying to describe chest pain, palpitations, and shortness of breath. As with anyone, this could be due to a range of medical diagnoses, e.g. heart attack, chest infection, pulmonary embolism.

His clozapine prescription is extremely important, as there are four main adverse effects to consider:

- Neutropenia or agranulocytosis—most common in first 18 weeks of treatment; can cause overwhelming infection. Be aware of possible benign ethnic neutropenia (BEN) in Emmanuel's case (**Box 10.9**).
- Benign, resting tachycardia—especially in the first 4–6 weeks; usually resolves.
- Myocarditis—most common in first 8 weeks.
- Cardiomyopathy—usually after 8 weeks; asymptomatic *or* insidious cardiac failure.

Emmanuel is in the high-risk period for myocarditis and neutropenia: have a low threshold for concern. If neutropenic, a chest infection may account for his presentation.

Myocarditis can present with chest pain, dyspnoea, palpitations, and 'flu-like symptoms (fever, fatigue). Signs include tachycardia/arrhythmia, hypotension, and evidence of acute heart failure on examination, e.g. peripheral oedema. Be wary—sometimes the presentation is very mild.

Essential investigations

Following a full history and physical examination, the key initial investigations are:

- Neutropenia/agranulocytosis:
  - FBC.
  - CRP—raised.
- Myocarditis:
  - CRP—raised, typically >100mg/L.
  - Troponin—raised, especially if double the upper limit of the normal range.
  - ECG—ST changes (often depression or saddle ST segments) ± diffuse T-wave flattening or inversion.

Immediate management

Emmanuel's FBC is normal, but CRP and troponin are raised, suggesting myocarditis.

Discuss Emmanuel's case with the medical registrar or cardiologist. Slightly raised CRP or troponin—in the absence of cardiac symptoms—can sometimes be closely monitored on the psychiatric unit. However, Emmanuel's presentation suggests greater urgency, and you'll probably be advised to stop clozapine and transfer him to the general hospital for an urgent echocardiogram and further evaluation by cardiology. Strike off his clozapine *now*, to prevent medication errors.

The nursing team will help you by arranging an ambulance, copies of his medication and observation charts, and a registered mental health nurse (RMN) to accompany Emmanuel to hospital. You should write a cover letter, including:

- Emmanuel's psychiatric and medical diagnoses.
- Medications (noting clozapine and that this is now being withheld).
- Examination findings ± investigation results.
- Suspected myocarditis.
- That Emmanuel is under S2 MHA, will be accompanied by an RMN, and that he *must not be allowed to leave the hospital (staff should involve security if required)*.
- Risks—particularly his recent statement that he wants to dig out the microchip from his heart (suicide/self-harm).
- Contact details for you and his regular team.

Emmanuel may be very frightened; don't forget to explain what's happening and check if he'd like you to contact any relatives or friends. Discuss his case with your on-call senior to ensure you haven't missed anything important. Then contact liaison psychiatry, so that they can proactively review Emmanuel.

Longer-term management

Cardiology will work with liaison psychiatry to manage Emmanuel's care while in the general hospital.

Emmanuel will have been on clozapine due to resistant psychotic symptoms, suggesting he'll get only limited benefit from other antipsychotics. Nonetheless, he's likely to need some medication to try and decrease his current degree of distress and risk. This should be discussed with cardiology and pharmacy, and might include an antipsychotic with few cardiac side effects (e.g. aripiprazole) or sedative medication (e.g. benzodiazepines).

Once the emergency has passed, it *may* be possible to rechallenge with clozapine, but this needs a full risk/benefit discussion with Emmanuel, as myocarditis can recur. Any rechallenge would be in collaboration with the cardiologists, and would require close monitoring with echocardiogram, CRP, and troponin.

If clozapine is felt to be too dangerous, Emmanuel might benefit from a range of other measures to combat distressing psychotic symptoms, e.g.

- Alternative medications or medication combinations, e.g. high-dose olanzapine ± amisulpride.
- Psychology input, e.g. CBT, ACT.
- Substance misuse work.
- Reduction of social stressors.

There's always *something* that can be done, and the team will need to work with Emmanuel to ensure he doesn't lose hope, and learns how best to cope with any residual symptoms.

> 💡 **Good psychiatric care requires medical *and* psychological skills; with only one, you're only half a doctor.**

Movie buff
K-PAX (2001): persistent delusional disorder? Suspend your disbelief (and don't emulate the psychiatrist's boundaries)!.

Spider (2002): a harrowing portrayal of Patrick McGrath's novel of the same name (1990). This follows Denis Cleg's release from a long-stay institution, and his ongoing struggle with psychotic symptoms

Revolution #9 (2003): a young journalist's life descends into psychosis.

The Soloist (2009): Jamie Foxx transforms himself into Nathaniel Ayers, a Julliard-trained musician whose battle with hallucinations render him homeless.

Book shelf
Amis, M. (1987) 'Insight at Flame Lake'. In *Einstein's Monsters*: charts Dan's relapse of schizophrenia, narrated through his and his uncle's alternating diaries, taking a critical look at clinical and lay notions of insight.

Cockburn, P. and Cockburn, H. (2011) *Henry's Demons*: true account describing Henry Cockburn's experience of schizophrenia, written by Henry and his journalist father. Illustrates the dilemmas of enforced treatment and concept of recovery.

Crawford, P. (2002) *Nothing Purple, Nothing Black*: beautiful novel exploring schizophrenia. Crystal is taken out of the asylum during a transition to community care, but is unable to cope, resulting in a terrifying relapse with command hallucinations.

Diski, J. (1990) *Then Again*: Katya's mother struggles to accept her psychotic illness. A striking feature of this sensitive novel is its graphic but not sensationalized account of the vulnerability of people with psychotic disorders.

Perkins Gilman, C. (1892) *The Yellow Wallpaper*: a feminist text and account of the historical use of 'rest cure' for mental illness. One of the key images throughout the book is the barred yellow wallpaper through which the narrator begins to claw, seeking freedom at the cost of psychosis.

Schiller, L. and Bennett, A. (1994) *The Quiet Room: A Journey Out of the Torment of Madness*: autobiographical account of psychosis told from the perspectives of the patient, doctors, parents, siblings, and friends, examining the impact of psychosis on the family and social network.

Note

1. McGrath, P. (1990) *Spider*. London: Penguin.

Journal club

Barnes, T.R.E., Schizophrenia Consensus Group of British Association for Psychopharmacology (2011) Evidence-based guidelines for the pharmacological treatment of schizophrenia: recommendations from the British Association for Psychopharmacology. *Journal of Psychopharmacology*, **25**(5), 567–620.

Cantor-Graae, E., Selten, J.-P. (2005) Schizophrenia and migration: a meta-analysis and review. *American Journal of Psychiatry*, **162**, 12–24.

Fearon, P., Kirkbride, J.B., Morgan, C., et al. (2006) Incidence of schizophrenia and other psychoses in ethnic minority groups: results from the MRC AESOP Study. *Psychological Medicine*, **36**, 1541–50.

Jackson, H.J., McGorry, P.D. (2009) *The Recognition and Management of Early Psychosis: A Preventive Approach* (2nd ed.). Cambridge: Cambridge University Press.

Leff, J., Vaughn, C. (1981) The role of maintenance therapy and relatives' expressed emotion in relapse of schizophrenia: a two-year follow-up. *British Journal of Psychiatry*, **139**, 102–4.

National Institute for Health and Care Excellence (NICE) (2014) *Psychosis and Schizophrenia in Adults: Prevention and Management*. Clinical Guideline 178. London: NICE.

Pharoah, F., Mari, J., Rathbone, J., et al. (2006) Family intervention for schizophrenia. *Cochrane Database of Systematic Reviews*, **12**, CD000088.

Read, J., van Os, J., Morrison, A.P., et al. (2005) Childhood trauma, psychosis and schizophrenia: a literature review and clinical implications. *Acta Psychiatrica Scandinavica*, **112**, 330–50.

Resources

BMJ Best Practice information sheets on schizophrenia: www.bestpractice.bmj.com/

Go to www.oup.com/uk/stringer2e for a wealth of additional resources, including an OCSE mark scheme, filmed scenarios, and self-assessment questions.

11 Substance use Disorders

True or false?

Answers on p. 277

1. Binge drinking contributes around 10% of UK alcohol consumption.
2. Alcohol dependence is 75% genetically inherited.
3. A woman's maximum safe daily alcohol intake is 2 units.
4. Alcohol is a stimulant, which inhibits the GABA system.
5. 'Dual diagnosis' means substance misuse combined with alcohol dependence.
6. 'Snowballing' means using crack with cocaine.
7. Alcohol directly causes more deaths annually than recreational drugs.
8. Hallucinogens are commonly smoked.
9. The CAGE questionnaire screens for drug problems.
10. If dependence causes physical harm, it is considered 'harmful use'.

Contents

Principles
Introduction
Epidemiology
Aetiology
- Genetics
- Childhood and life experiences
- Occupation
- Psychiatric illness

Theories of dependence
- Learning theories
- Neurobiological models

Alcohol: clinical presentation
- Intoxication
- Withdrawal
- Complications

Drugs: clinical presentation
- Opioids
- Cannabinoids
- Stimulants
- Hallucinogens
- Sedatives
- Inhalants
- Novel psychoactive substances

Differential diagnosis
Investigations
Management
- Biological interventions
- Psychological interventions
- Social interventions

Prognosis

Reality
General approach: tips, tricks, and cautionary tales

The interview
- Alcohol history
- Opioid history

Next steps
Aggression: 72 hours after a road traffic accident
- Differential diagnosis
- Preparation
- Assessment
- Management

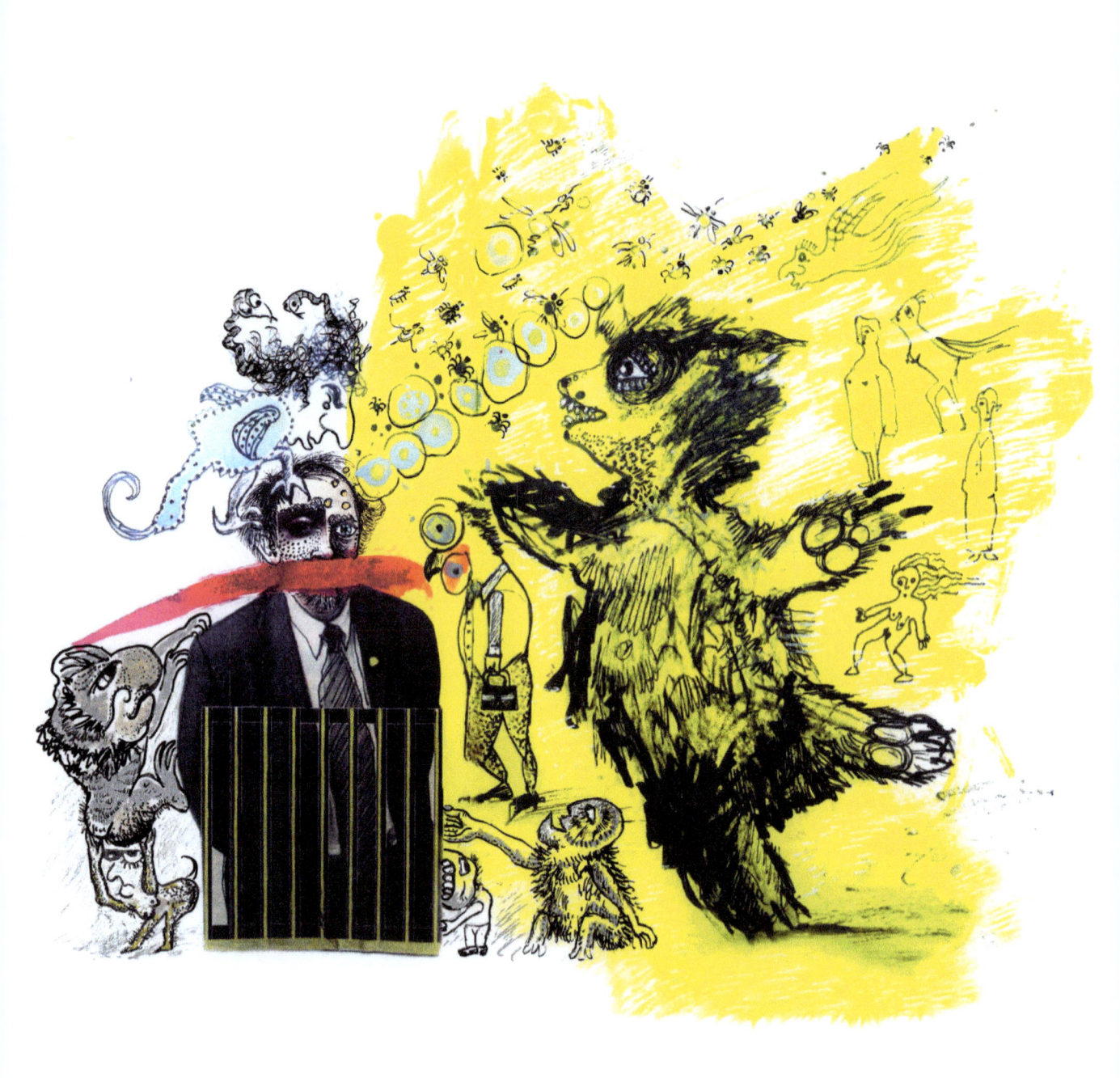

PRINCIPLES

If he had been able to hold off through yesterday, today he would have been normal again; and he knew himself and his habits well enough to know that that would have lasted some days, held possibly even two or three weeks, for he was a periodic drinker, with intervals of sobriety between. At the same time, he knew himself well enough also to know that once started, he had to go through it to the end, there was no stopping now, he could not prevent the downward curve to the final state of danger, destruction, or collapse. Short of being locked up, nothing could help him now till it had played itself out, safely or otherwise.

Charles Jackson, *The Lost Weekend*[1]

Introduction

People start using alcohol or drugs for many reasons: curiosity, peer pressure, thrill-seeking, to relax, get high, forget problems, or *self-medicate* pain or uncomfortable emotions (e.g. anxiety). Whatever the reason for starting, some people reach a point where the substance dominates their life and they can't function without it. Problematic substance use carries a massive social burden—causing physical and mental illness, accidents, crime, and social problems. Despite its overt presence in police stations and hospitals, substance use is often invisible: a secret problem for which people are too ashamed to seek help.

Disorders due to substance use encompass drug or alcohol use that causes physical, mental, or social dysfunction. This divides into:

- **Intoxication:** a dose-dependent, transient state following drug use.
- **Harmful use:** a pattern of use likely to cause physical or psychological damage.
- **Dependence:** *needing* to use a substance to feel or function normally, after a period of regular use. It's recognized by a cluster of symptoms (**Table 11.1**). Addictive substances cause *physical* dependence, evidenced by physiological *withdrawal* symptoms when stopping them (e.g. nicotine cravings relieved by patches). This is distinct from *psychological* dependence: emotional and motivational difficulties when stopping an addictive behaviour (e.g. substituting the *habit* of smoking with an inhalator or e-cigarette).

Epidemiology

Young men (late teens to early twenties) are the heaviest drinkers, although alcohol misuse is increasing among women. Male-to-female ratios are:

- 2:1 for alcohol use disorders.
- 4:1 for substance use disorders.

Prevalence rates are shown in **Table 11.2**. Problematic substance use is highly comorbid with mental health problems; having *both* is called *dual diagnosis*. Using multiple substances (which may include alcohol) is not uncommon.

Binge drinking (>8 units for men or >6 units for women in one session) constitutes 27% of UK alcohol consumption.

Aetiology

Substance use disorders have complex biopsychosocial aetiologies; many causative factors are common to both alcohol and drugs.

Genetics

Family, twin, and adoption studies suggest that substance use disorders have a heritability of 40–60%. Some of this genetic vulnerability may be mediated by personality traits, e.g. impulsivity, anxiousness/avoidance, reward-seeking. Though multiple genes are implicated, interest has focused on those involved in dopamine 'reward' pathways (see p. 80). For example, reduced

Table 11.1 Features of dependence

Feature	Explanation	Example
Tolerance	Bigger doses are increasingly needed to get the same effect	The amount of heroin needed for an opioid-dependent person to get 'high' would easily kill a new user
Withdrawal	Physiological state when the substance is stopped/decreased, causing: (a) A characteristic withdrawal syndrome for that substance, or (b) Substance use to prevent/relieve withdrawal symptoms	(a) Alcohol withdrawal, e.g. shaking, retching, sweating, seizures (b) Early morning drinking
Compulsion	Strong desire to use	Craving a cigarette
Loss of control	Difficulty controlling starting, stopping, or amount used	Can't refuse a drink
Continued use despite harm	Can't stop using, despite clear mental/physical health consequences	Injecting heroin despite developing abscesses
Salience (primacy)	Obtaining and using the substance becomes so important that other social priorities are neglected	Dropping out of university as smoking cannabis becomes more important than studying
Reinstatement after abstinence	Tendency to return to previous pattern and level of use after abstinence	After not smoking for a year, a single cigarette triggers a quick return to the previous 20/day habit
Narrowing of repertoire	Loss of variation in use of the substance	Drinking the same amount of the same drink in the same way, every day

dopamine-2 receptor levels may make people compensate for low endogenous dopamine stimulation, by seeking out external pleasures ('rewards'). Genes involved in serotonin and gamma-aminobutyric acid (GABA) pathways play a role.

Table 11.2 Prevalence of substance use disorders

Disorder	12-month prevalence[a]	Lifetime prevalence[b]
Alcohol dependence	1.3%	5.4%
Drug dependence	0.4%	3.0%
Any substance use disorder	3.8%	14.6%

Data from: (a) Kessler, R.C., et. al. (2005) Prevalence, severity, and comorbidity of twelve-month DSM-IV disorders in the National Comorbidity Survey Replication (NCS-R). *Archives of General Psychiatry*, **62**, 617–27; (b) Kessler, R.C., et al. (2005a) Lifetime prevalence and age-of-onset distributions of DSM-IV disorders in the National Comorbidity Survey Replication (NCS-R). *Archives of General Psychiatry*, **62**, 593–602.

Ethanol is metabolized to acetaldehyde, which is broken down by aldehyde dehydrogenase. Some East Asian populations have less effective enzymes, causing acetaldehyde accumulation, which causes unpleasant facial redness, palpitations, and nausea ('flush reaction'); due to this, affected people tend to avoid alcohol. Cirrhosis and cancer risks are raised if they *do* drink.

Childhood and life experiences

Risk factors include lower parental socioeconomic group and educational achievement, parental substance dependence, ineffective parenting, family breakdown, and childhood abuse. Affected adults more commonly had conduct disorder as children, achieved poorly in school, experienced bullying, and were involved in antisocial peer groups or gangs.

Adolescence is a high-risk period, not only because of vulnerability to stress and risk-taking behaviour, but also because the developing brain is sensitive to modification of dopamine reward pathways.

If you and your patient swapped the first 10 years of your lives, would you still be the medic?

Occupation

Stress and socially sanctioned drinking increase the risk of alcohol use disorders in certain occupations, e.g. publicans, journalists, doctors, military personnel, people in the entertainment industry.

Psychiatric illness

Substance use disorders are associated with personality disorders, depression, BPAD, ADHD, psychosis, and anxiety disorders (particularly social anxiety disorder).

Theories of dependence

Learning theories

Social learning theory

'Vicarious learning' explains how substance dependence can develop following *observation* of behavioural rewards in others (e.g. social acceptance following alcohol consumption) as well as direct experience (e.g. numbing of distress following drug use).

Operant (Skinnerian) conditioning

In *positive reinforcement*, behaviours that are rewarded are repeated, e.g.:

- Rats keep pressing levers that supply food.
- People keep using drugs that feel pleasurable.

In *negative reinforcement*, behaviours are repeated if they *relieve* unpleasant experiences, e.g.:

- Rats keep pressing levers that end electric shocks.
- People keep using:
  - Paracetamol to relieve headaches.
  - Drugs to escape the unpleasant reality of their lives.
  - Drugs to end unpleasant withdrawal states, once dependent.

Classical (Pavlovian) conditioning

Pavlov's famous experiment showed that by presenting the natural stimulus for salivation (food) with the sound of a bell, dogs were conditioned to salivate to the bell alone. In substance dependence, cravings become conditioned to 'cues' (e.g. needles for heroin users), so the cue itself can trigger craving, causing drug-seeking behaviour.

> 💡 Some American soldiers became dependent on heroin during the Vietnam War. On returning to the USA, many gave up heroin almost effortlessly—the loss of cues removed many of the withdrawal phenomena.

Motivational theory

The Stages of Change model[2] explains *motivation to change* as a stepwise process.

- **Pre-contemplation:** can't see a problem or need to change, e.g.:
  - 'I just like a drink—it's normal.'
- **Contemplation:** recognizes the problem but doesn't want to change *yet*; open to discussing the pros and cons of change, e.g.:
  - 'I should cut down, but not today . . .'
- **Preparation:** wants to change and planning to do this soon, e.g.:
  - 'I want to get pregnant. I'll stop drinking next month.'
- **Action:** cuts down or stops altogether, e.g.:
  - 'Just a lemonade, thanks.'
- **Maintenance:** remains abstinent (or maintains an agreed low level of use), e.g.:
  - 'I really crave a beer sometimes, but it passes.'
- **Relapse:** starts using again, e.g.:
  - 'I thought I'd have *one* drink, but I couldn't control it. I'm drinking daily again'

Relapse isn't 'failure', but a learning opportunity: understanding the triggers for relapse helps the next attempt at abstinence.

Neurobiological models

The brain's dopaminergic 'reward' pathways start in the ventral tegmental area, projecting onto the nucleus accumbens, prefrontal cortex, and limbic system ('the emotional brain').

- Dopamine release in the nucleus accumbens is central to the sensation of pleasure, which drives the search for rewarding experiences.
- The prefrontal cortex has a role in motivation and planning, and can encourage or 'rationally' inhibit reward-seeking.

Most addictive drugs strongly increase synaptic dopamine levels in the reward pathway. The brain adjusts by reducing natural dopamine production; addiction may then develop as the brain becomes dependent on the drug for the dopamine 'rush'. Alcohol and opioids also affect other neurotransmitters, e.g. mimicking GABA's soothing, inhibitory action.

Alcohol: clinical presentation

Intoxication

Alcohol is relaxing, lowering inhibitions and making people feel sociable and cheerful. Higher levels cause drunkenness: slurred speech, poor coordination, and exaggerated emotions (hilarity, tearfulness, misery, irritability). Disinhibition, impulsivity, and poor judgement can cause risky or aggressive behaviour. *Blackouts* may occur: amnesia for the drinking period, despite normal consciousness. Severe intoxication ('alcohol poisoning') can cause vomiting, ataxia, respiratory depression, confusion, coma, and death. **Box 11.1** gives a guide to units.

Withdrawal

As blood alcohol levels fall, withdrawal symptoms can emerge, e.g. headache, nausea, retching, vomiting, tremor, sweating, anxiety, and insomnia (familiar, if you've ever had a hangover). Examination signs include agitation, tachycardia, and hypotension. Alcohol is a central nervous system (CNS) depressant, stimulating the GABA inhibitory system to reduce brain excitability. When people who are alcohol dependent suddenly stop drinking, their neural pathways become hyper-excitable, risking seizures. Severe withdrawal causes delirium tremens (**Box 11.2**) or death.

💡 **Don't advise alcohol-dependent people to suddenly stop drinking. It's well-meaning, but potentially fatal advice.**

BOX 11.1 Alcohol units

Alcohol is measured in units: 1 unit is 8g of pure alcohol.
   To calculate units exactly = volume (litres) × alcohol by volume (ABV; %)
   Roughly speaking, 1 unit =

- ½ pint of ordinary strength beer (284mL, 3.5–4%).
- 1 small glass of lower-strength wine (125mL, 10%).
- 1 standard measure of spirits (25mL, 40%).
- 1 standard measure of sherry/port (50mL, 20%).

UK low-risk drinking guidelines are the same for men and women:

- Maximum 14 units a week.
- Spread drinking evenly over at least 3 days a week.
- Drink-free days can help people cut down.

💡 **Drinks are often stronger than these examples, and 'home measures' are usually more generous than pub measures.**

BOX 11.2 Delirium tremens (DTs): a medical emergency

- Onset ~48 hours into abstinence; duration 3–8 days.
- Symptoms:
  - Confusion.
  - Hallucinations, especially visual (insects, tiny people) and tactile (itch, burn, crawling skin).
  - Affective changes, e.g. terror, hilarity, anger.
  - Gross tremor, especially hands.
  - Autonomic disturbance: sweating, tachycardia, hypertension, dilated pupils, fever.
- Mortality: 5%, rising to 30% if untreated or complicated, e.g. sepsis.
- Management: reducing regimen of benzodiazepines; parenteral thiamine (to prevent Wernicke's encephalopathy; Box 11.3); correct potentially fatal dehydration and electrolyte abnormalities.

Complications

See **Figure 11.1**.

Physical

- **Liver:** fatty liver, the first stage of alcoholic liver disease, is usually asymptomatic. It may progress to alcoholic hepatitis, with malaise, hepatomegaly, and ascites. End-stage liver disease (cirrhosis) develops in 10–20% of alcohol-dependent people; complications include ascites and hepatic encephalopathy.
- **Gastrointestinal:** pancreatitis, oesophageal varices, Mallory–Weiss tear, gastritis, and peptic ulceration.
- **Neurological:** increased risk of cerebrovascular disease, peripheral neuropathy, myopathy, seizures, dementia, Wernicke–Korsakoff syndrome (**Box 11.3**), and cerebellar degeneration.
- **Cancers:** mouth, pharynx, larynx, oesophageal, breast, bowel, liver, and pancreas.
- **Cardiovascular:** increased risk of ischaemic heart disease, hypertension, and cardiomyopathy.
- **Head injuries/accidents** while intoxicated, e.g. fractures, subdural haematoma.
- Foetal alcohol syndrome (Table 19.3).

Psychiatric

- **Depression, anxiety, self-harm, and suicide** are increased in alcohol dependence.
- **Cognitive impairment:** due to dementia or Korsakoff syndrome (**Box 11.3**).

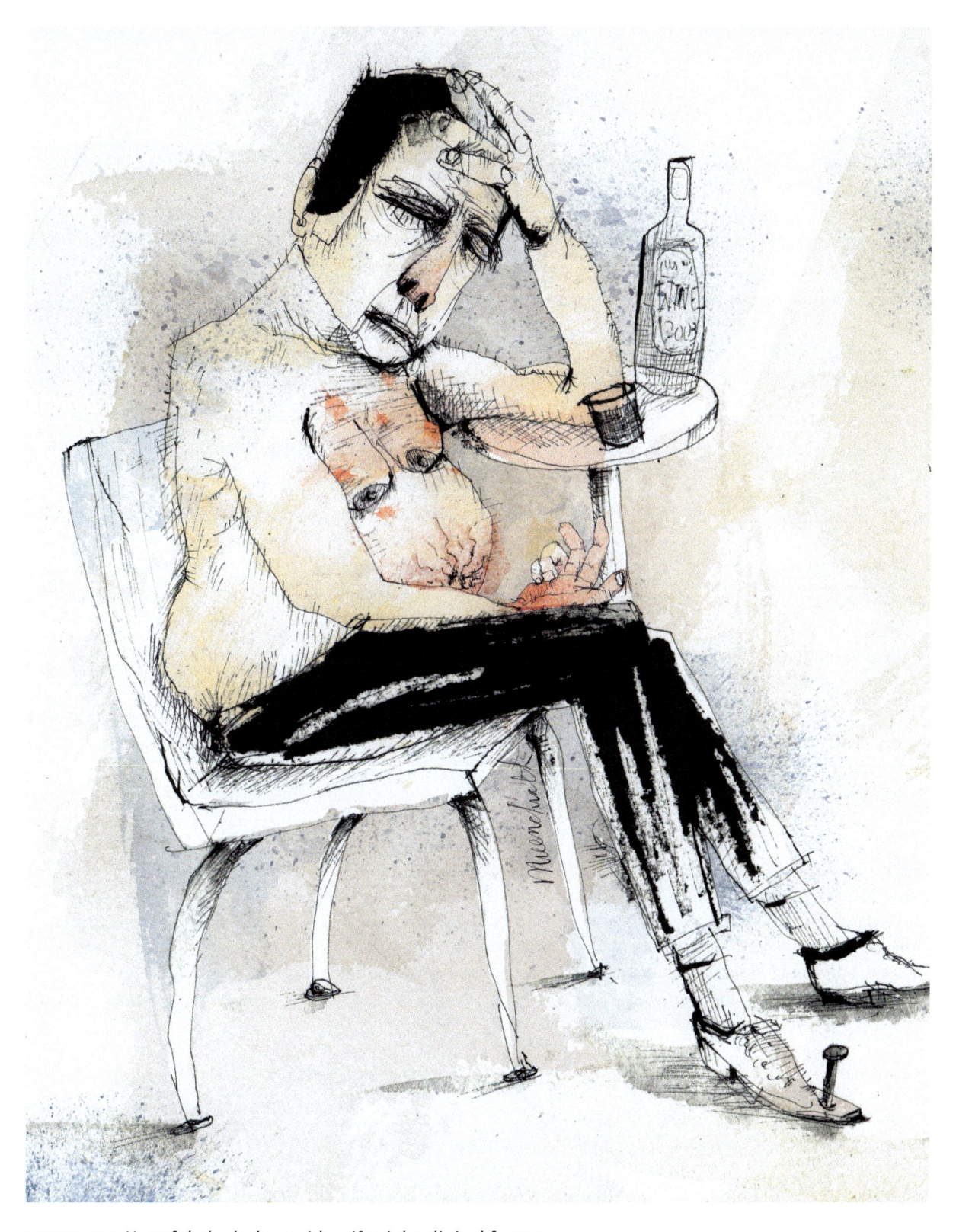

FIGURE 11.1 Harmful alcohol use: identify eight clinical features

Alcohol: clinical presentation 107

BOX 11.3 Wernicke–Korsakoff syndrome

Wernicke encephalopathy
- A medical emergency!
- Caused by acute thiamine (vitamin B$_1$) deficiency, due to inadequate intake, absorption, and cellular utilization in chronic alcohol use.
- Classically presents with the triad of confusion, ataxia, and ophthalmoplegia.
- Treat urgently with parenteral (IM/IV) thiamine (Pabrinex®) for 3–5 days; oral thiamine absorption is poor.
- Untreated, can progress to . . .

Korsakoff syndrome
(See p. 136.)
- Irreversible anterograde amnesia (and some retrograde amnesia).
  - Can register new events, but can't recall them within a few minutes.
- People may confabulate to fill gaps in their memory.

- **Alcoholic hallucinosis:** auditory hallucinations in clear consciousness during or after heavy drinking. Hallucinations often have persecutory or derogatory content.
- **Morbid jealousy:** overvalued idea/delusion of a partner's infidelity. It's associated with alcohol dependence, impotence, and violence.

Social
Alcohol use disorder can become a vicious circle: social problems trigger drinking and are then created and perpetuated by continued use. Problems include unemployment, absenteeism/poor work attendance, domestic violence, sexual exploitation, and divorce. Crime may occur while intoxicated (e.g. drink-driving, physical/sexual assault) or to fund the habit (e.g. theft). Children are at increased risk of neglect, abuse, and conduct disorder.

Drugs: clinical presentation

Illicit drugs were traditionally grouped into six categories: opioids, cannabinoids, stimulants, hallucinogens, sedatives, and solvents (see **Table 11.4**, p. 116). More recently, *novel psychoactive substances* (NPS) have been developed in laboratories worldwide, hitting the market faster than they can be classified or fully understood.

The social consequences of alcohol are true for many drugs, especially in dependence. Funding a habit can be expensive and may lead to theft, drug dealing, or commercial sex work.

Opioids
Heroin (diamorphine, *brown, gear, H, horse, smack*) is the most notorious opioid. Others include **morphine**, **pethidine**, **codeine**, and **dihydrocodeine**. Heroin is a μ (mu) opioid agonist, stimulating brain and spinal cord receptors normally activated by endogenous endorphins (the body's natural painkillers).

Initially, people usually smoke (*chase*) heroin, but progress to intravenous (IV) injection (*mainlining*) as tolerance builds. Pure heroin can be snorted; tablets like dihydrocodeine and codeine are swallowed. See **Figure 11.2**.

To inject heroin, people heat and dissolve it with water in a *spoon* (small container, e.g. bottle cap, actual spoon). They draw it into the syringe through a *filter* (cotton bud or cigarette filter), removing solid particles that could clog the needle. People usually first inject into the antecubital fossa, but repeated injections damage veins, so they have to inject in other veins (e.g. feet, groin), subcutaneously (*skin popping*) or intramuscularly.

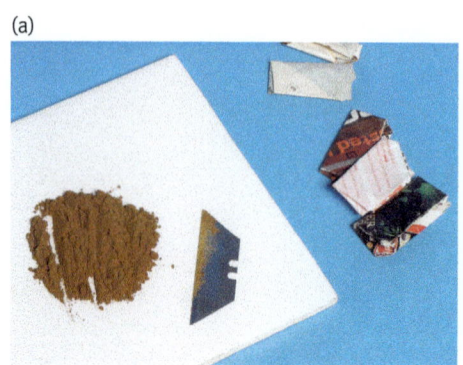

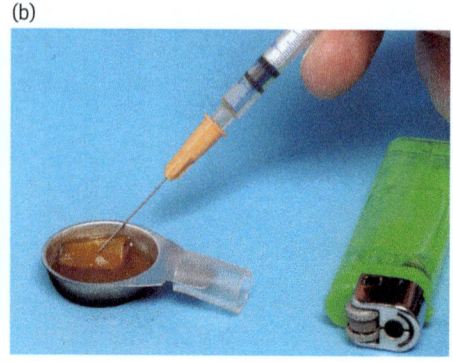

FIGURE 11.2 Heroin: (a) powder and wraps, (b) spoon, filter, syringe.
Photographs courtesy of TICTAC Communications Ltd.

Intoxication

IV opioid use produces an intense rush or buzz, with feelings of euphoria, warmth, and well-being. Other effects are sedation, bradycardia, respiratory depression, 'pinpoint' (constricted) pupils, and analgesia, and some people vomit or feel dizzy (especially the first time). Non-IV use causes milder effects.

> 💡 *Speedballing* combines heroin with cocaine, for a bigger rush.

Withdrawal

Withdrawal typically begins around 6 hours after injecting heroin, peaking at 36–48 hours (**Figure 11.3**). It's extremely unpleasant but *not* life-threatening. People have dilated pupils, and feel dysphoric (miserable), sick, and restless. They yawn irresistibly but can't sleep. As the effects on opioid receptors reverse, everything 'runs': diarrhoea, vomiting, sweating, lacrimation, and rhinorrhoea. People feel feverish with aching joints/muscles, abdominal cramps and piloerection (causing goosebumps, hence *going cold turkey* or *clucking*). For withdrawal in neonates, see **Box 11.4**.

Complications

Overdose can kill through respiratory failure or aspiration of vomit while sedated. Constipation, anorexia, and low libido are side effects. IV use causes numerous problems (**Table 11.3**).

Cannabinoids

Cannabis (*bud, dope, ganja, marijuana, pot, puff*) comes from the *Cannabis sativa* plant:

- *Grass/weed*—from leaves and flowers.
- *Hash/hashish*—from the resin.
- *Skunk*—newer, stronger strains of cannabis.

The main psychoactive components, delta-9-tetrahydrocannabinol (THC) and cannabidiol (CBD), act on cannabinoid receptors in the brain. People usually smoke cannabis in *spliffs/joints* (with tobacco) or through a *bong* (water pipe). It can be *inhaled* (*vaped*) via an e-cigarette or vaporizer, eaten in cakes or biscuits, or drunk as a tea (**Figure 11.4**). (*Spice* is a synthetic cannabinoid, a type of NPS; see p. 115.)

Intoxication

Effects vary with expectations and original mood state (which cannabis tends to enhance). However, higher CBD levels cause relaxation, contentment, giggling, and talkativeness, while higher THC levels cause anxiety, panic, and paranoia. People may feel inspired or enlightened, find profundity in the mundane, and experience time as having slowed down. Hunger pangs (*munchies*) can trigger overeating of sweet foods. Nausea and vomiting (*a whitey*) can happen, especially when combining cannabis with alcohol. Other signs include bloodshot eyes, tachycardia, poor coordination, and a dry mouth.

Withdrawal

It was thought that cannabis didn't cause physiological dependency, but a withdrawal syndrome has been identified in some people after heavy and prolonged use. Symptoms include anxiety, irritability, restlessness, nausea, headaches, and poor sleep, appetite, and concentration.

Complications

Physical

Smoking cannabis aggravates asthma and risks lung disease and cancer.

Psychiatric

Cannabis can trigger psychosis, especially in vulnerable people using it heavily from a young age, particularly high-potency cannabinoids like skunk (see p. 80). Lethargy and poor motivation are recognized features of chronic, heavy use. Regular use of high-THC cannabis is associated with depression, anxiety, ADHD, and PTSD. See **Box 11.5**.

Stimulants

Stimulants (**Figures 11.5 and 11.6**) potentiate the effects of the monoamine neurotransmitters dopamine, noradrenaline, and sometimes serotonin. They include cocaine, crack cocaine, amphetamine-type stimulants (e.g. amphetamine, methamphetamine, ecstasy, methylphenidate) and khat.

Cocaine (*C, charlie, coke, snow, toot, wash, white*) is a white powder, usually arranged in lines and snorted, e.g. using a rolled-up bank note. It can also be dissolved and injected. **Crack cocaine** (*crack, rocks*) is a concentrated form, made by heating cocaine in a baking soda solution until the water evaporates, leaving rocks which are heated and smoked (making a *crack*ing noise, hence the name).

Amphetamine (*speed, uppers, whizz*) is a tablet, or pinkish-white paste/powder. It's snorted, rubbed on the gums, swallowed in cigarette paper (*parachuting/bombing*), dissolved in drinks, or injected. **Methamphetamine** is similar, but also available as highly addictive, smokeable, glassy rocks known as *crystal meth* (*ice*).

Ecstasy (3,4-methylenedioxymethamphetamine; *E, MDMA*) is usually a tablet, but can be purer, crystalline powder (1g can contain as much MDMA as ten tablets). Use is usually confined to dance and party circuits. Ecstasy's

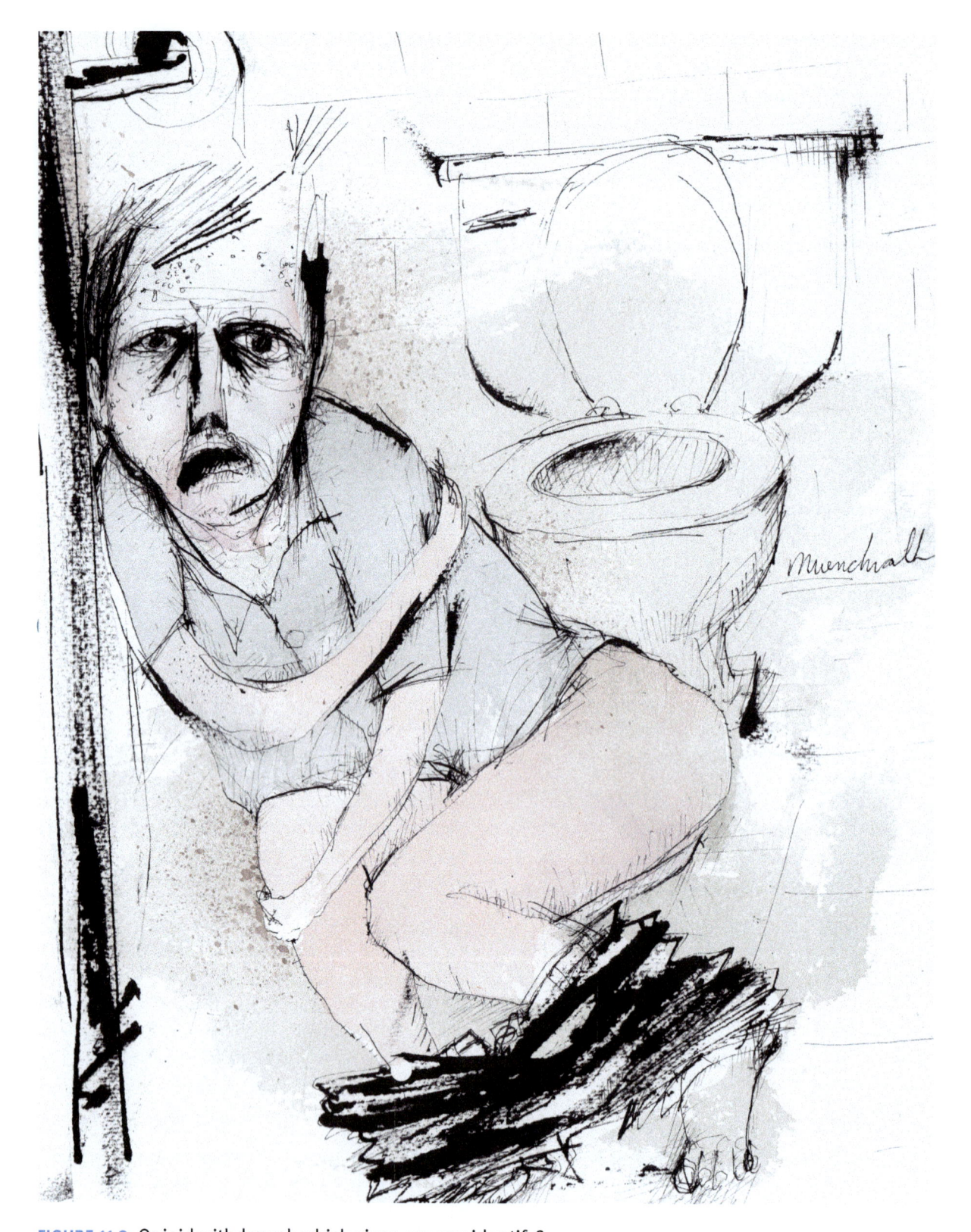

FIGURE 11.3 Opioid withdrawal: which signs can you identify?

> **BOX 11.4** Neonatal abstinence syndrome
>
> Babies of opioid-dependent mothers suffer withdrawal symptoms within hours of birth:
>
> - High-pitched crying.
> - Loose stools, vomiting.
> - Sweating, fever, tachypnoea.
> - Restlessness, tremor.
> - Hypertonia, convulsions.
>
> Treatment involves paediatric opioid preparations, anticonvulsants, and supportive measures. Opioids also cause intrauterine growth restriction, low birth weight, and prematurity. Sudden infant death syndrome (SIDS) is increased.

chemical structure and action—of serotonin release and reuptake inhibition—make it a cross between a stimulant and a hallucinogen (although hallucinations are rare).

Khat (*chat, qat*) is a leafy green plant. People from the Arabian Peninsula and North-East Africa (especially Yemen, Somalia, and Ethiopia) chew khat leaves for their mild stimulant effects.

Intoxication

All stimulants speed up the mind and body: making people energetic, alert, excited, and euphoric (*high*). They may be chatty and show frenzied or prolonged activity, e.g. dancing all night. Stimulants suppress appetite and sleep, and cause tachycardia and raised blood pressure. Excessive confidence and impulsivity, combined with poor judgement, can cause risky behaviour, e.g. unsafe sex. *Ecstasy* additionally produces a sense of empathy and closeness to others, and sometimes bruxism (teeth-grinding).

Most stimulants start working within a few minutes and last up to 3 hours, depending on the drug and administration route. Part of the addictive appeal of smoking crack or crystal meth is the almost immediate and *extremely* intense high (sometimes likened to an 'all body orgasm'); this ends after a few minutes with crack, but lasts a few hours with crystal meth.

Withdrawal

There's often an unpleasant comedown ('crash') within 24 hours of stopping stimulants, followed by several weeks of withdrawal. Symptoms include depression, irritability, lethargy, and cravings.

Ecstasy and khat *don't* cause withdrawal, but can lead to psychological dependence. Khat is rarely dangerous in overdose.

Complications

Physical

Stimulant use is associated with insomnia, weight loss, arrhythmias, and hypertension. In overdose, stimulants can cause multiorgan failure (particularly renal failure from rhabdomyolysis), seizures, stroke, coma, and death. Mixing stimulants with alcohol increases the risk of fatal cardiac events, and IV use can cause the complications noted in **Table 11.3**.

- *Cocaine* is a vasoconstrictor: snorting it damages the nasal mucosa, causing necrosis and septal perforation. Sharing 'snorting equipment' can spread BBVs.
- Tooth decay and loss occur with *methamphetamine* ('*meth mouth*') and *khat*.
- *Ecstasy* has caused deaths from overheating and dehydration in clubs.

Psychiatric

Anxiety, panic, aggression, and psychosis can occur. Cocaine can produce formication (*cocaine bugs*)—the sensation of insects crawling on/below the skin.

Hallucinogens

Drugs in this group (**Figure 11.7**) affect dopamine, serotonin, and glutamate neurotransmitters.

LSD (lysergic acid diethylamide; *acid, Lucy, trips, window*) is a liquid usually impregnated on *tabs* or *blotters* (tiny paper squares with pictures on them). **Psilocybin**

Table 11.3 Complications of IV drug use

Infection	Injection introduces bacteria, causing cellulitis (infection under the skin) or abscess (accumulation of pus)
Deep vein thrombosis (DVT)	Repeated femoral vein injection damages valves, slowing venous return and facilitating DVTs
Emboli	Septic emboli cause gangrene or pulmonary emboli
Infective endocarditis	Injected microorganisms settle on cardiac valves
Sepsis	From direct injection of contaminating bacteria *or* spread from abscesses or cellulitis
Blood-borne viruses (BBVs)	Needles, water, filters, and spoons can transfer blood; sharing *any* of these risks BBVs, e.g. hepatitis B/C, HIV
Increased overdose risk	IV use causes sudden, potentially overwhelming effects (smoking allows greater control over the 'dose')

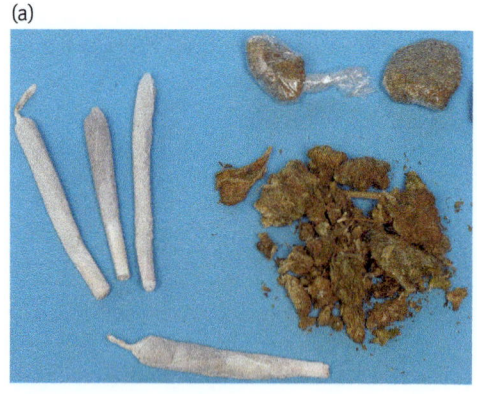

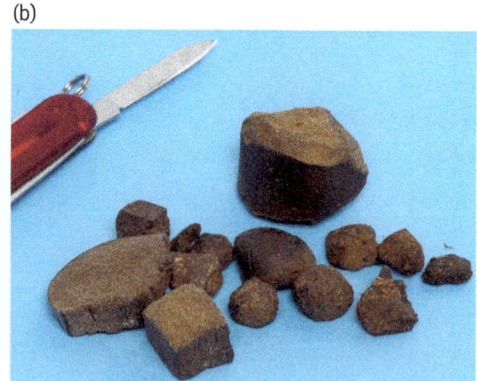

FIGURE 11.4 Cannabis: (a) grass, (b) hash.
Photographs courtesy of TICTAC Communications Ltd.

(in *magic mushrooms* e.g. the liberty cap) is eaten or drunk, and has effects similar to LSD but milder.

PCP (phencyclidine; *angel dust, hog*) and **ketamine** (*K, Vitamin K, Super K, Special K, donkey dust*) are anaesthetics, which cause hallucinations and dissociative symptoms. They come as liquid, powder, or pills and both can be snorted.

Intoxication

Intoxication lasts a few hours. Hallucinogens cause altered mood (e.g. euphoria) and sensory experiences, e.g. visual illusions and hallucinations, distortions of sound, time, colour, and everyday objects. Synaesthesia (experiencing a sensation in another modality, e.g. hearing a smell), depersonalization, and derealization may occur. Ketamine and PCP also cause anaesthesia, and feelings of dreaminess, floating, and detachment from reality (ketamine's extreme dissociative effects are called *going down the K-hole*).

Complications
Physical
People can suffer accidents while acting on hallucinogenic experiences (e.g. jumping from a window while feeling they can fly), or may not realize they're causing damage due to ketamine/PCP anaesthesia (e.g. nonchalantly plucking out teeth). PCP can cause dangerous hyperthermia, and prolonged use of ketamine causes bladder ulceration and frank haematuria. The main risk from magic mushrooms is mistakenly eating poisonous species.

BOX 11.5 THC and CBD

Newer, high-potency cannabinoids are associated with the highest risk of psychosis, due to high THC and low CBD levels. This supports the theory that CBD protects against harmful psychiatric effects of THC; its potential antipsychotic properties are now being researched.

Psychiatric
Bad trips are when hallucinogenic experiences become frightening and unpleasant. Anxiety and depression may result. LSD users may experience disturbing *flashbacks* to trips, even years later. PCP's effects are particularly unpredictable, and associated with violent outbursts.

Sedatives

Sedatives are depressant drugs which enhance the inhibitory effect of GABA transmission. **Benzodiazepines** (*downers, sleepers, tranx*) are prescribed for insomnia and anxiety, but have a high potential for misuse and dependency. They're usually swallowed as tablets, but can be dissolved and injected. **Alcohol** and **barbiturates** are also included in this class, although barbiturates aren't seen much now (they're rarely prescribed due to lethality in overdose).

GHB (gamma hydroxybutyrate; *G, liquid ecstasy*) is a strongly sedative anaesthetic, mainly used on the club scene. It's a white powder or colourless, oily liquid, and usually sipped or mixed with soft drinks. **GBL** (gamma butyrolactone) and **1,4-BD** (1,4-butanediol) are chemicals which convert to GHB after ingestion; originally legal alternatives to GHB, they've now also been outlawed. GHB and GBL have been used to facilitate sexual assaults ('date rape'): their salty taste can be hidden in soft drinks, and make the victim disinhibited or unconscious, often with amnesia for the assault (**Figure 11.8**).

Intoxication
Sedatives cause a feeling of calm, mild euphoria, loss of inhibitions, and sedation (though GHB is a mild stimulant at low doses).

Withdrawal
Withdrawal symptoms include nausea, vomiting, headaches, anxiety, depression, and uncomfortable body

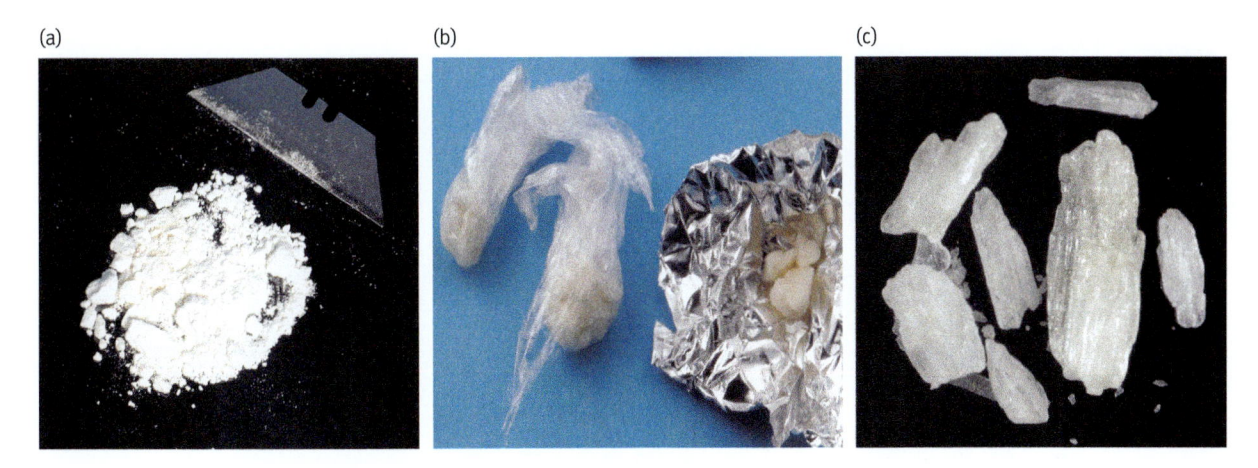

FIGURE 11.5 Stimulants: (a) cocaine, (b) crack, (c) methamphetamine.
Photographs courtesy of TICTAC Communications Ltd.

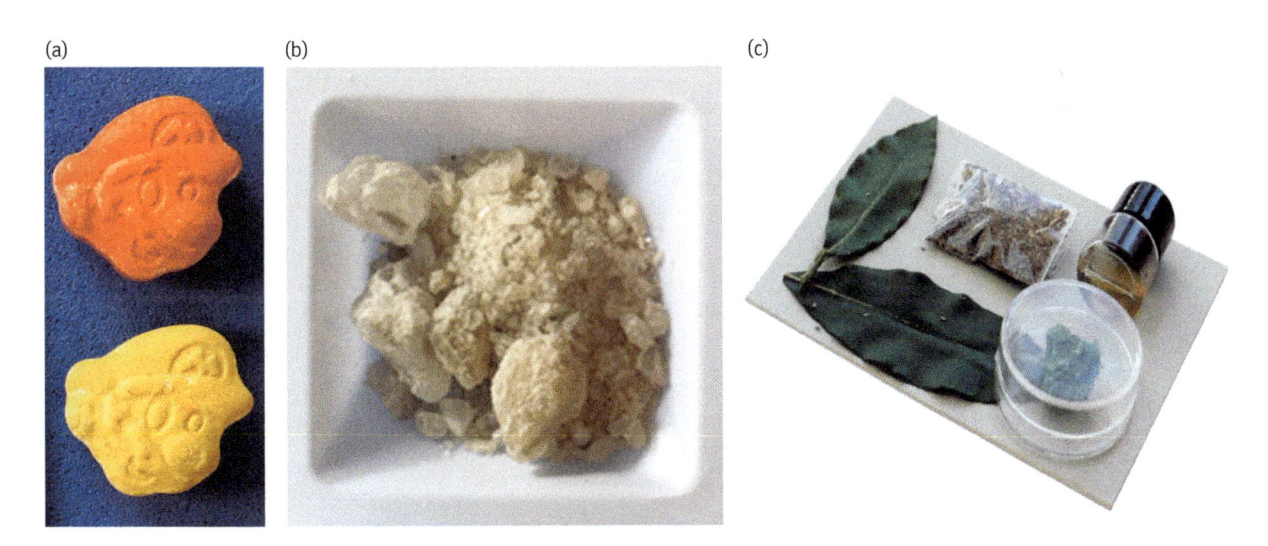

FIGURE 11.6 Stimulants: (a) ecstasy tablet examples, (b) crystal MDMA, (c) khat. (a) and (b)
Photographs courtesy of TICTAC Communications Ltd. (c) by Oli Butterworth

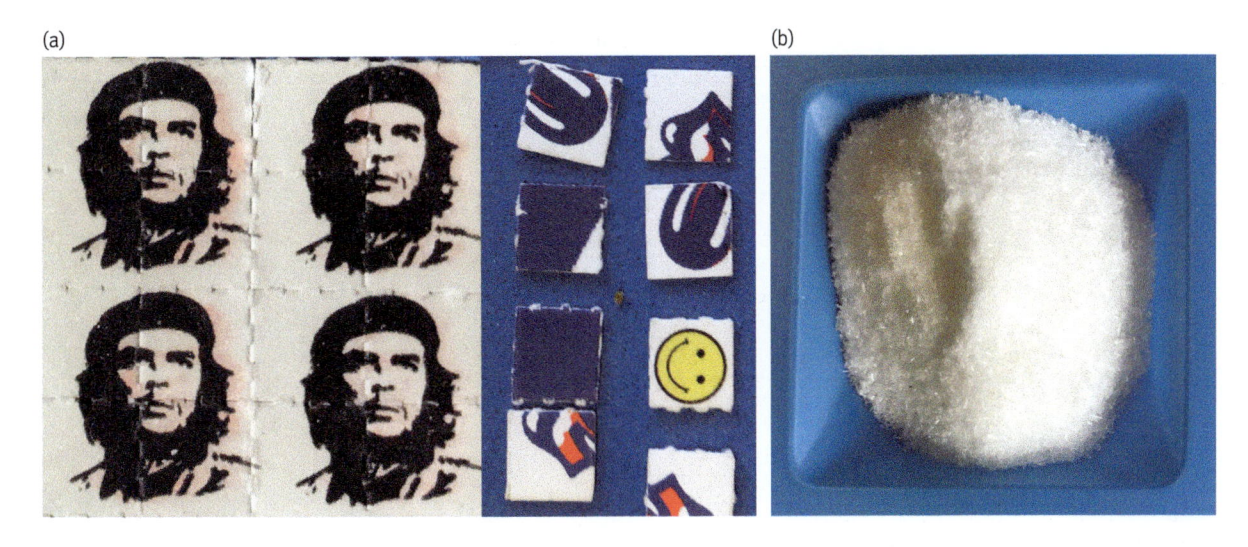

FIGURE 11.7 Hallucinogens: (a) LSD blotters examples, (b) ketamine.
Photographs courtesy of TICTAC Communications Ltd.

Drugs: clinical presentation   113

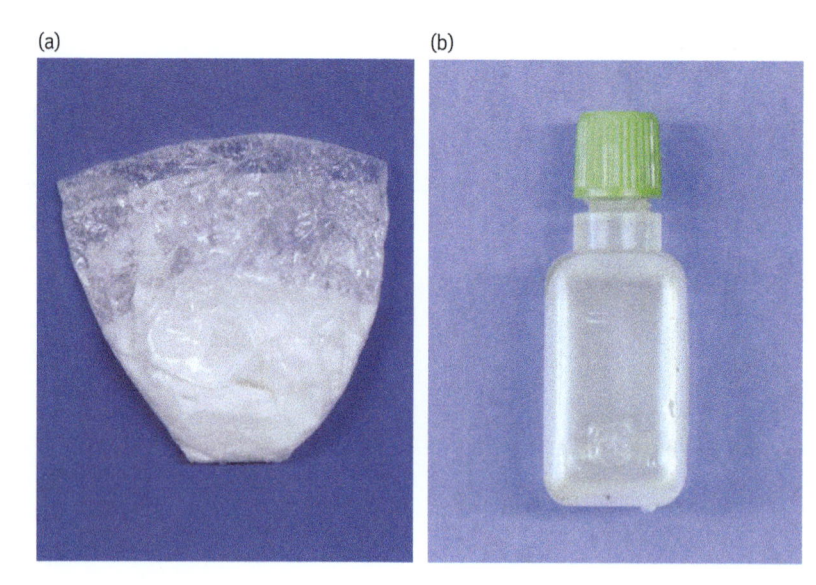

FIGURE 11.8 (a) GHB as powder, (b) GBL as liquid.
Photographs courtesy of TICTAC Communications Ltd.

sensations; in severe cases confusion and seizures can occur. Abrupt discontinuation of dependent use is discouraged without medical supervision. GHB dependence can develop after a relatively short period of use, and can be life-threatening.

Complications

At higher doses, sedatives cause slurred speech, ataxia, vomiting, coma, and respiratory collapse. Overdose can kill through respiratory arrest, particularly in combination with alcohol or opioids.

Inhalants

These compounds produce vapours which are inhaled (**Figure 11.9**).

Volatile solvents (glue, gas)

Solvents are found in many products such as paint, glue, nail varnish remover, cigarette lighter refills, paint, petrol, and aerosols. Use is more common in younger teenagers. They're inhaled directly (*huffing*), squirted into the throat, sniffed from an impregnated cloth/sleeve, or sprayed into a plastic bag which the person puts over their head to breathe

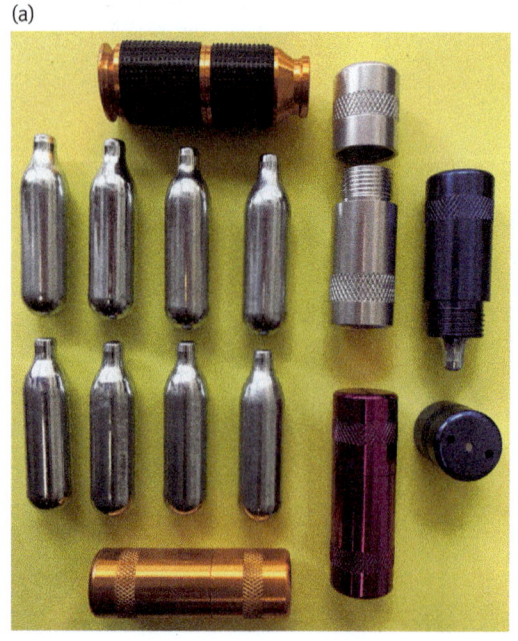

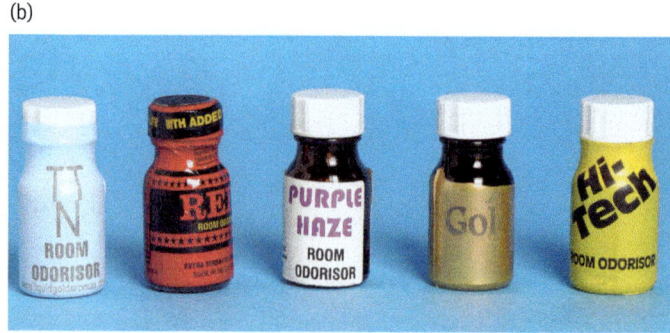

FIGURE 11.9 Inhalants: (a) nitrous oxide, (b) nitrites.
Photographs courtesy of TICTAC Communications Ltd.

from. Intoxication is similar to alcohol, causing euphoria and disinhibition. Some people report hallucinations.

Volatile anaesthetics

The commonest is **nitrous oxide** (N_2O, *laughing gas, hippy crack, whippets*), a depressant used as a dental anaesthetic and an aerosol propellant. It's usually inhaled from a balloon inflated from a canister; and often passed around in groups. Intoxication causes euphoria and uncontrollable fits of laughter.

Nitrites (poppers, TNT, rush)

Amyl nitrite and **butyl nitrite** are the commonest and used medically as vasodilators. They're volatile liquids, usually inhaled from bottles. Intoxication causes a sudden euphoric 'rush', and enhancement of sexual experience; use is associated with the male gay club scene.

Withdrawal

Inhalants may cause psychological rather than physical dependence.

Complications

Some people experience hangovers, with severe headaches, fatigue, and depression. At higher doses, inhalants cause ataxia, vomiting, dizziness, muddled thinking, and sometimes hallucinations. Heart failure, coma, and death (from vomit aspiration) can all occur. Squirting solvents into the throat can cause swelling and asphyxiation. Inhalation from bags risks suffocation: tell-tale signs are blistering and redness around the mouth and nose. Heavy nitrous oxide use is linked to vitamin B_{12} deficiency and anaemia.

Novel psychoactive substances

NPS are chemicals synthesized to mimic standard recreational drugs (**Figure 11.10**). New NPS are constantly being developed, and there are hundreds of varieties. Though hard to categorize, they can be roughly placed in the same overall groups as established drugs, giving similar effects and risking similar complications (**Table 11.4**). However, risks are greater, since users and clinicians understand them less, and their effects can be more toxic and unpredictable. They're also more difficult to accurately detect on urine drug screen. The most common NPS are cannabinoids and stimulants.

Synthetic cannabinoid receptor agonists (**SCRAs**), known as **spice** or **noids** are usually smoked in herbal mixtures, or as liquids via e-cigarettes or vaporizers. Being often more potent than cannabis (**Box 11.5**), SCRAs' resultant agitation and psychosis is unpredictable, and they can cause more severe dependence and withdrawal. They can also cause confusion, hypertension, seizures, and stroke.

Stimulants, e.g. **mephedrone** (*meph, m-cat, miaow*). Chemical structures can be tweaked to produce different combinations of euphoric, empathic, or hallucinogenic effects. As well as the usual routes, they can be injected or taken rectally.

> 💡 The UK *Misuse of Drugs Act 1971* groups most traditional drugs into classes (A, B, C), and guides penalties for manufacturing, possessing, or supplying them. Class A (e.g. heroin, cocaine) attracts the toughest penalties. Classes don't necessarily relate to the dangerousness of the drug. The *Psychoactive Substances Act 2016* legislates against NPS (they're no longer called *legal highs*).

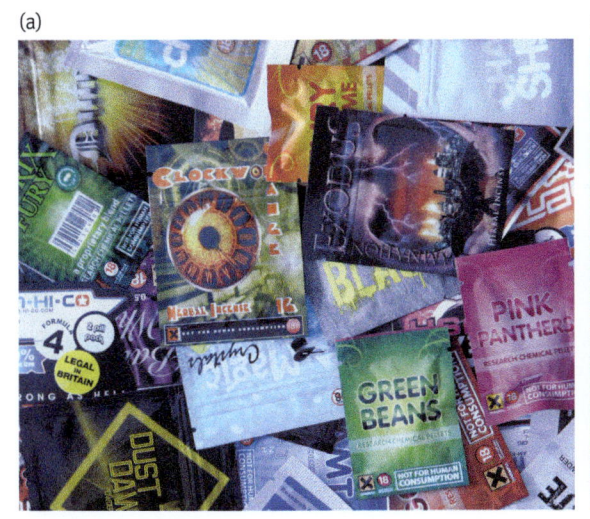

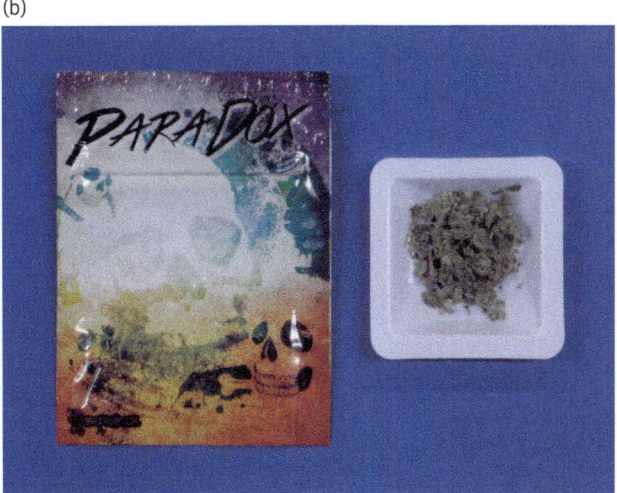

FIGURE 11.10 NPS: (a) various, (b) synthetic cannabinoid example.
Photographs courtesy of TICTAC Communications Ltd.

Table 11.4 Illicit drug summary

Drug class and examples	Route of administration	Intoxication ⇒ complications	Withdrawal
Opioids			
Heroin Morphine Pethidine Codeine Dihydrocodeine NPS, e.g. MT-45, novel fentanyls	Smoked IV/IM/SC Snorted Swallowed	Euphoria Sedation Analgesia Pinpoint pupils ⇩ Respiratory depression Bradycardia Death	Everything 'runs': • Diarrhoea • Vomiting • Lacrimation • Rhinorrhoea • Sweating Dysphoria Cramps, aches Fever Insomnia, agitation Yawning Piloerection Dilated pupils
Cannabinoids			
Cannabis NPS, i.e. SCRAs	Smoked Eaten Drunk Vaped	Relaxation Euphoria Anxiety Hunger Perceptual changes ⇩ Paranoia/ psychosis Lethargy SCRAs: seizures, tachycardia, hypertension, hyperthermia, agitation, aggression	Restlessness Irritability Insomnia Anorexia
Stimulants			
Cocaine Crack Amphetamine Methamphetamine Ecstasy Khat NPS, e.g. mephedrone	Snorted Swallowed Smoked IV Chewed (khat)	Energy Euphoria Insomnia Anorexia ⇩ Disinhibition Anxiety Psychosis Arrhythmia, stroke Agitation/psychosis	'Comedown': • Depression • Lethargy
Hallucinogens			
LSD Psilocybin PCP Ketamine NPS, e.g. methoxetamine (*mexxy*), 2C-series	Swallowed	Euphoria Visual distortions Hallucinations Synaesthesia ⇩ Anxiety Disinhibition Psychosis	Nil

Table 11.4 Continued

Drug class and examples	Route of administration	Intoxication ⇒ complications	Withdrawal
Sedatives			
Alcohol Benzodiazepines Barbiturates GHB/GBL/1,4-BD NPS benzos, e.g. diclazepam, flubromazepam	Swallowed Injected	Euphoria Disinhibition Sedation ⇩ Slurred speech Ataxia Respiratory depression Unconsciousness, coma	Anxiety Insomnia Confusion Seizures
Inhalants			
Solvents Nitrous oxide Nitrites	Inhaled	Disinhibition Euphoria Hallucinations ⇩ Dizziness Vomiting Coma	'Hangover' headache

Differential diagnosis

This applies for alcohol *and* drugs. Substance use disorders may trigger, mask, coexist with, or be mistaken for other physical and psychiatric illnesses.

- **Organic illness:** don't assume that confusion, ataxia, or psychotic symptoms are solely due to intoxication or withdrawal; there may be an underlying physical cause, e.g. head injury and subdural haematoma from falls.
- **Psychiatric illness** (see **Box 11.6**), e.g.:
  - Depression/mania.
  - Psychosis.
  - Anxiety disorder.
  - Personality disorder.

> **BOX 11.6** Questions to help distinguish substance use from psychiatric disorders
>
> - Which problem came first?
> - Do psychiatric symptoms 'fit' with known symptoms of that substance?
> - Do psychiatric symptoms stop once abstinent?
> - Is there a personal or family history of the psychiatric illness?

Investigations

- **Physical health screening:** people may neglect themselves, so examine fully, think broadly, and be opportunistic. Investigations will be guided by the history, examination, and clinical presentation, e.g. general observations, weight; ECG if history of chest pain or using stimulants; TB testing in high-risk populations; routine screens (e.g. cervical).
- **Blood tests** include:
  - FBC, MCV, *vitamin B_{12}*—alcohol use disorder may cause a macrocytic anaemia due to vitamin B_{12} deficiency.
  - *LFTs*—raised transaminases suggest hepatocellular damage (from alcohol /hepatitis); *GGT* rises with *recent* heavy alcohol use.
  - *U&Es*—several drugs affect the kidneys and bladder, e.g. cocaine, ecstasy, ketamine. Electrolyte disturbances may precipitate arrhythmias.
  - *BBV screening* if IV drug use.
- **Drug screens:** useful when drug use is uncertain or disputed. A *urine drug screen* (UDS, **Box 11.7**) or *saliva drug screen* can identify some common drugs, but doesn't routinely spot NPS. *Hair samples* provide data on repeated drug or alcohol use for the last 90 days or more, but are expensive and take time to process, so are mainly used in legal settings.

> **BOX 11.7** Urine drug screen (UDS)
>
> Although not 100% sensitive, a UDS can detect drugs for some days after last use:
> - Heroin: 1–2 days.
> - Amphetamine: 2 days.
> - Cocaine: 2–4 days.
> - Methadone: 7 days.
> - Cannabis: up to 1 month (heavy, daily use).

Management

Before trying to manage a substance use problem, always check whether someone *wants* to change (see 'Stages of Change', p. 105). If not, they'll seek treatment for complications (e.g. abscess) but continue using. Don't get frustrated! They're just not ready to stop yet, but may still benefit from *harm reduction* approaches (see p. 119). *Addictions services* can support people to change and offer specialist prescribing, psychology input, and advice to service users, carers, and professionals.

Biological interventions

General healthcare

Physical health should be optimized, e.g. dental care, management of diabetes or asthma. Injecting drug users and commercial sex workers can be offered vaccinations, testing, and treatment for BBVs; risk is reduced through needle exchanges and free condoms. Likewise, it's important to identify and treat mental health problems.

Alcohol

Withdrawal and detoxification

'Detox' minimizes discomfort and risk during alcohol withdrawal. It may be planned (e.g. with an addictions team), or unplanned (e.g. after emergency hospital admission). It involves the following:

- *Long-acting benzodiazepines* (e.g. chlordiazepoxide) replace alcohol and prevent withdrawal symptoms, including seizures and DTs. They're gradually withdrawn and stopped.
- *Parenteral thiamine* (vitamin B_1) is prescribed to prevent Wernicke's encephalopathy.

Community (home) detoxification can be offered for uncomplicated alcohol dependence, using a fixed dose-reducing regimen of benzodiazepines over 5–7 days. *Inpatient detoxification* is needed if there's a history of withdrawal seizures, comorbid medical or psychiatric illness, or nobody at home to observe and support the person. Hospital staff grade withdrawal symptoms using objective scales, e.g. the Clinical Institute Withdrawal Assessment for Alcohol (CIWA) scale. Benzodiazepines are given in response to symptoms; the total dose at 24 hours guides the reducing regimen.

Relapse prevention

Acamprosate is an anticraving drug, thought to act on the midbrain; it can support people recovering from alcohol dependency. *Disulfiram* (Antabuse®) may discourage drinking. It inhibits acetaldehyde dehydrogenase, so that drinking causes acetaldehyde accumulation, with almost immediate unpleasant flushing, throbbing headache, and nausea/vomiting.

Drugs

Acute withdrawal

Opioid withdrawal is deeply unpleasant but—unlike alcohol withdrawal—can't kill. Even without access to substitute prescribing (see below), withdrawal symptoms may be eased with antidiarrhoeal medications (loperamide), antiemetics (metoclopramide), and non-opioid painkillers. Withdrawal from other substances may also be palliated, e.g. nicotine replacement in cannabis use and benzodiazepines in stimulant withdrawal.

Abrupt withdrawal in benzodiazepine dependence carries a high risk of seizures. This can be avoided by switching to an equivalent dose of a benzodiazepine with a longer half-life (often diazepam); it's patiently reduced, sometimes with anticonvulsants to prevent seizures. GHB withdrawal is extremely dangerous and may need detoxification with very high benzodiazepine doses.

> 💡 **Naltrexone** is an opioid antagonist, competitively displacing opioids from receptors to remove their euphoric effects. It can aid relapse prevention after opioid detox. It also decreases the enjoyment of drinking, so can help people remain abstinent from alcohol.

Substitute prescribing

Substitute prescribing swaps harmful street opioid use for safer (usually oral) alternatives. Benefits include breaking links with dealers, cutting injection risks, and offering stability to enable employment. *Methadone* (liquid) is a full agonist at opioid receptors with a longer half-life than heroin (so withdrawal is longer but milder). *Buprenorphine* (sublingual tablet) is a partial agonist at the μ receptor, blocking the euphoric effects of heroin while preventing withdrawal symptoms.

Methadone or buprenorphine are initially taken in a supervised environment, and doses gradually titrated until the person experiences *no* withdrawal symptoms. They can be slowly weaned down and stopped over weeks or months. Although complete abstinence is possible, it's not always realistic: some people thrive on substitute prescribing regimens but deteriorate when detoxing. For them, long-term methadone/buprenorphine maintenance enables them to get on with life, with minimal risks.

💡 **The RIOTT study found that supervised injection of 'medical' grade heroin (diamorphine) caused greater reductions in street heroin use than supervised injectable methadone or optimized oral methadone, in people for whom conventional treatment was ineffective.**

Overdose

For most drug overdoses, the treatment is supportive: body temperature regulation; intubation and ventilation in respiratory suppression (e.g. opioids, GHB); correction of hypotension and arrhythmias. Some drugs have antidotes for use in overdose, e.g.:

- Benzodiazepines: *flumazenil* (benzodiazepine antagonist).
- Opioids: *naloxone* (opiate antagonist) reverses heroin's effects, plunging people into immediate withdrawal; lifesaving, but distressing. Its short half-life means that repeated injections or continuous infusion may be needed.

Psychological interventions

Brief interventions

In harmful alcohol use, *brief interventions* (non-judgemental, motivational conversations) can help people reduce their drinking to safer levels, e.g. explaining safe drinking limits and the effects of alcohol. Simple measures to reduce units or the risks of getting drunk include keeping a drink diary, choosing lower ABV drinks, eating before drinking, and alternating alcoholic drinks with soft drinks.

Motivational interviewing (MI)

MI is a therapeutic approach which aims to empower people to change a behaviour. It can be provided as a course of therapy, but is more usually incorporated into everyday work; the style is sometimes described as 'dancing not wrestling' with people who misuse substances. It often incorporates the Stages of Change model (see p. 105) to understand how ready someone is to change.
Key concepts include:

- *Empathy*: build rapport and identify someone's *own* goals and reasons for change.
- *Developing discrepancy*: help somebody recognize the *gap* between where they are now and where they want to be.
- *Rolling with resistance*: avoid disagreement and conflict, as these undermine the relationship and distract from the goal (change).
- *Encouraging change talk*: explore ambivalence and help people talk themselves into change.
- *Supporting self-efficacy*: build someone's belief in their ability to change and empower them to take small steps to change.

Realistic, personalized goals are created, e.g.:

- Short term: reduce alcohol consumption.
- Medium term: detox.
- Long-term: attend university.

Cognitive behavioural therapy

CBT can help people develop effective alternative coping strategies for substance misuse. Pros and cons are explored, learning to recognize cravings and high-risk situations posing risks of relapse. However, most CBT evidence is for alcohol dependence, with some evidence for benzodiazepine and cannabis misuse.

Social interventions

In addition to trying to resolve social stressors that may be driving or exacerbating substance misuse, there are specific substance use interventions.

Harm reduction approaches

When someone wants to keep using a substance, they may accept support to help them use more safely. Harm reduction approaches include:

- Providing naloxone to heroin users and their family, friends, hostel staff (etc.) in case of overdose.
- Providing needle exchanges (where people can swap used needles for clean ones) and sharps boxes to prevent needle stick injuries.
- Teaching basic life support, including the recovery position.

Advice can save life (and sometimes limb), e.g.:

- Safer injecting practices, e.g. sterilizing equipment, no sharing, safer vein choice.
- Use in a safe environment, in the company of trusted friends who'll keep them safe while under the influence.
- Not combining drugs (especially opioids and sedatives, due to the risk of respiratory depression).
- Legal highs and stimulants: try a small test dose, and wait at least 2 hours to see the response before trying more (formulations can vary wildly, even from the same dealer).

- Ecstasy: stay hydrated by sipping non-alcoholic drinks, but no more than 1 pint an hour.

Peer support

Twelve-step programmes are peer led, global support networks that recognize 12 steps towards recovery, e.g. accepting powerlessness over the addiction, surrendering to a 'higher power'. *Alcoholics Anonymous* (AA) was founded in 1935 and has around 2 million members who attend regular groups; experienced members often 'sponsor' newer attendees. *Narcotics Anonymous* (NA) and *Cocaine Anonymous* (CA) evolved from AA and operate in a similar way. *Al-Anon* and *Nar-Anon* are related groups, offering mutual support to the relatives and friends of people with substance use problems.

Self-Management and Recovery Training (SMART) meetings are also peer-led and offer alternatives to AA/NA/CA.

Rehabilitation

Whether as a residential or day programme, the aim is to initiate a complete restructuring of the person's life. Residential (living on-site) options offer a more complete break for people whose lives and friendships have revolved around substance misuse. Structured groups focus on areas such as relapse prevention, problem-solving, skills development (e.g. IT training), and accessing training or employment.

Prognosis

Drug and alcohol disorders tend to follow a relapsing–remitting course; people may relapse several times before eventually becoming abstinent. After a period of alcohol dependence, complete abstinence is often necessary, as 'controlled drinking' (trying to drink within healthy limits) often leads to relapse. Substance misuse is associated with significant morbidity and mortality. Alcohol harm costs the UK £21 billion annually. In 2016, there were 7327 UK alcohol-specific deaths, 3744 drug poisoning deaths, and 1,135,709 alcohol-related hospital admissions. IV administration, chaotic use, and polydrug use are poor prognostic factors. It's *always* worth taking the time to ask every patient about smoking, drinking, and drug use.

> **Loss of judgement and increased impulsivity due to intoxication with drugs or alcohol is important when assessing risk of harm to self or others. A few drinks could be the deciding factor for someone who's been considering suicide...**

REALITY

General approach: tips, tricks, and cautionary tales

1. Don't judge

People who use alcohol or drugs are often treated with disdain or irritation, and judged as 'bad patients' who cause their own problems (interestingly, someone who breaks their leg snowboarding is often treated compassionately). There's no evidence base to support a judgemental approach—it *doesn't* make people change. So, don't:

- Lecture, scold, or blame them for their problems.
- Tell scare stories to 'put them off' using the substance.
- Use offensive labels, e.g. calling them 'alcoholics', 'addicts', or 'junkies'.

If you're condescending, self-righteous, and rude, they won't return, and you'll prevent them accessing help.

2. Motivate without 'trying'

It's an interesting paradox: the harder you try to change someone, the more stubbornly they'll stay the same. So, instead of *trying* to make someone change, surprise them with compassionate acceptance: *respect their right to continue* using drugs or alcohol. It's absolutely their choice, and *not* your responsibility to fix. What a relief! You *don't* have to find the magic words to make them see sense and change the habit of a lifetime.

Instead, concentrate on building rapport and listening empathically: people often talk themselves into change when they don't have to defend themselves against criticism. Ultimately, if someone knows you want the best for them, they'll approach you for help when they're ready.

3. On tact and tarrying

Barking 'Tell me about your drug use!' generally makes people edge away; use a more diplomatic approach. For example, if blood tests show a raised GGT and you suspect heavy drinking, gently bring the conversation round to alcohol, giving someone the *chance* to raise any worries they have themselves, e.g.:

> You: Your blood tests suggest your liver's been under stress recently. Can you think of any reason for that?
>
> Sam: Um ... No ...
>
> You: Well, lots of things affect the liver, including alcohol. Do you ever drink alcohol?
>
> Sam: Yes ... Maybe a bit too much, sometimes ...
>
> You: OK. Can we talk about that first?

On the other hand, if you've been asked to take a substance misuse history (in real life or OSCEs), don't tiptoe around the subject—just get on with it, kindly and without embarrassment:

- I've been asked to find out about your alcohol use—would that be OK?
- I understand you use speed. Can you tell me more about that?

4. Don't bat an eyelid

Don't show shock or disgust at someone's substance misuse—they may close down and minimize their use out of embarrassment. Be unflappable but not cold, e.g. listen curiously as someone describes injecting into their groin, but wince and show concern if they disclose an abscess.

5. Clarify jargon

Drug street slang varies widely, so don't be afraid to clarify terms, and consider using them with the person, e.g.:

> Tracey: Cat valium's awesome!
>
> You: Sorry, what's cat valium?
>
> Tracey: Ketamine.
>
> You: Ah! How much cat valium do you use?

You'll feel silly for demanding a UDS for someone blissed out on Bach Flower Remedies.

6. Don't ignore the signs

If someone's intoxicated, you won't have a useful conversation—agree to talk later. Alternatively, if they're obviously withdrawing, alert staff to their symptoms. This relieves discomfort, and may be life-saving in the case of alcohol or GBL withdrawal.

7. Personal disclosures

Don't divulge your *own* substance misuse to try and gain rapport with patients. It won't help them to know about it, they'll rarely respect you for it, and you'll get into trouble if they tell your colleagues. If you have problems with drugs or alcohol, get some help (see p. 186).

The interview

• = Example question. ∗ = Question linking to other parts of the history. [x] = The substance.

Current use

Type, Route, Amount, Pattern = TRAP.

- *Do you use any drugs or alcohol? Tell me about that ...*
- What do you use? *[Type of drug]*
- How do you use it? *[Route of administration]*
- How much do you use? *[Amount]*
- How often do you use [x]? *[Pattern]*
  - *[If daily]* Talk me through a typical day.
  - *[Not daily/no 'typical' day]* Is there a pattern?
    - When did you last use [x]?
    - Talk me through *that* day (*or the last week/month*).
- *Do you use anything else? [Screen: alcohol, drugs, tobacco, prescription and over-the-counter medications, 'herbal' preparations]*

Daily use suggests dependence. Asking someone to take you through a 'typical day' will often tell you all you need to know about dependence, e.g. nobody *starts* drinking 50 beers a day—this comes through *tolerance*; morning use is often to stop or prevent *withdrawal* symptoms, and may be a time of intense *craving*; using repeatedly in a day suggests *loss of control*.

💡 Try to record alcohol in units and drugs by weight, e.g. grams. Though people may describe use in financial terms, prices vary across the country.

Positives and negatives

People usually have good reasons for substance misuse, at least initially. Being curious about the 'positives' lets the person know you're not judging them:

- *What do you like best about [x]?*

Now you're in a better position to ask about negatives:

- *Is there anything you don't like about [x]?*

This links with dependence (*salience* and *continued use despite harm*).

Diagnosis: harmful or dependent use

Not everything is harmful (e.g. people *can* drink alcohol safely), but continued use despite harm suggests *harmful use* and three or more dependence criteria in the past year suggest *dependent use*. The CAGE questionnaire relates to alcohol and can be accessed via www.patient.co.uk/doctor/cage-questionnaire. Two positive answers suggest a possible drinking problem, and the need for a full alcohol history (don't use CAGE *after* exploring someone's drinking).

Continued use despite harm

- *Has [x] affected your health in any way?*
  * Has [x] caused any physical health problems? *[Screen relevant symptoms, e.g. alcohol: seizures, heartburn, liver problems, accidents]*
  * Has it affected your mental health? *[Screen: mood, psychosis, memory]*
  * Have you ever injected [x]? Ever shared needles?
    – Has that caused any problems? *[Screen: abscess, infection, BBVs, DVT]*

Salience (primacy)

- *Are there things you don't do now because [x] is more important?*
  * How does [x] affect your work/studies/relationships?
  * How would life have been different without [x]?
  * Do you miss out on anything because of [x]?
  * How do friends or relatives view your [x] use?

Tolerance

- *How has your use of [x] changed over time?*
- Do you need to use more than you used to, to get the same effect?

Withdrawal

- *How do you feel before your first [x] of the day?*
- How do you feel if you haven't had [x] for a while?
  – How do you make yourself feel better?

Compulsion to use

- *Do you ever really crave [x]?*
- Does [x] ever feel irresistible, even if you don't really want to use it?

Loss of control

- *Does your use of [x] ever feel out of control?*
- Is it hard to stop using [x] once you've started?
- Could you ever have *just one* [x] in a day?

Past use
Main substance

- *How old were you when you first tried [x]?*
- Were there times you used more than you do now?
- *Have you ever tried to stop using [x]?*
  * What happened? *[Withdrawal/reinstatement after abstinence?]*
  * What was the longest you managed to stop?
  * What helped the most?
  * When you tried [x] again, how quickly did you return to your usual levels? *[Reinstatement after abstinence]*
  * Have you ever overdosed? *[Opioids/sedatives]*
  * Have you ever injected? *[Drugs]*

Other substances

- *What else have you tried in the past?*
  – How old were you? *[Each substance]*
  – Do you still use it now?

Future use
Motivation to change

- *You've said there are lots of things you like about [x], and that it has some drawbacks. What do you think you'll do, longer term?*
- What are you most *worried* about, if you keep using x?
- It can be hard to change... Would you like any help with that?

💡 The Alcohol Use Disorders Identification Test (AUDIT) is a screening tool developed by the World Health Organization. It helps identify alcohol misuse, but can't replace a thorough history.

1. Alcohol history (15 minutes)

Candidate's instructions

John Darwin is a 40-year-old builder whose manager has instructed him to see the GP. You're a medical student at the surgery. Please take an alcohol history.

Patient's brief

Key characteristics
- I didn't drink this morning, but *need* to: I'm shaky, sweaty, restless.
- I'm cooperative, but annoyed about being 'made' to come in.

History

My boss will sack me if I don't deal with my 'drink problem'. He wouldn't even have noticed if he hadn't confused our water bottles—he took a sip of mine and found I wasn't drinking water. I don't operate heavy machinery but he's afraid I'll fall off the scaffolding.

Mum and Dad were both drinkers. She left us when I was little and Dad took his anger out on me, beating me 'til I left home at 15. I stayed with friends and found I'd forget everything with a few beers, but needed to drink *more* to forget as time went on. I was detoxed in hospital 5 years ago, after breaking both arms while drink-driving. I then joined AA and didn't drink again until 2 years ago when I heard Dad had died and the old memories flooded back. I was soon drinking at my old levels.

Each day's the same. I wake feeling shaky and sick each morning until I drink the vodka I keep by my bed. That first drink is like medicine for my body and I've had fits when I've missed it. I get through a bottle of vodka each day (70cl). I take some to work, hidden in a water bottle, but I'm desperate for a drink by the end of the day and always go down the pub after work. I can't stop at one drink, though—it's always 5 or 6 pints (5.2% ABV). I get vodka for the next day on my way home and finish off the rest of the day's supply before bed. There isn't room in my life for anything but drinking and working to pay for my drinking. I've lost my close friends, haven't had a girlfriend in years, and have been banned from most pubs for fighting. I get blackouts so I can't remember most of the fights.

The pub landlady says I drink too much, but it just annoys me—she's got no right to judge me. Why should I feel guilty? My Dad's to blame for my drinking. I don't *want* to cut down, but I know I must to keep my job.

Other history
- I have indigestion. A few days ago I vomited up some blood.
- My GP prescribed antidepressants for depression 6 months ago but they made me feel sick so I stopped them.
- I take indigestion and vitamin tablets.
- I smoke 40 cigarettes a day. I've never tried other drugs.
- I feel depressed and don't enjoy anything anymore. I'm tired and feel like I'm dragging myself about at work. I'm not suicidal but feel hopeless.
- I no longer drive.

Questions
Can I get a detox?

Worries
I'll lose my job/The blood I vomited could be a sign of cancer.

💡 John is alcohol dependent, and drinking around 45 units a day (more than triple the 'safe' *weekly* allowance). He *mustn't* suddenly stop drinking (risks seizures and DTs) but shouldn't be working on scaffolding (time off or less risky work would be helpful). John needs a physical health review (oesophageal varices/peptic ulcer/Mallory–Weiss tear) and referral to the local Addictions Service. They can assess his motivation to change and organize for a detox, probably as an inpatient, given his history of seizures and living alone. Longer-term rehabilitation will be essential.

2. Opioid history (15 minutes)

Candidate's instructions
Elaine Smith is 23 and uses heroin. She was admitted with a groin abscess. She's preoperative and wants a doctor to prescribe methadone, but the surgical team is in theatre. You're a medical student on the team. The registrar has asked you to take a substance use history so that she can address the situation quickly, once out of theatre.

Patient's brief

Key characteristics
- I'm tense and irritable, but can be calmed down and will then talk openly.
- I just want methadone, the operation, and to get home.
- I'm not currently in much pain from the abscess.

History
I first smoked smack (heroin) at 17. I'd got a modelling contract and drugs were everywhere. Smack made me happier and calmer than I'd ever felt, but after a while I couldn't get the hit I wanted, no matter how much I smoked. My boyfriend, Mark, helped me inject: the high was *amazing*, like falling in love. I just wanted that hit again, but it quickly stopped being about the high and became more about stopping the withdrawal. You feel sick and shivery, like you've got 'flu—then there's diarrhoea, vomiting, goosebumps, and cramps.

I spend £60 on 1.5g of smack every day. I inject three times a day to feel normal, and use sleepers to get through the night (3×10mg diazepam). I've used up my arms (veins) and inject in my groin. Heroin's the most important thing in my life and I've done stuff I'm not proud of to get it . . . (After I lost my modelling contract, Mark pimped me out. He takes the cash and pays me in smack. It doesn't sound fair, but he looks out for me. Sometimes I steal stuff to sell, but I haven't been caught.)

I know it's wrecked my life. I've lost my family and friends; I had a leg blood clot last year and I've accidentally overdosed twice. I've shared needles when desperate and got Hep B. Smack controls me now—I lost control of *it* years ago. I detoxed 2 years ago, but Mark wouldn't give up and tempted me back. I went to the addictions team a couple of times for methadone, but they wanted meetings and urine samples and it was just easier to carry on. I want a detox, just not *yet*.

Other history
- I've tried most things (E, coke, crack, weed, speed) but smack and sleepers are all I use now. I don't drink, but smoke 20 fags a day.
- Mum was a drinker. My childhood was great until I was 12, when she got a new boyfriend. He was horrible—that's all I'm saying.
- I'm not depressed or suicidal, but I OD'd with paracetamol a few years ago.
- I use inhalers for asthma.

Questions
Can I have methadone now? When will I see the doctor?

Worries
I won't make it through the night without methadone.

💡 Don't promise Elaine methadone. The team needs to make this decision, having seen clear evidence of withdrawal symptoms, a positive UDS, and spoken with liaison psychiatry and the anaesthetist. If she *hasn't* recently used heroin, methadone could kill her. Meanwhile, symptomatic treatment can make her more comfortable, e.g. loperamide, metoclopramide, paracetamol.

NEXT STEPS

Aggression: 72 hours after a road traffic accident

You're an orthopaedic FY1. The ward manager calls, requesting help with Terry Harrison. He's 28 and was admitted 3 days ago after crashing his car while drunk; he required open reduction internal fixation of bilateral femoral fractures. Terry seems confused today and is shouting aggressively and waving his crutches.

- What's the differential diagnosis?
- How will you assess and manage Terry?

Differential diagnosis

- Alcohol related: intoxication, withdrawal, DTs, Wernicke's encephalopathy.
- Other causes of confusion: delirium (e.g. postoperative sepsis), missed head injury.
- Shouting and distress: psychosis, personality disorder, extreme pain, communication difficulties.

Preparation

On the phone, advise the ward manager to contact security and safeguard other patients and staff. Say how soon you'll attend.

Assessment

On arrival, don't immediately prescribe sedatives—assessment will be much harder if you've knocked Terry out. Talk to staff and quickly review his notes for evidence of substance misuse, a past psychiatric history, or head injury (e.g. lowered Glasgow Coma Scale score on admission). Clues to heavy alcohol use include the drink-driving history, examination findings (e.g. ascites), and blood results (macrocytosis, raised GGT/LFTs). Check whether he's shown withdrawal symptoms (e.g. CIWA scale) or received any benzodiazepines or thiamine. If withdrawing, he's at risk of seizures; agitation could represent *post*-ictal confusion.

Assess Terry with security staff present if needed. Using de-escalation techniques to defuse the situation (see p. 18), find out what's upsetting Terry, and whether you can negotiate with him or meet his needs (e.g. analgesia). Then:

- Observe for signs of alcohol withdrawal (e.g. sweating, tremor), DTs (clouding of consciousness, hallucinations) or Wernicke's encephalopathy (confusion, ataxia, ophthalmoplegia).
- Assess orientation and attention.
- Examine him for other causes of confusion, e.g. postoperative infection, focal neurology.

Management

Investigate and treat causes of delirium as quickly as possible, e.g. CT head, antibiotics for sepsis. Treat alcohol withdrawal and DTs with benzodiazepines and parenteral thiamine. Have a low threshold for suspecting Wernicke's encephalopathy: the classic triad (confusion, ataxia, and ophthalmoplegia) is *rare*, so even *one* of these symptoms should make you consider parenteral thiamine. Discuss doses and duration with the liaison psychiatrist or medical registrar.

Liaison psychiatry may advise as-needed benzodiazepines as rapid tranquillization for agitation, or an antipsychotic for problematic psychotic symptoms (low dose and titrated up slowly, as this can lower the seizure threshold).

Terry should be nursed one-to-one in a well-lit side room, with security present as necessary. He will remain in hospital, receiving immediate urgent treatment under the MCA if he lacks capacity. If he resists or refuses treatment, liaison psychiatry may organize a MHA assessment.

> 💡 **Once the situation's under control there's an opportunity for psychoeducation: for Terry to address his alcohol use and for the admitting doctor to address their reluctance to prescribe a detox for someone with clear alcohol problems. This situation can be avoided in the majority of cases.**

Movie buff

A Scanner Darkly (2006).
Breaking Bad (TV, 2008–2013): a chemistry teacher starts manufacturing methamphetamine after a terminal diagnosis.
Drugstore Cowboy (1989).
Human Traffic (1999).
Long Day's Journey into Night (1962).
Pure (2002).
Requiem for a Dream (2000).
T2 Trainspotting (2017).
The Basketball Diaries (1995).
The Wolf of Wall Street (2013).
Trainspotting (1996).
Walk the Line (2005).
Withnail & I (1987).

Book shelf

Burroughs, A. (2004) *Dry*: second in his memoir trilogy, Dry relates Burrough's real-life battle with alcohol dependence, as a young advertising executive.

Doyle, R. (1998) *The Woman Who Walked Into Doors*: Roddy Doyle's brutal text explores domestic violence, depression, and alcohol dependence. Acutely realistic, it ultimately champions survival beneath its bleak narrative.

Welsh, I. (1999) *Trainspotting*: this cult classic examines the bleak reality of heroin and other addictions.

Wurtzel, E. (2003) *More, Now, Again*: following up *Prozac Nation* (on the rise of depression diagnoses and lifestyle use of Fluoxetine), Wurtzel descends into cocaine and methylphenidate abuse, before documenting her recovery.

Footlights

Macmillan, D. (2015) *People, Places and Things* (Oberon Modern Plays). Actress Emma's inpatient detox and rehabilitation showcases the fine line between staff, patients, and carers; the roles of family, trauma, and coping in addiction; and facing up to reality sober.

O'Neill, E. (1991 edition) *Long Day's Journey into Night* (Nick Hern Books). In this autobiographical tale, Mary Tyrone's return from the sanatorium for treatment of morphine addiction is mirrored in her children's alcohol misuse, and husband's financial control.

Notes

1. Jackson, C. (1994) *The Lost Weekend*. New York: Syracuse University Press.
2. Prochaska, J.O., DiClemente, C.C. (1982) Transtheoretical therapy: toward a more integrative model of change. *Psychotherapy: Theory, Research & Practice*, **19**(3), 276–88.

Journal club

Tracy, D.K., Wood, D.M., Baumeister, D. (2017) Novel psychoactive substances: types, mechanisms of action, and effects. *BMJ*, **356**, i6848.

Williams, A.V., Marsden, J., Strang, J. (2014) Training family members to manage heroin overdose and administer naloxone: randomized trial of effects on knowledge and attitudes. *Addiction*, **109**, 250–9.

Resources

www.drinkaware.co.uk
www.talktofrank.com
www.tictac.org.uk

Go to www.oup.com/uk/stringer2e for a wealth of additional resources, including an OCSE mark scheme, filmed scenarios, and self-assessment questions.

12 Organic Psychiatry

True or false?

Answers on p. 277

1. Left frontal lobe lesions cause expressive dysphasia in right-handed people.
2. Pick disease is characterized by rounded collections of hyper-phosphorylated tau protein.
3. Normal pressure hydrocephalus is the triad of dementia, tremor, and urinary incontinence.
4. Sporadic Creutzfeldt–Jakob disease (CJD) has earlier onset and more prominent psychiatric symptoms than variant CJD.
5. Half of people with epilepsy develop depression.
6. Verbal fluency indicates temporal lobe function.
7. Doctors inform licensing authorities whenever patients are medically unfit to drive.
8. Tumours may cause autoimmune encephalitis.
9. Amnestic disorders are characterized by profound retrograde amnesia.
10. Risk of delirium is increased in people with dementia.

Contents

Principles
Introduction
Neuroanatomy
Delirium (acute confusional state)
- Aetiology
- Clinical presentation
- Investigations
- Management
- Prognosis

Dementia
- Frontotemporal dementia (FTD)
- Huntington disease (HD)
- HIV-associated neurocognitive disorder (HAND)
- Normal pressure hydrocephalus (NPH)
- Transmissible spongiform encephalopathies (TSEs)

Amnestic disorder
- Pathology
- Clinical presentation
- Treatment

Transient global amnesia
Frontal lobe syndrome
Traumatic brain injury
- Clinical presentation
- Psychiatric sequelae
- Management

Parkinson disease
- Pathology
- Clinical presentation
- Psychiatric sequelae

Multiple sclerosis
- Psychiatric sequelae

Stroke (cerebrovascular accident)
- Psychiatric sequelae

Epilepsy
- Psychiatric sequelae

Autoimmune encephalitis
Miscellaneous systemic illnesses

Reality
General approach: tips, tricks, and cautionary tales
- Assess cognition
- Frontal lobe testing

Next steps
MS and fitness to drive
- Differential diagnosis
- Management
- Driving

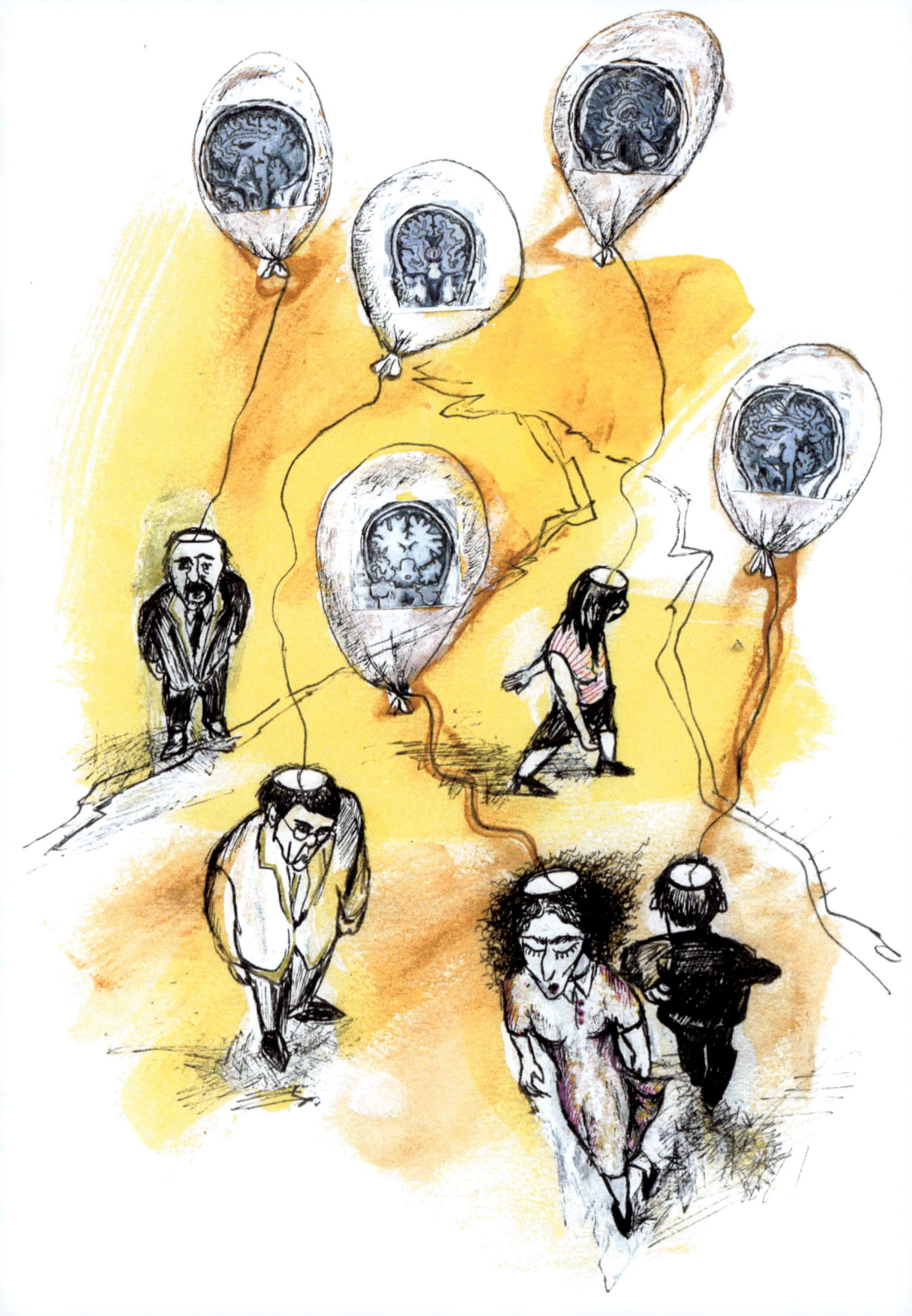

PRINCIPLES

I had amnesia . . . I didn't have a surname, or parents with faces, or even a good idea of my age. And now the means to end that uncertainty was in my hands. The papers in the briefcase would tell me what I had been doing and thinking about in the very last hour before the attack. At the very least, they would reveal my profession, and I felt sure that from that basic piece of information, the remaining secrets of my history would fall quite naturally into place.

Alex Garland, *The Coma*[1]

Introduction

Organic psychiatric disorders are directly caused by demonstrable physical illnesses or structural problems of the brain, e.g. space-occupying lesions, hyperthyroidism. By contrast, *functional* psychiatric disorders lack a clear physical cause (e.g. schizophrenia). Liaison and neuropsychiatry (**Box 12.1**) grapple with the interface between mind and body, making them compelling subspecialties.

Neuroanatomy

Knowing the roles of different parts of the brain gives you clues to the areas affected by local disease or damage. More generalized involvement produces a wide variety of symptoms (e.g. delirium) due to 'whole-brain' effects. Although a simplification, **Figure 12.1** and **Table 12.1** should nudge your neocortex to recall some basic neuroanatomy.

Delirium (acute confusional state)

Delirium is acute and transient confusion due to an underlying physical problem. It affects up to:

- 30% of medical inpatients.
- 50% of postoperative patients.
- 80% of people admitted to intensive care.

Risk factors include older age, male sex, pre-existing physical/mental illness (especially dementia), substance misuse, polypharmacy (multiple medications), malnutrition, pain, sensory impairment, and immobility. See **Table 12.2** for a comparison of delirium with dementia.

Aetiology

Delirium is caused by physical illness—when you see it, seek the underlying organic problem (often multifactorial). *Causes* include (mnemonic: VITTAMIN):

- *Vascular*, e.g. stroke, heart attack.
- *Infectious*, e.g. urinary tract/chest infection, encephalitis, sepsis.
- *Traumatic*, e.g. head injury, burns, fractures.
- *Toxic*, e.g. drug or alcohol intoxication/withdrawal, poisoning, overdose.
- *Autoimmune*, e.g. systemic lupus erythematosus, multiple sclerosis (MS).
- *Metabolic*, e.g. liver/renal failure, electrolyte imbalance, hypoglycaemia.
- *Iatrogenic*: 'deliriogenic' medications, e.g. sedatives, anticholinergics, opiates, steroids.
- *Neoplastic*, e.g. space-occupying lesion.

BOX 12.1 Liaison psychiatry and neuropsychiatry

People with organic psychiatric disorders present to all medical specialties. Liaison and neuropsychiatrists have specific skills to assist in their diagnosis and management and play key roles in managing often distressing behavioural, cognitive, and psychiatric symptoms of these disorders.

Management includes both treating the organic disorder itself where possible, and providing tailored treatment for the psychiatric symptoms. Neuropsychiatrists, for example, may advise neurologists on the safest antipsychotics in epilepsy, suggest medical or psychological factors influencing seizure frequency, and recommend non-pharmacological management strategies for staff and carers. Organic disorders can profoundly affect a person's behaviour and personality, so families often need support, education, and advice.

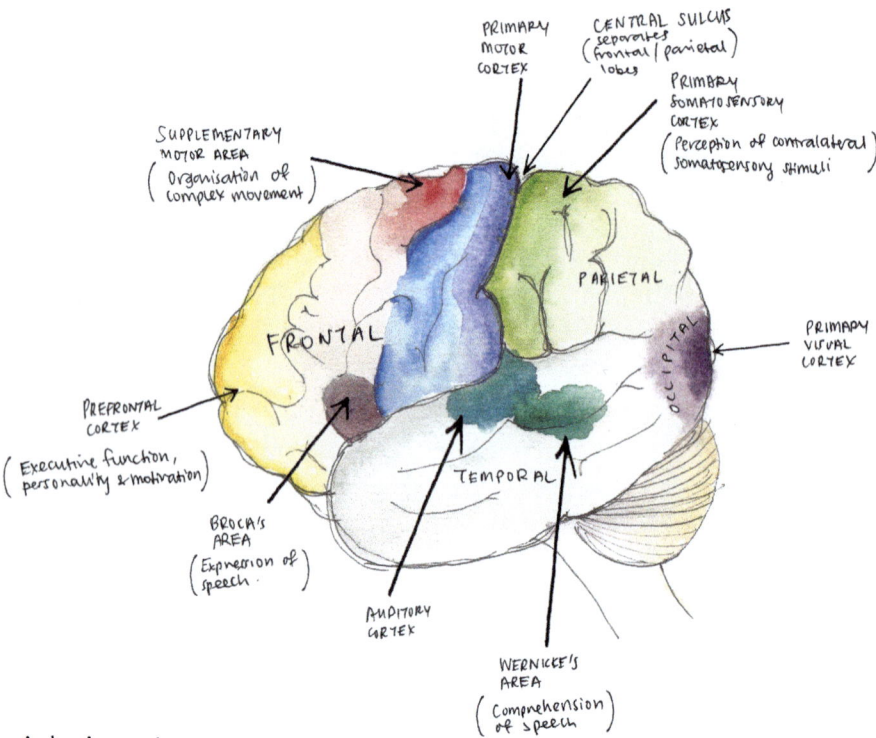

FIGURE 12.1 Basic brain anatomy.

Even seemingly minor problems can tip vulnerable people into delirium, e.g. constipation, pain.

💡 *Any* change in an older person's mental state should make you consider delirium.

Clinical presentation

See **Box 12.2**. Onset is *sudden* (hours to days), and symptoms *fluctuate*, with brief, lucid moments when the person seems fine; it's often worse at night. *Altered consciousness* ranges from drowsiness or stupor to *clouded consciousness* ('fogginess', inability to focus) to vigilance or hyper-alertness.

Global cognitive impairment includes *inattention*, disorientation, and poor memory. *Thinking* may be *disorganized* (illogical/rambling) or impoverished. Being delirious is usually extremely frightening, but mood changes can also resemble depression or mania. People can experience transient, often persecutory delusions, illusions, and hallucinations (most commonly visual). Insomnia or a reversed sleep–wake cycle are both common. You may hear people talking about patients being 'CAM positive',[2] meaning that they probably have delirium from bedside testing (www.hospitalelderlifeprogram.org/uploads/disclaimers/Short_CAM_Training_Manual_8-29-14.pdf).

Delirium can be:

- **Hyperactive**—hyper-alert and agitated, e.g. wandering, screaming, pulling out catheters.

- **Hypoactive**—drowsy, lethargic, withdrawn. This '*quiet delirium*' is easily missed in busy wards or care homes: sufferers may simply seem peaceful or undemanding.

- **Mixed**—fluctuating between the two (commonest).

💡 Recent confusion *never* diagnoses dementia!

Investigations

- **Full physical examination and observations** (BP, HR, RR, SpO_2, temperature). Include digital rectal examination if there's a history of constipation.

- **Mental state examination**: differential diagnoses for delirium include depression (if hypoactive), mania (if hyperactive), and negative symptoms of schizophrenia.

- **Medication chart review**: recent changes, deliriogenic medications.

- **Cognitive assessment** (see p. 144): delirium is commoner in people with dementia.

- **Collateral history**, especially, whether the person is *usually* forgetful.

- **Essential blood tests:**
  - *FBC*—infection/anaemia/haematological malignancy.
  - *U&Es*—electrolyte disturbance, especially hyponatraemia, acute or chronic kidney injury.

Table 12.1 Lobes, functions, and lesions

Region	Functions	Symptoms of dysfunction
Frontal lobe		
Prefrontal cortex	'Executive' function Social behaviour and personality	*Frontal lobe syndrome* (p. 137): • Executive *dysfunction*, i.e. *impaired*: attention, judgement, planning • Socially inappropriate behaviour, personality change
Broca's area (dominant hemisphere)	Language production	*Expressive dysphasia* (difficulty *producing* language): *telegraphic speech*, with short words and sentences, e.g. 'Want cake' for 'I want some cake'. Comprehension largely intact
Motor, premotor, and supplementary motor cortex	Contralateral motor function Suppression of 'primitive' reflexes	*Contralateral spasticity, hemiparesis, gait disturbance, apraxia* *Frontal release signs* (reflexes from early infancy re-emerge), e.g. sucking, 'rooting' (p. 147)
Temporal lobe		
General	Auditory, olfactory, gustatory perception	*Auditory impairment/agnosia.* *Auditory, olfactory, gustatory hallucinations* (e.g. in temporal lobe epilepsy)
	Memory	*Amnestic disorder* (p. 136): profound anterograde amnesia (can't form new memories)
	Emotional regulation	*Lability*
Wernicke's area (dominant hemisphere)	Language comprehension	*Receptive dysphasia* (difficulty *understanding* language). Fluent but nonsensical speech, with mistakes, additional sounds, words, and neologisms, e.g. 'I filly iver want a gar some cakes'
Parietal lobe	Somatosensory perception Integration of sensory perception, for bodily attention Calculation	*Contralateral sensory impairment* *Apraxia*: difficulty performing skilled tasks (e.g. drawing, dressing) despite normal sensory and motor function *Agnosia*: difficulty recognizing stimuli, despite normal sensation, e.g. objects by touch or sight *Contralateral neglect*: inattention to one side of the perceptual field, despite normal sensation *Dyscalculia*: problems understanding and using numbers
Occipital lobe	Visual perception and interpretation	*Contralateral visual defects* *Visual agnosia* *Cortical blindness*: loss of vision despite normal eyesight
Arcuate fasciculus (dominant hemisphere)	Communication between Broca's and Wernicke's areas	*Conduction (associative) dysphasia*: intact comprehension, but impaired repetition of speech

NB: language production and comprehension occur in the 'dominant' side of the brain: *l*anguage is on the *l*eft in right-handed people *and* most left-handed people.

Table 12.2 Comparison: delirium versus dementia

Feature	Delirium	Dementia
Onset	Sudden (hours–days)	Gradual (weeks–months) *Exception: large ('strategic') stroke in vascular dementia*
Course	Fluctuant	Slowly progressive *Exceptions:* • *Stepwise decline in vascular dementia* • *Fluctuating presentation in dementia due to Lewy body disease (DLB)*
Duration	Short (days–weeks) <6 months (ICD-10)	Lifelong >6 months (ICD-10)
Consciousness	Impaired	Unaffected
Attention	Impaired	Unaffected
Thinking	Disorganized (hyperactive delirium) Impoverished (hypoactive delirium)	Impoverished
Delusions	Common, simplistic, changeable	Sometimes (later in illness), systematized
Hallucinations	Common (as are illusions)	Sometimes (later in illness) *Exception: visual hallucinations are a central feature of DLB*
Prognosis	Recovery, once underlying cause resolves (though may leave residual deficits)	Deterioration

---

BOX 12.2 Delirium: example mental state examination (MSE)

- *Appearance and behaviour*: agitated, elderly woman, wearing a hospital gown, smelling of urine. Frightened expression. Plucking at cubicle curtains, and brandishing her walking stick.
- *Speech*: incoherent mumbling/shouting.
- *Mood*: (subjective) unable to comment; (objective) frightened, irritable.
- *Thought*: persecutory delusions ('They've stolen my handbag!').
- *Perception*: visual hallucinations (insects) and illusions (misidentifying curtains as ghosts).
- *Cognition*: can't engage in formal assessment. Disorientated to time, place, and person. Poor attention and concentration. Unable to retain information, e.g. current location.
- *Insight*: doesn't believe she's unwell. Refusing interventions.

- *LFTs*—liver damage (e.g. hepatic encephalopathy); abnormalities may suggest alcohol misuse (risk factor for falls, subdural haematomas, alcohol-related dementia, and Korsakoff syndrome, p. 136).
- *TFTs*—hypothyroidism can mimic dementia.
- *CBG*—hypoglycaemia and hyperglycaemia cause confusion.
- *Vitamin B_{12}, folate*—deficiencies can cause reversible cognitive impairment.
- *Bone profile*—calcium abnormalities in parathyroid and other disorders can affect cognition.
- *HIV and syphilis serology*—HIV and neurosyphilis can cause cognitive impairment.
• **Additional tests as clinically indicated (not exhaustive!):**
- *Septic screen*: MSU (exclude UTI); CXR, blood cultures, wound swabs, sputum/stool samples as suggested by symptoms.
- *Neurological investigations*, e.g. CT/MRI head, anti-NMDA and voltage-gated potassium channel (VGKC) antibodies, lumbar puncture, EEG.
- *Substance use*: breathalyser, UDS.

Management

1. **Treat the cause and exacerbating factors**, e.g. dehydration, pain, constipation. Stop unnecessary medications. Optimize nutrition and ensure any dentures fit.
2. **Behavioural management:**
   - Address sensory problems, e.g. hearing aids, spectacles.
   - Frequently reorientate, e.g. clocks, calendars, verbal reminders, photos.
   - Good lighting: gloomy conditions worsen hallucinations and illusions. Ensure sufficient night-time lighting to see where they are, without keeping them awake.
   - Sleep hygiene (see p. 44).
   - Avoid over- *or* under-stimulation. If the ward is noisy, a side room may help, but isolation can worsen disorientation.
   - Minimize change:
     - Avoid unnecessary moves.
     - One nurse to engage the person each shift.
     - Establish routines, including toileting.
     - Remove items which can be thrown or tripped over.
     - Silence unnecessary noises, e.g. alarms.
     - Encourage visits from family and friends.
     - Allow safe or supervised wandering: restraint increases accidents.
3. **Medication** can increase confusion and risk of falls. If agitated behaviour is risky (e.g. aggression), or there's extreme distress, *consider* short-term, low-dose medication, e.g. antipsychotic (haloperidol or olanzapine) or a benzodiazepine if antipsychotics are contraindicated.
4. **Consider referral** to a geriatrician or old age psychiatrist, to manage ongoing physical or psychiatric problems once delirium has resolved. Remember, people who suffer delirium are at increased risk of subsequent dementia.

💡 The best teams *prevent* delirium by proactively optimizing physical health and routinely using behavioural management in vulnerable adults. About 30–40% of deliriums are preventable.

Prognosis

Delirium is associated with increased mortality, longer and repeated admissions, and subsequent nursing home placement. It may take days, weeks, or even months to completely resolve after treating the underlying cause. Some people never fully recover, often because chronic physical and mental health comorbidities limit full recovery. This change in loved ones is frightening, so it's important to take time to explain symptoms and prognostic uncertainty.

💡 The brain is like a jelly being 'poked' by a physical problem; delirium is the resultant 'wobble'. When the poking stops, the jelly wobbles for a while afterwards: don't expect delirium to resolve as soon as the physical cause is treated.

Dementia

Chapter 13 covers dementia management, Alzheimer disease (AD), vascular dementia (VD), and dementia due to Lewy body disease (DLB). Here, we review some *rarer* causes of dementia arising in younger people (under 65s). See **Box 12.3**.

💡 These dementias are particularly tragic: imagine receiving a dementia diagnosis in your forties, knowing your personality may change, and you'll lose the ability to work and look after yourself and your family.

Frontotemporal dementia (FTD)

FTD is most commonly diagnosed in 45- to 65-year-olds. Most cases are 'sporadic' (no known cause) but around a third are familial, showing autosomal dominance inheritance. Key mutations affect three genes: those coding for microtubule-associated protein tau and progranulin, and a gene on chromosome 9.

Pathology

The hallmarks of FTD are asymmetrical anterior temporal and/or frontal lobe atrophy: cortical atrophy, neuronal loss, and gliosis are characteristic. There's no clear correlation between pathological severity and clinical symptoms.

BOX 12.3 Cortical versus subcortical dementia

The cortex (grey matter) is the outermost brain area, made of neuronal cell bodies. The subcortex (white matter) is deeper, formed from neuronal axons, and includes structures such as the basal ganglia and thalamus. Although features overlap, dementias are sometimes subdivided into:

- *Cortical*, e.g. AD, frontotemporal dementia:
  - Symptoms affect cortical functions, e.g. memory, language.
- *Subcortical*, e.g. dementias due to PD or HD:
  - Symptoms include *bradyphrenia* (mental slowing), depression, bradykinesia, other movement disorders, and executive dysfunction (due to connections between the basal ganglia and frontal lobes).

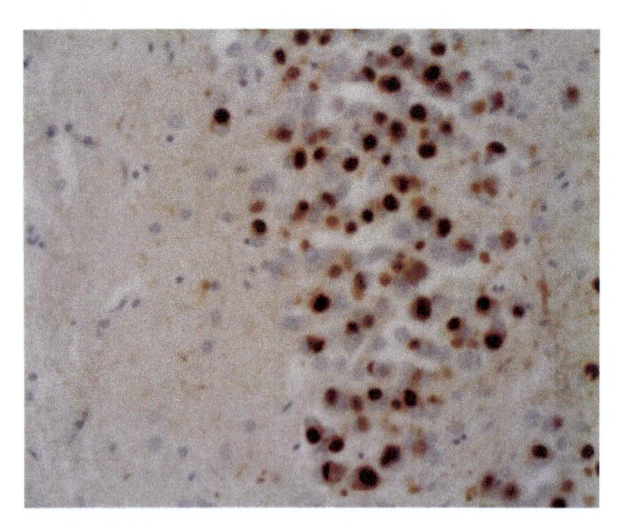

FIGURE 12.2 Pick bodies stained with anti-tau antibodies.

By kind permission of Dr Andrew King

Pick disease is a type of FTD. Biopsy shows characteristic 'Pick bodies' (collections of hyper-phosphorylated tau protein; **Figure 12.2**) and 'Pick cells' (ballooned neurons).

Clinical presentation

Initially, there are two main FTD subtypes:

- *Behavioural variant FTD*: prominent disinhibition and personality change (frontal lobe syndrome (FLS), p. 137).
- *Primary progressive aphasia:* worsening speech and language problems.

These often overlap, particularly later on, when memory problems emerge. Executive dysfunction, binge eating, and other compulsive behaviours can affect all sufferers. Death is usually within 5–10 years.

Huntington disease (HD)

HD is an autosomal dominant disease, causing dementia and chorea (rapid, 'dancing' movements). Its causative mutation is a trinucleotide cytosine–adenine–guanine (CAG) repeat in the huntingtin gene on chromosome 4. The longer the CAG repeat, the earlier and more severe the presentation. Though onset is usually in early middle age, each inheritance lengthens the repeat, causing earlier onset with each generation (*anticipation*).

Pathology

The caudate, putamen, and deep cortex show neuronal loss, gliosis, and deposits of abnormal huntingtin protein. Neuroimaging sometimes shows caudate atrophy with lateral ventricle dilatation (**Figure 12.3**). The EEG may be flat.

Clinical presentation

Personality and behavioural changes include depression, euphoria, irritability, and aggression; subcortical dementia emerges later (**Box 12.3**). Chorea affects the person's limbs, trunk, face, and speech muscles, and produces a wide-based, lurching gait.

Though gene therapy trials show promise, there's currently no cure. Relatives may want genetic testing

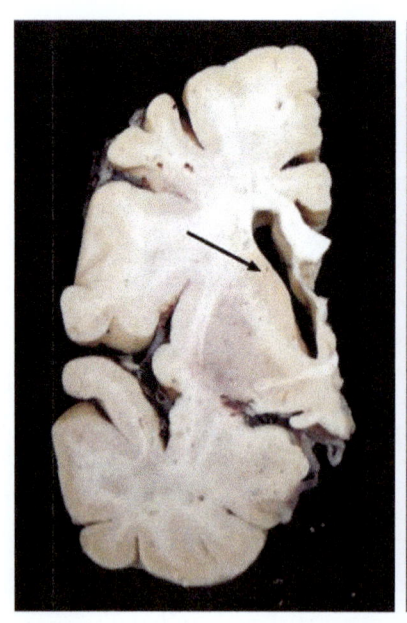

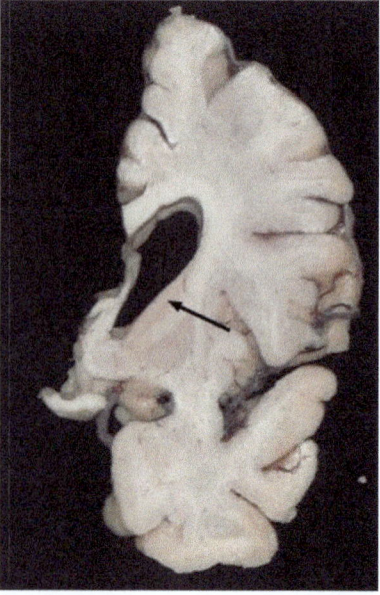

FIGURE 12.3 Coronal slices from cerebral hemispheres: healthy control (left) and HD (right). The caudate nucleus (arrows) is flattened in HD.

By kind permission of Dr Andrew King

to see if they carry the mutation. Death is usually from an intercurrent illness (e.g. pneumonia), but *suicide* is the second commonest cause of death.

💡 Chorea may be due to a relative dopamine excess in the atrophied basal ganglia, and as such, can be thought of as the 'opposite' of parkinsonism. Antipsychotics or tetrabenazine may help.

HIV-associated neurocognitive disorder (HAND)

HAND encompasses a range of neurocognitive disorders caused by HIV infection of the CNS. The risk of developing HAND increases with age, cardiovascular risk factors, hepatitis C infection, and substance use disorder (e.g. methamphetamine).

Clinical presentation

- *Asymptomatic cognitive impairment (ACI)*: although the person doesn't notice problems, formal testing shows mild cognitive deficits. Affects 30% of people taking antiretrovirals.
- *Mild neurocognitive disorder (MND):* objective cognitive deficits are accompanied by noticeable problems with memory, concentration, executive function, processing speed, and sometimes motor difficulties (e.g. bradykinesia). Affects 20–30% of people taking antiretrovirals.
- *HIV-associated dementia (HAD;* also known as *AIDS dementia complex (ADC)* or *HIV encephalopathy)*: may occur after progression from HIV to AIDS. Early apathy and withdrawal progress to subcortical dementia, with neurological symptoms, e.g. ataxia, tremor, seizures, myoclonus. MRI may show generalized atrophy and diffuse white matter changes. Affects 2–8% of people taking antiretrovirals.

💡 Depression, suicidal thoughts, anxiety, mania, and psychosis are all increased in HIV, *and* can be triggered by some antiretrovirals, e.g. efavirenz (depression, suicidal thoughts).

Normal pressure hydrocephalus (NPH)

NPH is a potentially reversible cause of dementia, usually affecting older adults. Up to 50% of cases are idiopathic, but known causes include head injury, subarachnoid haemorrhage, meningitis, and tumours. CSF absorption in the subarachnoid space is obstructed, leading to ventricular CSF accumulation (hydrocephalus) but *without* raised intracranial pressure (**Figure 12.4**); the mechanism remains poorly understood. Distorted periventricular white matter tracts produce a classic symptom triad:

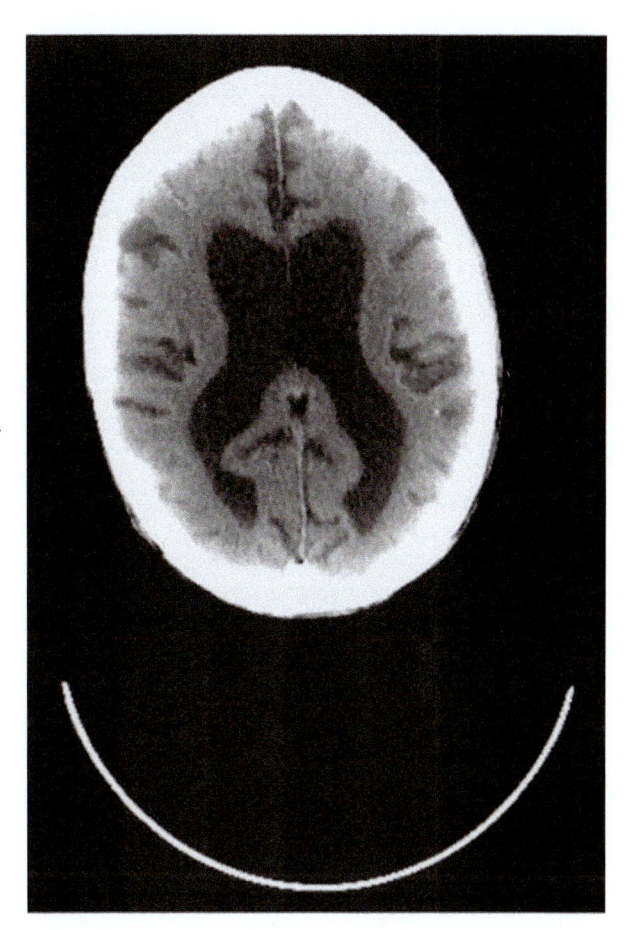

FIGURE 12.4 NPH: CT shows dilated ventricles, disproportionate to the degree of involutional changes or cortical atrophy.
By kind permission of Dr Mona Sriharan

- Dementia (subcortical).
- Unsteady gait.
- Urinary incontinence.

Treatment involves surgically placing a shunt to drain CSF from the ventricles to an area where the body absorbs it, e.g. peritoneum, atrium.

Transmissible spongiform encephalopathies (TSEs)

Cell membranes contain normal prion protein (PrP^c). If this changes into a misfolded, insoluble form (PrP^{Sc}), it causes TSEs, or *prion diseases*. A domino effect occurs as PrP^{Sc} turns other PrP^c into PrP^{Sc}. Animal prion diseases include *scrapie* in sheep and *bovine spongiform encephalopathy* (BSE) in cattle. The main TSE in humans is *Creutzfeldt–Jakob disease* (CJD); the commonest type is *sporadic* CJD (sCJD), due to spontaneous PrP^c misfolding. *Variant* CJD (vCJD) results, rarely, from eating BSE-infected beef (**Table 12.3**). CJD can also be *iatrogenic* (e.g. following blood transfusion) or *familial*.

Table 12.3 Comparison of sporadic (sCJD) and variant CJD (vCJD)

	sCJD	vCJD
Trigger	Unknown	Eating BSE-infected beef
Onset	Older: 40–60 years	Younger: mostly in twenties
Presentation	Neurological signs: extrapyramidal, pyramidal, cerebellar, myoclonus Dementia	Psychiatric symptoms: dementia, depression, irritability, psychosis, behavioural changes Ataxia, myoclonus, and sensory symptoms
EEG	Typically, triphasic sharp wave complexes	No specific findings
MRI	Normal, atrophy or high signal in *anterior* basal ganglia	'Pulvinar' sign: high bilateral signal in *posterior thalamus*
CSF	Raised 14-3-3, tau, S100, NSE proteins; positive RT-QuIC test	No specific findings
Biopsy	Not recommended unless alternative differential likely	'Daisy' or 'florid plaques' (**Figure 12.5**) Tonsil biopsy shows PrP^{Sc}
Prognosis (once symptomatic)	Death within 1 year, usually from heart/respiratory failure, or pneumonia	Death within 12–14 months

All types cause prion accumulation, leading to spongiform and amyloid changes in the cerebrum, basal ganglia, and cerebellum (**Figure 12.5**).

After up to 20 years' incubation, a rapidly progressive and fatal illness is marked by dementia, motor abnormalities (e.g. ataxia), and myoclonus (**Table 12.3**).

Prions are extremely resistant to disinfectants, heat, formalin, and ultraviolet and ionizing radiation, so transmission risks must be considered before *exposure-prone procedures*, e.g. diagnostic brain and tonsil biopsies. Additionally, brain biopsy risks lasting damage, so is only used when there's diagnostic uncertainty.

Amnestic disorder

Amnestic disorder is characterized by relatively circumscribed and *profound anterograde amnesia*—the inability to lay down new memories from the brain insult, onwards.

Pathology

Amnestic disorders are caused by damage to limbic structures dealing with *explicit memory* (**Box 12.4**): the hippocampus, mammillary bodies, parts of the thalamus, and surrounding cortex. As *implicit memory* is handled by a separate system (involving the basal ganglia and cerebellum), people with amnestic disorders usually have normal procedural memory and can even learn new skills.

Causes include trauma (e.g. brain injury), infection (e.g. herpes simplex encephalitis), tumours, carbon monoxide poisoning, and hypoxia. The commonest amnestic disorder is that due to *Korsakoff syndrome* (KS), caused by thiamine (vitamin B$_1$) deficiency, usually secondary to chronic alcohol misuse, or sometimes anorexia nervosa.

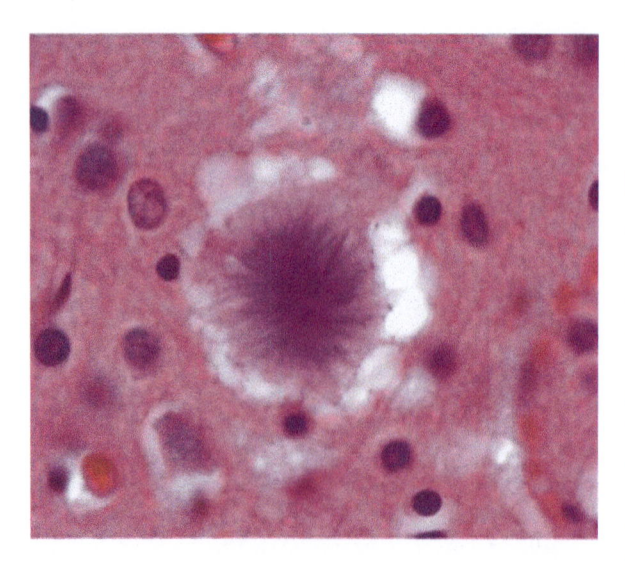

FIGURE 12.5 vCJD is characterized by *florid plaques* ('daisy plaques'): abnormal proteins surrounded by vacuoles in rounded deposits.
By kind permission of Dr Andrew King

> **BOX 12.4 Memory**
>
> Memory can be classified by duration or content.
>
> **Duration**
>
> - *Working memory (immediate memory/registration)*: briefly holding information in its original state. It's fleeting (while attending to the information) and limited (classically to 7 ± 2 items), e.g. checking lottery numbers.
> - *Short-term memory* processes initially consolidate new information by turning it into 'memorable' constructs, e.g. symbols, words.
> - *Long-term memory*: rehearsal consolidates important memories for retrieval, even years later.
>
> **Content**
>
> - *Explicit (declarative) memory*: memories that can be put into words. It's divided into *episodic* (autobiographical) and *semantic* (general knowledge) memory.
> - *Implicit (non-declarative) memory*: memories that are hard to verbalize, and are learned and accessed unconsciously. The main type is *procedural memory*: knowing *how*, e.g. to ride a bike.

Clinical presentation

See **Box 12.5**. No new explicit memories are laid down. Working memory is intact, but information is lost once it's no longer being actively used. Some people *confabulate*, describing things they 'remember' but which never happened; they're not deliberately lying, but trying to make sense of confusing memory gaps, using any memories that come to mind. There may be some retrograde amnesia (loss of memories *before* the damage), but other brain functions are relatively intact (unlike in delirium or dementia).

Treatment

Amnestic disorders are very disabling, and people often need intensive residential support. Prompt parenteral thiamine may prevent *Wernicke encephalopathy* (see p. 108: acute confusion, ataxia, and ophthalmoplegia) from developing into KS. Once KS is established, thiamine may prevent further progression, but can't reverse damage.

Transient global amnesia

Like amnestic disorders, people with transient global amnesia (TGA) suffer abrupt-onset anterograde amnesia, but it lasts less than 24 (usually 1–8) hours. They're usually aged over 40 and otherwise cognitively intact, feeling well throughout the episode. TGA is often precipitated by physical stress (e.g. swimming in cold water) or emotional upset. The cause is unclear, though ischaemic, migrainous, and epileptic mechanisms have been suggested. People with TGA are alert but bewildered, and aware that they're disoriented. They may repeatedly ask 'Where am I?' without retaining information. In contrast to *dissociative amnesia* (see p. 192), people with TGA *don't* forget their identity. Neurological examination is *normal* (intoxication, head injury, seizure, transient ischaemic attack or stroke must be excluded). Prognosis is good, though episodes sometimes recur.

Frontal lobe syndrome (FLS)

The frontal lobes are the brain's *brakes*: the part which shouts 'Wait! Do you *really* want to do that?' Rather than reacting to situations with basic impulses (e.g. *eat it, fight it, have sex with it*), the frontal lobes weigh up all available information, to select and carry out a reasoned response. Any damage (e.g. head injury, dementia, stroke) can cause FLS:

- *Executive dysfunction*:
  - Poor attention and working memory.
  - Poor reasoning and problem-solving.
  - Poor planning, decision-making, and judgement.

> **BOX 12.5 A hypothetical patient with amnestic disorder**
>
> Chatting normally, they'd score full marks for *immediate* recall on formal testing, but would be disorientated, with poor *delayed* recall. At the next meeting, they wouldn't remember you, but might tell nostalgic stories of your 'holiday together in Spain'. You could teach them to dance, and although they'd forget the lesson, they'd find they could dance a mean tango.

> **BOX 12.6 The frontal lobes of Phineas Gage**
>
> Phineas Gage was a railway worker in Vermont in 1848; his job involved packing sand over gunpowder with a metal rod (tamping iron). One day, the gunpowder exploded unexpectedly, shooting the rod through his left cheek, frontal lobes, and out the top of his head (Figure 12.6). He survived the accident *and* wound infections, but his doctor described a subsequent, drastic personality change: Phineas allegedly changed from being capable and conscientious, to impulsive, rude, bad-tempered, stubborn, distractible, and unable to finish tasks. His friends said he was 'no longer Gage'.

- Loss of flexibility.
- Difficulty inhibiting habitual responses.
- *Social behaviour and personality change* (**Box 12.6**):
  - Inappropriate behaviour (e.g. irresponsible, disinhibited, aggressive).
  - Impulsivity.
  - Euphoric or 'fatuous' mood; lability.
  - Apathy, no motivation/initiative.
  - Self-neglect.
  - Repetitive or compulsive behaviours (e.g. compulsive eating).

People with FLS tend to be *either* apathetic (dorsolateral damage) *or* impulsive and disinhibited (orbitofrontal damage). Speech and motor function may be affected, and frontal release signs can re-emerge (**Table 12.1**). They

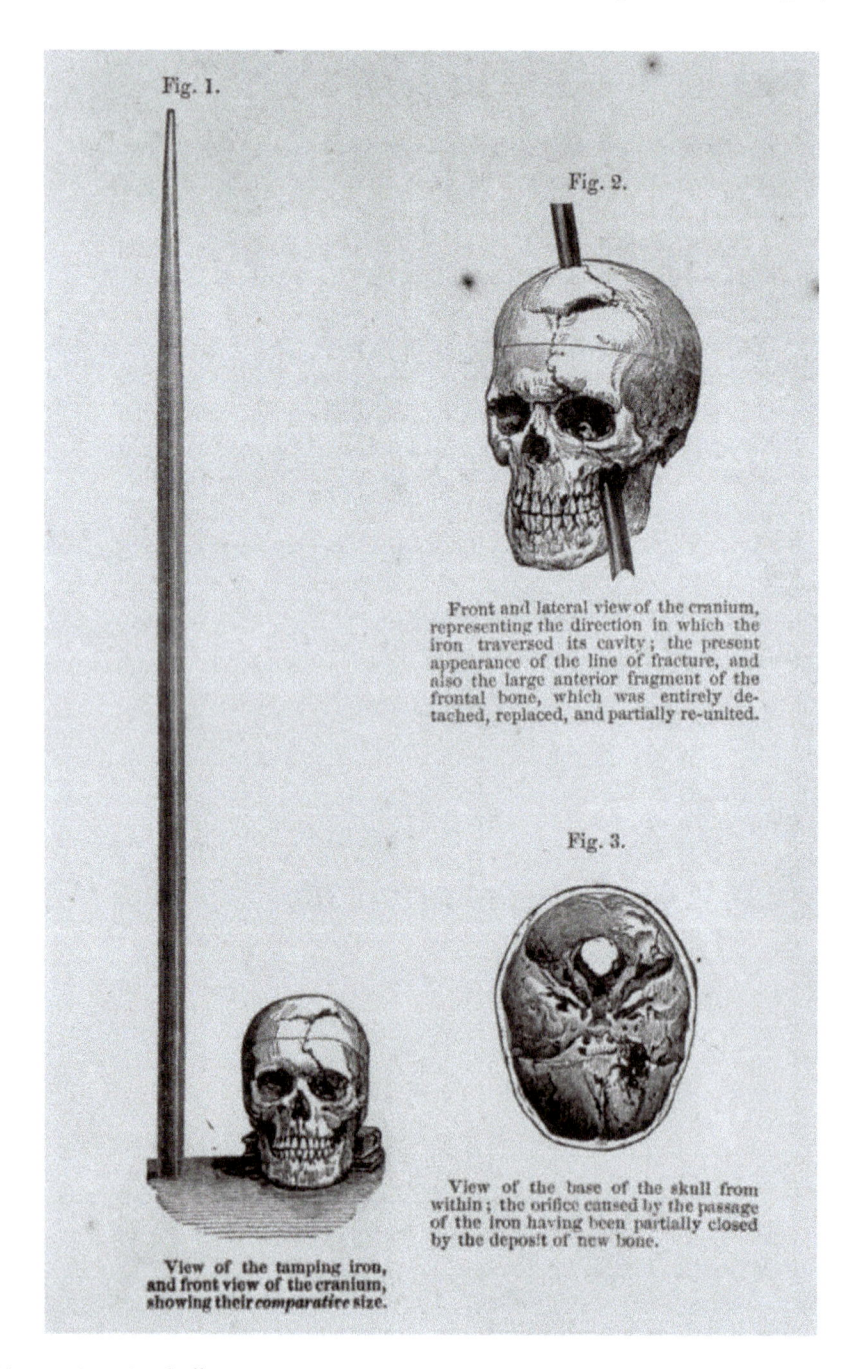

FIGURE 12.6 Phineas Gage's skull.

Reproduced from Harlow, J.M. (1869). Passage of an iron rod through the head. Read before the Massachusetts Medical Society, June 3, 1868. David Clapp & Som, Boston, MA, USA. Courtesy of the National Library of Medicine. www.resource.nlm.nih.gov/66210360R

may show *utilization behaviour* (inability to resist manipulating objects), e.g. grabbing and wearing someone else's glasses. They may also show *perseveration*: repeating a word or action, despite losing the original stimulus, e.g.:

> You: Where were you born?
> Stephen: Paris.
> You: Do you work?
> Stephen: Paris.
> You: What do you mean?
> Stephen: Paris.

Diagnosis requires neuroimaging (e.g. identifying atrophy, lesions), plus specialist neuropsychological testing and occupational therapy assessment of functional impairment (see p. 146 for bedside frontal lobe tests). Unless the cause is treatable, management is through rehabilitation and supportive care.

Traumatic brain injury

Head injuries are either *open* (where the skull is penetrated, causing local cerebral damage) or *closed* (skull intact, but brain damage is caused by acceleration, deceleration, and shearing forces). Traumatic brain injury (TBI) severity is graded as mild, moderate, or severe, often using the Glasgow Coma Scale, duration of coma, and duration of post-traumatic amnesia.

Clinical presentation

Immediate effects include *concussion* (brief loss of brain function), with delirium or coma in severe cases (especially closed injuries). Once normal consciousness is regained, memory problems are common:

- *Post-traumatic amnesia*: anterograde amnesia with disorientation and confusion. The longer it lasts, the greater the risk of complications.

- *Retrograde amnesia:* amnesia for events *before* the injury (from the last clear memory until the injury occurred). It doesn't predict outcome.

Psychiatric sequelae

Ongoing cognitive impairment

Deficits range from mild to severe, and are more likely to be *focal* (e.g. frontal, parietal) following open head injuries and *global* after closed head injuries. Typically, attention, concentration, memory, processing speed, and problem-solving are affected. Circumscribed and permanent anterograde amnesia can occur (amnestic syndrome).

Personality change

This can occur after any TBI, and is often frustrating or heartbreaking for loved ones. Changes may be subtle (e.g. exaggeration of premorbid traits) or disabling (e.g. FLS).

Post-concussion syndrome (PCS)

Concussion can cause PCS. Symptoms occur in 20–50% of people with a mild head injury; they usually last a few weeks, but persist in 10% for over a year. People become preoccupied with distressing symptoms:

- Somatic, e.g. headache, dizziness, fatigue, insomnia, noise sensitivity.
- Affective, e.g. depression, anxiety, irritability.
- Cognitive, e.g. poor concentration and memory.

Organic *and* psychological factors contribute to PCS, e.g. microscopic axonal injury is seen in even mild TBI; a history of mental health problems is a risk factor. PCS is more common in young men, sportspeople, and elderly or homeless people.

Other problems

Depression and anxiety affect up to 50% of TBI survivors, and can persist; there's an increased risk of attempted and completed suicide. TBI can also cause ongoing psychosis.

Management

Specialist brain injury services provide psychological and physical rehabilitation, and vital support for families. Any psychotropic medications are used with care due to side effects, e.g. antipsychotics increase the risk of seizures, benzodiazepines can cause paradoxical agitation.

Parkinson disease

Parkinson disease (PD) is a progressive CNS disorder. The cause is unknown (idiopathic), although genetic and environmental factors (e.g. exposure to pesticides) can increase the risk. For secondary parkinsonism, see **Box 12.7**.

Pathology

Dopaminergic cell degeneration in the substantia nigra causes dopamine depletion in dopaminergic tracts leading to the basal ganglia. Abnormal deposits of the

> **BOX 12.7** Secondary parkinsonism
>
> Parkinso*nism* (Parkinson *symptoms*) doesn't always mean PD; other causes include:
>
> - Medications, e.g. antipsychotics.
> - Toxins, e.g. cyanide, carbon monoxide.
> - Brain lesions, e.g. strokes, tumours.
> - Wilson disease.
> - Repeated head injury ('boxing encephalopathy'/'punch-drunk syndrome')
> - *Parkinson plus syndromes* (neurodegenerative disorders comprising PD, with additional deficits): progressive supranuclear palsy, corticobasal degeneration, multiple system atrophy, and DLB (see Chapter 13).

protein alpha-synuclein form in affected cells as Lewy bodies (p. 154).

Clinical presentation

The classic triad of symptoms is:

- *Tremor* ('pill-rolling' type).
- *Rigidity* (experienced as stiffness).
- *Bradykinesia* (slowed movement).

Other signs and symptoms include stooped posture and shuffling ('festinating') gait, recurrent falls, mask-like facial expression, speech and swallowing difficulties, constipation, and urinary problems. Mood symptoms commonly precede motor symptoms.

Psychiatric sequelae

Depression

Depression occurs in up to 45% of people with PD. It can be hard to diagnose since symptoms can overlap, e.g. lack of smiling (reduced facial expression) and psychomotor slowing. Treatment is as for primary depression (see p. 40).

> 💡 When physical illnesses resemble depression, focus on *cognitions* (e.g. hopelessness, guilt) and the *experience* of depression (e.g. sadness, anhedonia). This helps confirm a diagnosis of depression.

Parkinson disease dementia

Up to 80% of people with PD eventually develop dementia. It's associated with increased mortality, carer stress, and nursing home admission. An early symptom is *bradyphrenia*, which progresses to dementia. PD presents *before* cognitive impairment, in contrast to DLB, where cognitive impairment precedes parkinsonian symptoms. Acetylcholinesterase inhibitors can help both disorders.

Psychosis

Psychosis affects up to 40% of people with PD, and can also be a side effect of dopaminergic anti-parkinson medication. Visual hallucinations, often of animals or people, are common. Psychosis strongly predicts the need for nursing home care. Dopaminergic drugs can be slowly withdrawn, or cautious doses of atypical antipsychotics tried, but both can exacerbate parkinsonism; management involves striking a balance between too much dopamine (psychosis) and too little (parkinsonism).

Multiple sclerosis

MS is a chronic autoimmune disorder, characterized by demyelination, inflammation, and plaque formation in CNS white matter tracts. Pathology occurs at different sites at different times, causing various neurological symptoms. MS may be:

- *Relapsing–remitting* (80%) initially, though symptoms later become permanent (*secondary progressive form*).
- *Primary progressive* (10%), deteriorating without remission.
- *Benign* (<10%), relapsing infrequently, and never causing permanent symptoms.

Psychiatric sequelae

People may suffer embarrassing *pathological affect* ('emotional incontinence'): excessive emotional outbursts, e.g. suddenly laughing or crying for little reason.

Up to 50% of people with MS develop depression, secondary to the MS itself, disability and pain, or medication (e.g. steroids, baclofen, interferon). Treatment is as for primary depression. The risk of suicide is near double that of the general population.

MS relapses or medication can cause mania or psychosis.

Half of people with MS have cognitive problems, e.g. with memory and concentration. Dementia affects up to 60% of people with late-stage MS.

Stroke (cerebrovascular accident)

About 85% of strokes are ischaemic and 15% are haemorrhagic; symptoms lasting less than 24 hours are classed as transient ischaemic attacks (TIAs).

Strokes are the second leading cause of death worldwide. UK survival rates have improved due to better medical management (e.g. routine thrombolysis), but this has increased disability rates: half of survivors have a lasting disability, and a third are dependent on others.

Psychiatric sequelae

Cognitive and neurological symptoms correlate to the areas of brain damage, e.g. FLS, hemiparesis, dysphasia. Other psychiatric symptoms aren't reliably associated with specific stroke locations.

Depression affects up to a third of people post stroke, and impedes recovery. Severity is influenced by disability, previous mental illness, and the level of social support. Treatment is as for primary depression, with specialist rehabilitation. Other common symptoms include anxiety, apathy, and pathological affect.

Epilepsy

Epilepsy is characterized by recurrent, unprovoked seizures. It's associated with an increased risk of psychiatric disorders, particularly in treatment-resistant and temporal lobe epilepsy. Possible reasons include the psychosocial burden and stigma of epilepsy, its neurological sequelae, underlying brain abnormalities, and medication side effects.

Psychiatric sequelae

Depression affects up to 50% of people, and suicide rates are four times higher than in the general population. Psychosis (6% of people) may be 'inter-ictal' (temporally unrelated to seizures) or 'post-ictal' (occurring immediately after seizures). Other psychiatric issues include anxiety, dysthymia, cognitive impairment, and associated learning disabilities. Antidepressants and antipsychotics are prescribed with caution, as they can reduce the seizure threshold.

Autoimmune encephalitis

Encephalitis is inflammation of the brain parenchyma, either in response to an infectious pathogen (e.g. herpes simplex virus 1 or 2) or an autoimmune process. Symptoms of infectious encephalitis include 'flu-like symptoms, headaches, and altered consciousness level. These, coupled with symptoms of CNS infection such as fever, photophobia, neck stiffness, speech, motor, sensory changes and seizures, mean an organic cause should be strongly suspected.

In autoimmune encephalitis, an insidious onset of confusion, personality or behaviour change, psychotic symptoms, sleep disturbance, and memory loss, as well as movement disorders and seizures, can be mistaken for a psychiatric presentation. Autoimmune encephalitis is therefore a differential diagnosis for any first episode of psychosis, mania, or dementia. It's a potentially curable cause of psychosis, so must not be missed! Anti-NMDAr encephalitis is caused by antibodies to the

Table 12.4 Organic and iatrogenic causes of psychiatric symptoms

Psychiatric symptoms	Organic and medication causes
Depression	Addison disease (hypoadrenalism) Cushing syndrome (hyperadrenalism) Hypo/hyperparathyroidism Hypothyroidism Systemic lupus erythematosus (SLE) Vitamin B_{12} (cobalamin) or B_9 (folate) deficiency Corticosteroids, interferon, antihypertensives, beta-blockers
Mania	Cushing syndrome Hyper/hypothyroidism Neurosyphilis Corticosteroids, antidepressants
Anxiety	Hyperthyroidism Hypoglycaemia Phaeochromocytoma Corticosteroids, antidepressants, levothyroxine
Psychosis	Acute porphyria Cushing syndrome Encephalitis Hypothyroidism ('myxoedema madness')/hyperthyroidism Neurosyphilis SLE Corticosteroids, L-dopa, levetiracetam
Dementia	Addison disease Cushing syndrome Hypo/hyperparathyroidism Hypothyroidism Neurosyphilis (Box 12.8) Vitamin B deficiencies, e.g. thiamine, niacin, folate, cobalamin.

N-methyl-D-aspartate receptor, which are often generated in response to an underlying tumour (classically, an ovarian teratoma). Investigations include neuroimaging (CT/MRI), and blood/CSF auto-antibodies. If present, an underlying cause for autoimmune encephalitis must be treated, alongside supportive care and immune therapies such as steroids, immunoglobulins and plasma exchange. Residual psychiatric and memory problems can follow.

Miscellaneous systemic illnesses

In addition to the neurological disorders already described, many systemic illnesses and medications cause psychiatric problems. **Table 12.4** isn't exhaustive! (See also **Box 12.8**.)

> **BOX 12.8** Neurosyphilis
>
> Neurosyphilis is a tertiary presentation of syphilis, infecting the CNS. It presents 10–20 years after an untreated primary syphilis infection, and manifests as:
>
> - *General paresis:* elation/depression, delusions, cognitive decline, and neurological deficits. It was a common reason for admission to psychiatric asylums until penicillin was introduced in the early twentieth century.
> - *Meningovascular syphilis:* usually presents like a stroke, with subacute encephalitis, personality change, and labile mood.
>
> Rates are now rising again, possibly due to increasing casual, unprotected sex. Concurrent HIV infection increases the risk of developing neurosyphilis.

REALITY

General approach: tips, tricks, and cautionary tales

This section focuses on working with people suffering from *delirium*.

1. Behaviour is communication

If people can't express themselves verbally, they communicate *non-verbally*. When meeting a confused person, read their behaviour and wonder what they're trying to tell you—then engage them on *that* level. For example, a stick-wielding older person may feel threatened; asking, 'What's scaring you?' is more likely to address his aggression (and avert a fall) than confiscating his stick.

> 💡 Wandering may communicate anxiety, boredom, pain, a full bladder, or a search for someone/something that seems 'lost'.

2. Beat the competition

Delirium makes it hard to focus: information can't be filtered out or retained easily, making the ever-changing environment overwhelming and distracting. To help someone focus on *you* and your message, cut out competing stimuli (e.g. television) and make their environment stable, calm, and quiet.

3. Provide clues

Repeatedly reorientate the person. Each time you meet them, introduce yourself and gently remind them where they are. Ensure that they wear their watch, glasses, and hearing aid if available. Write down important information, e.g. *Henry will visit at 2pm* (leave the note near a clock).

4. Comfort always

Being confused is frightening. Gently but firmly reassure the person that they're safe and that you're there to help them. Explain their situation and your actions, speaking clearly and simply, communicating only one idea per sentence. Ensure they know how to get help: a call button may stop someone screaming, by reassuring them that nurses are contactable.

5. Recruit experts

Family and friends are often keen—but unsure how—to help. Explain the situation and what they can do, e.g. reassuring, reorientating, offering fluids. They may explain why certain staff or situations upset the person, e.g. because of cultural norms or past traumatic experiences.

6. Delirium's left hook

Confused and agitated people can lash out. Even a frail, elderly person can give you a lovely black eye, so be careful!

> 💡 People with delirium are temporarily not 'themselves'. Safeguard their values and dignity until they recover.

MINI – ADDENBROOKE'S COGNITIVE EXAMINATION
UK Version A (2014)

Name:
Date of Birth:
Hospital No. or Address:

Date of testing: ___/___/___
Tester's name:_____
Age at leaving full-time education:_____
Occupation: _____
Handedness: _____

ATTENTION

➢ Ask: What is the | Day | Date | Month | Year

Attention [Score 0-4]

MEMORY

➢ Tell: "I'm going to give you a name and address and I'd like you to repeat the name and address after me. So you have a chance to learn, we'll be doing that 3 times. I'll ask you the name and address later."

Score only the third trial.

Memory [Score 0 – 7]

	1st Trial	2nd Trial	3rd Trial
Harry Barnes			
73 Orchard Close			
Kingsbridge			
Devon			

FLUENCY – ANIMALS

➢ **Animals**
Say: "Now can you name as many animals as possible. It can begin with any letter. You have one minute. Go ahead."

Fluency [Score 0 – 7]

≥ 22	7
17-21	6
14-16	5
11-13	4
9-10	3
7-8	2
5-6	1
<5	0
total	correct

FIGURE 12.7 M-ACE UK Version A.

Reproduced from Hsieh H. et al. The Mini-Addenbrooke's Cognitive Examination: A New Assessment Tool for Dementia. *Dementia and Geriatric Cognitive Disorders* 39(1–2): 1–11.

CLOCK DRAWING

➢ Clock: Ask the subject to draw a clock face with numbers and the hands at ten past five. (For scoring see instruction guide: circle = 1, numbers = 2, hands = 2 if all correct).	**Visuospatial** [Score 0-5]

MEMORY RECALL

➢ Ask "Now tell me what you remember about that name and address we were repeating at the beginning"

		Memory [Score 0-7]
Harry Barnes	....	
73 Orchard Close	....	
Kingsbridge	....	
Devon	....	

TOTAL SCORE	**/ 30**

Updated 25/05/2014

Copyright © 2015, S. Karger AG, Basel. https://doi.org/10.1159/000366040. Distributed under the terms of the Creative Commons Attribution 3.0 Unported (CC BY 3.0). https://creativecommons.org/licenses/by/3.0/

1. Assess cognition (15 minutes)

Candidate's instructions
Joan Woodring is a 75-year-old widow. She was diagnosed with PD 3 years ago, and her son thinks she's becoming more forgetful. You're a medical student in general practice. Assess cognition, using the Mini-Addenbrooke's Cognitive Examination (M-ACE).

Patient's brief
Key characteristics
- I wear a fixed, blank expression; my speech and movements are slow.
- I know the month and year, but not the day or date.
- I make mistakes repeating the name and address, getting it mostly right on my third try. When asked later, I only remember the name.
- I name five animals, before getting stuck.
- I draw a *tiny* clock, with correct numbers, but hands at twenty-five past ten.

Candidate's guidance
Initially, use the M-ACE form (Figure 12.7) as guidance, but *learn* the test, in case you don't have forms on the wards or in OSCEs.
- Get paper and a pen, noting answers and scores as you go (this helps you spot gaps if you get muddled).
- Introduce the test, e.g. 'I understand your son's been worried about your memory. Is it ok if I ask you some questions to check your memory?'
- Explain: 'Some questions are easy, but others are hard, so just try your best.'
- Check: age and occupation for context (e.g. a youthful rocket scientist shouldn't drop *any* points); difficulties reading or writing; need for glasses; whether she can hear you clearly.
- Anxiety lowers scores, so be kind, warm, and smile supportively (without revealing or hinting at answers). Suggest Joan *guesses* if unsure.
- *Scoring*:
  - ≤25/30 strongly suggests cognitive impairment.
  - ≤21/30 likely dementia (once other diagnoses excluded).
  - A perfect clockface requires multiple cognitive skills, so almost certainly *excludes* dementia.

💡 The M-ACE is the short version of the *gold standard* Addenbrooke's Cognitive Examination III (ACE-III). Full instructions are available online: https://sydney.edu.au/brain-mind/resources-for-clinicians/dementia-test.html

💡 Other bedside tests include the Montreal Cognitive Assessment (MOCA), the Mini Mental State Examination (MMSE), and the Standardized MMSE (sMMSE).

2. Frontal lobe testing (15 minutes)

Candidate's instructions
Mehmet Kaya is a 35-year-old chemist who suffered a frontal subdural haematoma in a road traffic accident, 5 weeks ago. His wife says he's a 'changed man.' His consultant asks you to test frontal lobe function.

Patient's brief
Key characteristics
- I'm cheerful, enthusiastic, and unaware I'm making mistakes.
- Hand movements: I repeat the first movement, over and over.
- Finger pointing: I *copy* the examiner's pointing.
- Word testing: I manage three different words, then keep repeating them.

- Proverbs: I give literal interpretations, e.g. 'Birds of a feather flock together' = *'Birds with the same feathers stay together'*.
- My 'guesses' are *extreme*, e.g. 20,000 camels in Holland.
- When the examiner strokes my . . .
  - Palm: I grasp their finger.
  - Lip: I pout.
  - Cheek: I turn my head towards their hand.

Candidate's guidance

If Mehmet fails something, document *what* he did, since different errors can provide useful clinical insights. Although formal testing is useful, it's *essential* to observe Mehmet's behaviour and gain a collateral history. Actions are shown in italics.

Set-shifting

The **Luria test** assesses *set-shifting*: the ability to switch between actions/ideas (important in sequencing behaviours).

- Can you do this?

Hold one hand flat, palm upwards. With your other hand, make three movements onto it: a fist, slice ('karate chop'), and a slap.

- [Once mastered] Now keep going until I say stop. [Look for three perfect cycles]

Perseveration occurs with frontal damage.

Inhibitory control

The **go/no-go task** assesses set-shifting *and* the ability to stop inappropriate responses (i.e. to do the opposite, Mehmet must inhibit his urge to copy you).

- When I touch my nose, you raise your finger, like this.

Point to the ceiling.

- When I raise my finger, you touch your nose, like this.

Touch your nose with your finger.

- It's tricky! Can you explain what I just said? [Check understanding]
- OK. Let's go.

Start with either move and see what Mehmet does. Leave your finger in place while awaiting his response. Alternate without a clear pattern.

Verbal fluency

FAS testing assesses verbal ability (retrieving words from semantic memory) and executive function.

- I'll ask you to say all the words you can, beginning with a certain letter. You can't use people's names or place names. So, if the letter was B, you could say brave or boy, but not Brian or Berlin. The words must be different from each other, so you can't say brave *and* braver or bravest. Keep going until I say stop. Does that make sense? [Check understanding]
- Please tell me words beginning with *F*. Go.

Time 1 minute. Repeat for A and S.

Normal ranges vary with age and education, but <15 words for each letter is concerning.

Abstract thinking and reasoning

These are assessed with *proverb interpretation* and *cognitive estimates*.

Proverb interpretation

- Some phrases have hidden meanings. For example, *too many cooks spoil the broth* isn't actually about cooks. It means that things go badly when too many people get involved. Does that make sense? [Check] Can you think of a hidden meaning for these . . .?
  - Birds of a feather flock together.
  - A stitch in time saves nine.
  - Don't count your chickens before they hatch.

Concrete interpretation suggests frontal lobe pathology, but also occurs in psychosis, ASD, and intellectual disability. Remember that proverbs don't always translate across cultures, and some are simply hard for everyone!

Cognitive estimates

Mehmet must make *reasonable guesses* for things he's unlikely to know, using relevant general knowledge (e.g. that horses are slower than cars).

- Please *guess* the answers to these questions . . .
  - How many camels are there in Holland?
  - How fast is a racehorse?
  - What's the best-paid job in this country?
  - How many lashes are on your lower eyelid? [*80–100 is a good guess*]

Frontal lobe damage produces extreme answers.

> *Frontal release signs*
> The primitive reflexes we have as babies may re-emerge with frontal damage.
>
> - Please hold your hands out.
>
> *Stroke across his palm towards his thumb.* (Grasp reflex)
>
> - May I touch your face, please?
>
> *Lightly tap his lips or stroke down his philtrum.* (Suck/pout reflex)
>
> *Stroke his cheek with your finger.* (Rooting reflex)

💡 **Naming *animals* in a minute is a quick alternative to FAS.**

NEXT STEPS

MS and fitness to drive

You're an FY2 in general practice, reviewing Shivangi Sharma, a 38-year-old teacher. She has MS, and recently relapsed with diplopia, so the GP started high-dose oral steroids. Shivangi is ushered in early, as she's disrupting the waiting room. She's talkative, giggly, and restless, but able to sit throughout the appointment. She says she feels 'superb' after 5 days of steroids, and mentions she'd have been late, but managed to 'put her foot down' while driving here from school.

- What's the differential diagnosis?
- How will you manage her immediately and longer term?
- What are your responsibilities regarding her driving?

Differential diagnosis

Shivangi is probably *hypomanic* since she has elated mood without marked loss of function (see p. 45). This is most likely an organic mood disorder, secondary to the steroids, though possibly due to the MS, or other causes (e.g. substance use). A *functional* illness (i.e. hypomania *without* an organic cause) is less likely, given the timing coincides with active MS and steroids.

Management

Undertake a psychiatric history, MSE, and physical examination; exclude other organic causes, e.g. infection. Explore risks associated with hypomania, e.g. progression to mania, self-neglect, vulnerability to sexual exploitation, overspending. Consider whether Shivangi can manage at home with family support, or whether the risks or treatment require a medical or psychiatric admission. Involve Shivangi and her family in exploring options and concerns.

Discuss management with your GP supervisor, neurologist, and/or duty psychiatrist. Steroids can be stopped if her acute MS relapse has resolved. The psychiatrist will advise on treating mania (e.g. benzodiazepines, mood-stabilizing antipsychotic) and can involve community mental health services if Shivangi is going home, or organize a psychiatric admission.

In future, the GP, neurologist, and psychiatric services will need to liaise closely, as Shivangi will be very susceptible to steroid-induced mania. This drug reaction must be clearly documented in her notes, letters, and drug charts. Psychiatric services should provide psychoeducation and consider CBT for relapse prevention, e.g. sleep hygiene (see p. 44), identifying relapse indicators. She'll need time off work while hypomanic, as she won't teach effectively, and may behave unprofessionally or be bullied by students. Longer term, a care coordinator or vocational worker could support Shivangi to address issues with her employer, e.g. work–life balance, reasonable adjustments to address temporary or permanent disabilities.

Driving

Check Shivangi's understanding of the law regarding driving and MS, and any action she's taken. She should have notified the appropriate body of her MS, e.g. the Driver and Vehicle Licensing Agency (DVLA)[3] in the UK. If you believe she's been driving when she wasn't safe to do so (for physical *or* mental health reasons), you must tell her this, and encourage her to contact the DVLA.

If she continues to drive, explain your responsibility to contact the DVLA on her behalf, and then do so if she won't contact them herself. Many people don't know the law, but will stop driving upon realizing the potential consequences, e.g. invalid insurance when driving against medical advice; points on their licence/disqualification. In extreme cases, doctors may have to involve police to stop someone driving while medically unfit to do so.

Ensure that Shivangi makes arrangements to return home safely (e.g. by taxi; partner to collect her car), and advise her not to drive until authorized by the DVLA.

💡 **People may be fit to drive *until* they use your prescriptions! Always advise people don't drive if medication causes sedation or coordination problems. Many psychotropic medications are sedative.**

Movie buff
Awakenings (1990): catatonia and parkinsonism following encephalitis lethargica.
Hilary and Jackie (1998): cellist Jacqueline du Pre's FLS secondary to MS.
Memento (2000): anterograde amnesia following head injury.
Regarding Henry (1991): personality change following head injury.
The Madness of King George (1994): confusion, agitation, and acute porphyria.

Book shelf
Amis, M. (2003) *Yellow Dog*: ethical and personality changes post head injury.
Calahan, S. (2013) *Brain on Fire: My Month of Madness*: a journalist's experience of NMDAr encephalitis.
Dostoevsky, F. (1868) *The Idiot*: the experience of epilepsy.
Garland, A. (2004) *The Coma*: consideration of mind–brain differentiation post head injury.
McEwan, I. (2005) *Saturday*: a neurosurgeon's encounter with Huntington disease.
Sacks, O. (1985) *The Man Who Mistook His Wife for a Hat*: precise, patient-centred accounts of neuropsychiatric conditions.

Notes

1. Garland, A. (2004) *The Coma*. London: Faber & Faber.
2. Inouye, S.K., van Dyck, C.H., Alessi, C.A., et al. (1990) Clarifying confusion: the confusion assessment method: a new method for detecting delirium. *Annals of Internal Medicine*, **113**, 941–8.
3. DVLA (2018) Assessing fitness to drive: a guide for medical professionals. See www.gov.uk/dvla/fitnesstodrive

Journal club

Goldstein, S. (2005) Neuropsychiatric assessment. *Psychiatric Clinics of North America*, **28**, 507–47.

Harlow, J.M. (1848) Passage of an iron rod through the head. *Boston Medical and Surgical Journal*, **39**, 389–93.

O'Connell, H., Kennelly, S.P., Cullen, W., et al. (2014) Managing delirium in everyday practice: towards cognitive-friendly hospitals. *BJPsych Advances*, **20**, 380–9.

Rickards, H., Jacob, S., Lennox, B., et al. (2014) Autoimmune encephalitis: a potentially treatable cause of mental disorder. *Advances in Psychiatric Treatment*, **20**, 92–100.

Go to www.oup.com/uk/stringer2e for a wealth of additional resources, including an OCSE mark scheme, filmed scenarios, and self-assessment questions.

13 Old Age Psychiatry

True or false?

Answers on p. 277

1. Dementia due to Lewy body disease (DLB) is characterized by stable cognitive impairment with parkinsonism and psychotic symptoms.
2. Cognitive behavioural therapy is of limited value for older adults with depression.
3. Female sex, poor hearing, and social isolation increase risk of late-onset psychosis.
4. Short-term memory loss is a normal part of ageing.
5. Amyloid plaques and neurofibrillary tangles are features of Alzheimer disease (AD).
6. Dysphasia suggests DLB.
7. Low-dose antipsychotics may be useful in vascular dementia.
8. Trazodone is an acetylcholinesterase inhibitor which slows progression of AD.
9. Male sex, physical disability, and social isolation increase risk of elder abuse.
10. M-ACE contributes to capacity assessment.

Contents

Principles
Introduction
Depression
Anxiety disorders
Psychosis
Dementia
- Epidemiology
- Aetiology
- Pathology
- Clinical presentation: overview
- Clinical presentation: subtypes
- Differential diagnosis
- Investigations
- Management
- Prognosis

Reality
General approach: tips, tricks, and cautionary tales

The interview
- Memory loss history
- Cognitive impairment: collateral history

Next steps
Capacity and a dangerous discharge
- Immediate containment
- Preparation
- Assessment
- Management: has capacity
- Management: lacks capacity

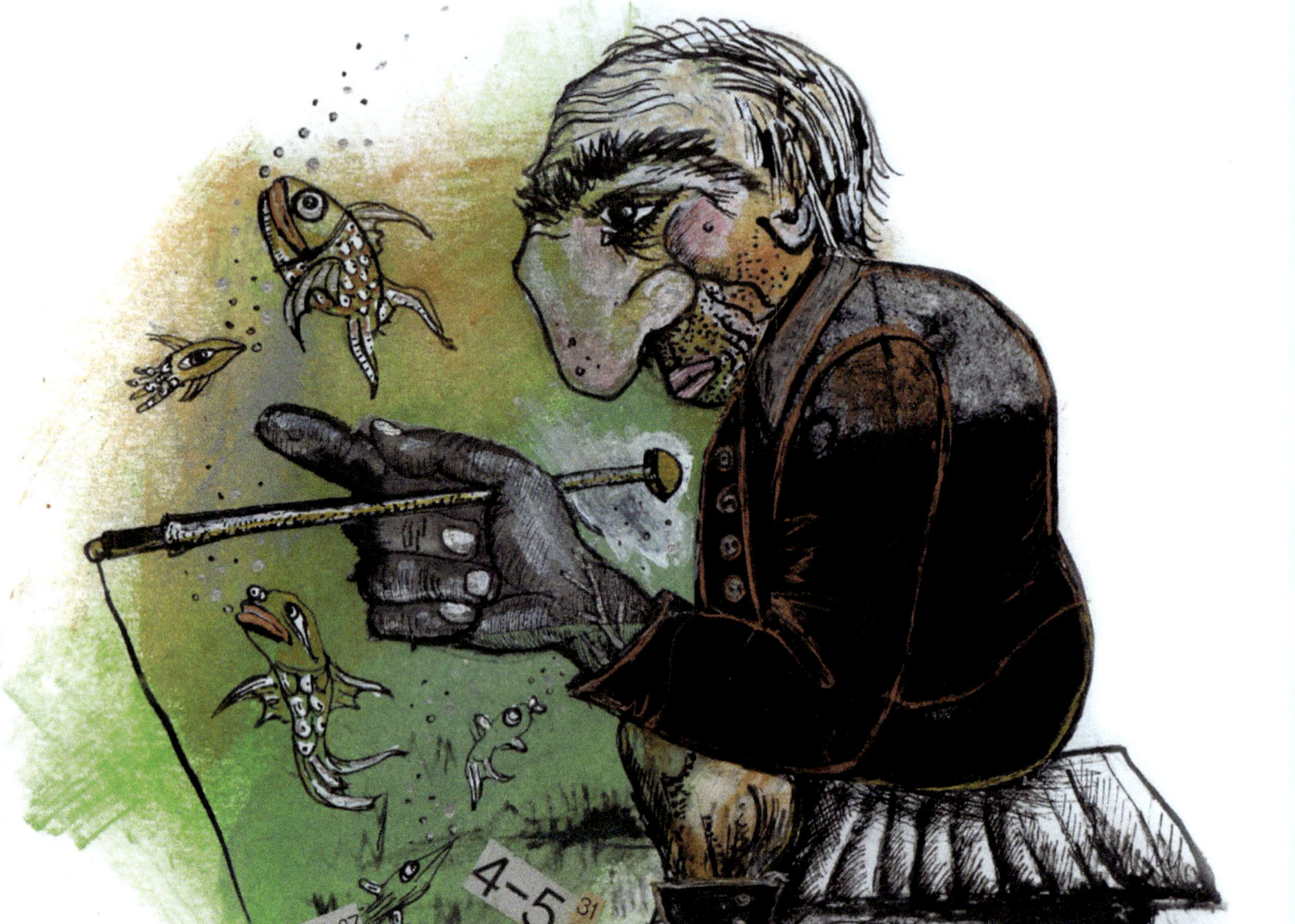

4–5
31
25-27
11
18
5
7
8
7
3
6
10
20
23
9
8
24

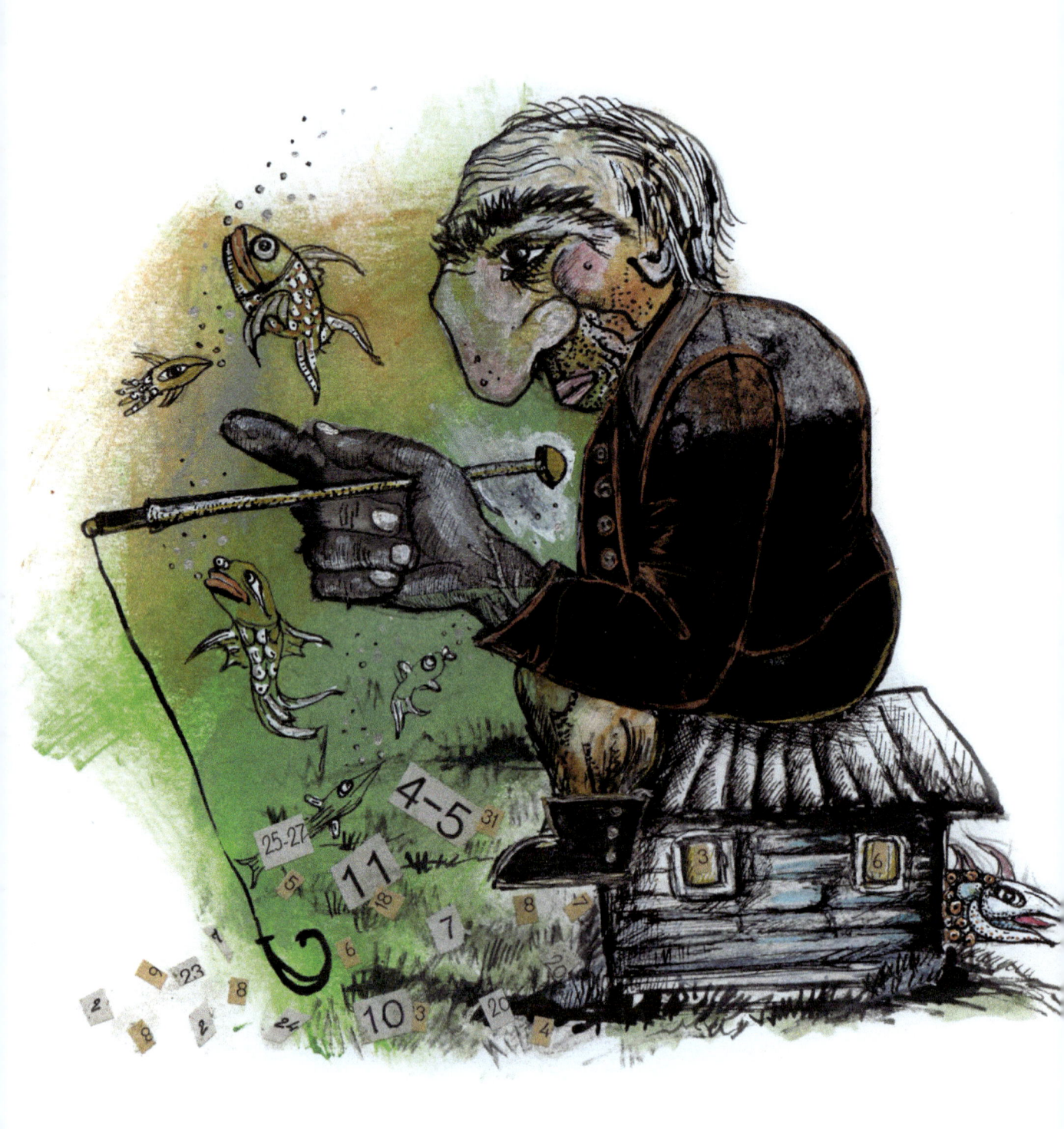

PRINCIPLES

'You're so beautiful,' said Alice. 'I'm afraid of looking at you and not knowing who you are.'
'I think that even if you don't know who I am someday, you'll still know that I love you.'
'What if I see you, and I don't know that you're my daughter, and I don't know that you love me?'
'Then, I'll tell you that I do, and you'll believe me.'

Lisa Genova, *Still Alice*[1]

Introduction

Mental health of older adults (MHOA) teams serve people aged 65 and over: they manage all new mental health problems, and are experts in dementia care. Teams consist of social workers, nurses, psychologists, occupational therapists, and psychiatrists—recognizing the particular needs of older people, including the often complex interplay between social, physical, and mental health problems.

MHOA teams focus less on symptoms *themselves* and more on how these symptoms affect everyday life and functioning; they often assess people *at home*, to understand how they're coping in a familiar environment. Working closely with carers, teams enhance quality of life and support people to stay in their own homes as long as possible.

> 💡 Optimize your reading! We'll cover depression, anxiety, and psychosis briefly, as they're discussed comprehensively in their respective chapters. For best effect, read them and Chapter 12 on organic psychiatry *with* this chapter as you explore older adult psychiatry.

> 💡 Organic causes *must* be ruled out whenever someone presents with mental health symptoms for the *first* time in *later life*.

Depression

About 15% of older people, and 30% of older hospital inpatients, are depressed at any time. Depression in later life (particularly a first episode) may be associated with cerebrovascular disease, vascular risk factors, and current or future cognitive deficits. Other risk factors more commonly affecting older people include bereavement, isolation, poverty, chronic pain, physical illness, and polypharmacy (multiple medications, making drug side effects and interactions more likely).

Older people present with depression similarly to younger people but may show more:

- Physical symptoms, e.g. constipation, insomnia, fatigue.
- Psychomotor agitation/retardation.
- Memory problems.
- Executive dysfunction.

Pseudodementia is when memory problems are so bad that depression resembles dementia.

Self-neglect and poor oral intake are important risks in older people and may be the first signs of depression. Suicide rates are higher (especially in men), so suicidal thoughts should be taken very seriously.

Depression management is similar to that of younger people:

- *Problem-solving, increasing socialization, and daytime activities.*
- *Psychological therapies*, e.g. CBT, psychodynamic, family, or couples therapy.
- *Antidepressants*—SSRIs are usually first line, though they may cause hyponatraemia, so monitor sodium levels. Mirtazapine can improve sleep and appetite, so may be preferred in frail, older people with insomnia.
- *Electroconvulsive therapy* (ECT) is sometimes needed for psychotic or life-threatening depression.

Anxiety disorders

The prevalence and incidence of anxiety disorders fall with age, possibly because of under-reporting. They're more common in women and in isolated people or those who've had adverse experiences. Some people with lifelong anxiety disorders may only access treatment when no longer able to maintain safety-seeking behaviours (see p. 169), e.g. avoidance, hoarding, rituals. Management is usually through CBT, although SSRIs can help.

Psychosis

Most older people with psychosis first became unwell in their youth. However, functional psychosis can develop for the *first time* in older people: it's called 'late-onset psychosis' after the age of 40, and 'very late-onset psychosis' after 60 (also known as *paraphrenia*/late-onset schizophrenia).

Women are more commonly affected, possibly due to loss of the protective effect of oestrogen after menopause. Risk factors include social isolation, sensory impairment, cerebrovascular pathology, being single/widowed, or (for women) without children. Positive symptoms (delusions and hallucinations) are often more prominent than negative symptoms.

Secondary psychotic symptoms also arise in other disorders affecting older people, including delirium, dementia, and mood disorders.

Management includes:

- Exclude organic causes (see p. 129).
- Optimize hearing and vision.
- *Low-dose* antipsychotic (older people are particularly prone to side effects).
- CBT.

💡 Blind or partially sighted people may 'see' patterns or complex images of people, objects, or landscapes (Charles Bonnet syndrome). They don't have other symptoms, and know the hallucinations aren't real.

Dementia

Dementia *isn't* a normal part of ageing. It's an acquired, chronic, usually progressive global cognitive impairment, interfering with activities of daily living (ADLs) (**Box 13.1**). Problems present in *clear consciousness for at least 6 months* distinguish dementia from delirium.

Epidemiology

The risk of dementia increases with age and the prevalence is:

- 5% of people aged 65 or over.
- 20% of people aged 80 or over.

The commonest types of dementia affecting older people are Alzheimer disease (AD), vascular dementia (VD), and dementia due to Lewy body disease (DLB).

BOX 13.1 Activities of daily living

- *Basic* (e.g. Barthel scale):
  - Bathing, dressing, grooming.
  - Toileting (including faecal/urinary incontinence).
  - Eating and drinking.
  - Mobility, e.g. walking, turning, transfers, using stairs.
- *Instrumental* (not necessarily daily, but enable independent living):
  - Meal preparation.
  - Housework.
  - Shopping.
  - Communicating, e.g. using telephones, email/internet.
  - Transportation, e.g. driving, using public transport.
  - Financial management.
  - Medication management.

See **Figure 13.1**. Early-onset (<65 years) dementias are discussed in Chapter 12.

Aetiology

Increasing age is a key risk factor for all causes of dementia.

Alzheimer disease

Risk factors include:

- Female sex (slightly commoner in women).
- Vascular risk factors, e.g. hypertension, smoking, diabetes.
- Low IQ/limited education.
- History of depression or head injury.

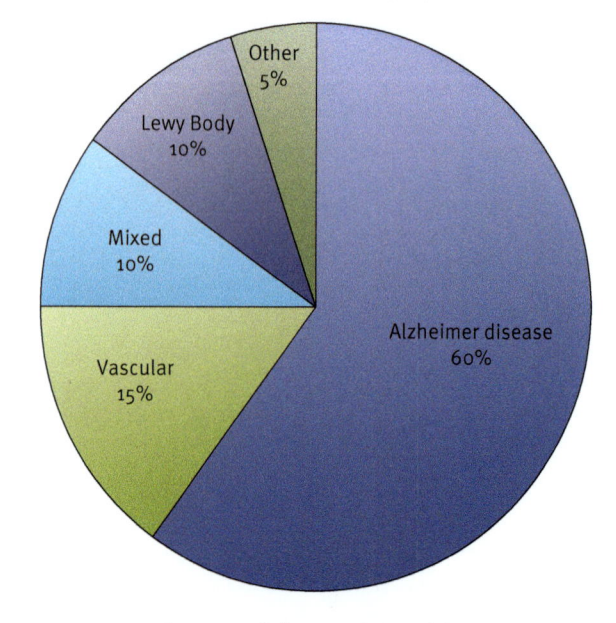

FIGURE 13.1 Causes of dementia in older people

- Alzheimer disease 60%
- Vascular 15%
- Mixed 10%
- Lewy Body 10%
- Other 5%

The heritability of AD is about 70%.

Late-onset or *sporadic* AD (65+ years) makes up 95% of cases. Multiple genes may be involved, but attention has focused on the apolipoprotein E (*APOE*) ε4 allele on chromosome 19. The APOE protein seems to be involved in breaking down β-amyloid (see later); the ε4 allele is less effective, so having one or two alleles increases the risk of AD.

Familial or *early-onset* AD (<65 years) is usually due to rare, autosomal dominant mutations affecting presenilin 1 (chromosome 14), presenilin 2 (chromosome 1), or amyloid precursor protein (*APP*; chromosome 21) genes. These influence the formation or breakdown of APP, predisposing to β-amyloid deposition.

> Relatives of people with familial AD require genetic counselling, unlike sporadic AD.

> People with Down syndrome (trisomy 21) have an increased risk of AD, connected to their *three* copies of the *APP* gene; a third develop AD in their 50s.

Vascular dementia

VD (or *multi-infarct dementia*) results from small strokes, caused by thromboemboli or arteriosclerosis. Risk factors are the same as for strokes (e.g. male sex, smoking, hypertension, diabetes, hypercholesterolaemia, atrial fibrillation), and there may be other signs of arteriosclerosis (e.g. cardiovascular disease, TIAs). VD may also be caused by amyloid angiopathy, so can occur with AD.

Multiple genes of small effect probably influence susceptibility to VD. Rare familial forms of VD can occur, e.g. cerebral autosomal dominant arteriopathy with subcortical infarcts and leucoencephalopathy (CADASIL).

Lewy body dementia

Men are more commonly affected, and although DLB doesn't seem strongly genetic, the risk increases in those with the *APOE* ε4 allele.

Pathology

Alzheimer disease

- *Plaques* (**Figure 13.2**): in neuronal cell membranes, APP influences cell growth and survival. When broken down abnormally, it forms insoluble extracellular plaques of β-amyloid which disrupt signalling between neurons, trigger immune-mediated inflammation, and damage blood vessels increasing the risk of haemorrhage ('amyloid angiopathy').
- *Neurofibrillary tangles* (NFTs) (**Figure 13.3**): plaques are also thought to trigger the abnormal phosphorylation of *tau* (an intracellular protein). Tau usually stabilizes microtubules (the cellular transport system), but when phosphorylated it collapses into twisted strands (NFTs), disrupting cell transport and causing neuronal death. The severity of dementia is most closely associated with the number of NFTs in the neocortex.
- *Cortical atrophy* follows from neuronal loss. The *hippocampus*, essential for short-term memory and visuospatial skills, is affected early, before temporal and parietal lobes. Neuroimaging shows enlarged sulci and ventricles (though this can also occur in normal ageing).
- *Cholinergic pathway loss*: AD is thought to mostly affect cholinergic neuronal pathways, causing symptoms such as memory loss. This theory was the rationale for developing acetylcholinesterase inhibitors (AChEIs) (see p. 159).

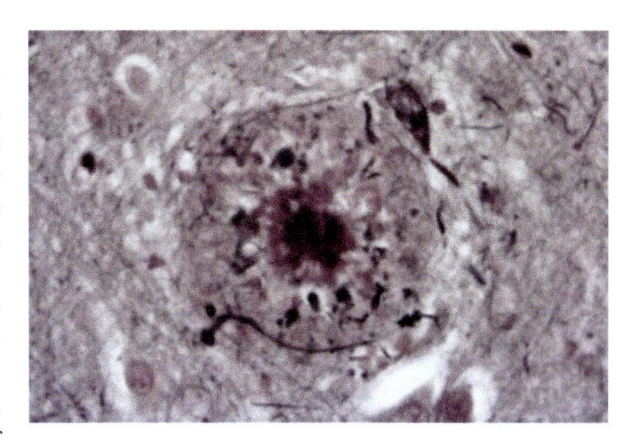

FIGURE 13.2 AD plaque (silver stain).
By kind permission of Dr Andrew King

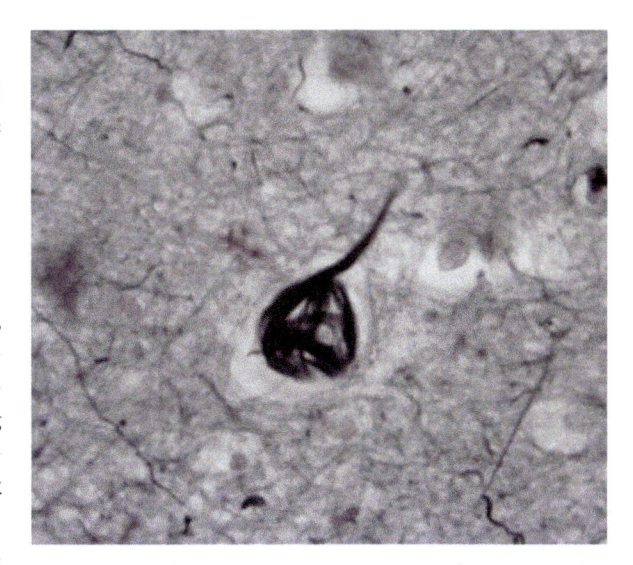

FIGURE 13.3 AD neurofibrillary tangle (silver stain).
By kind permission of Dr Andrew King

Vascular dementia

Arteriosclerosis, cortical ischaemia, and infarcts predominate. See **Figure 13.4**.

Lewy body dementia

DLB may be underdiagnosed, as it can only be confirmed postmortem. DLB and *Parkinson disease* (PD) are thought to be two expressions of a shared problem in metabolizing *a-synuclein* protein. This causes deposition of *Lewy bodies* (**Figure 13.5**): abnormal eosinophilic, intracytoplasmic neuronal structures composed of α-synuclein with ubiquitin.

- PD: Lewy bodies are found in the brainstem. Movement disorder (tremor, rigidity, bradykinesia) predates cognitive symptoms by at least a year.
- DLB: Lewy bodies are also seen in the cingulate gyrus and neocortex. Cognitive impairment precedes movement symptoms, or occurs *within a year* of their onset.

It's been suggested that DLB might be a variant of AD, as they share pathology, e.g. cholinergic loss in DLB, Lewy bodies in AD.

Clinical presentation: overview

Dementia affects multiple cognitive domains, though specific dementias often initially cause problems in particular areas (see later). Problems are often attributed to 'normal ageing' or absent-mindedness at first.

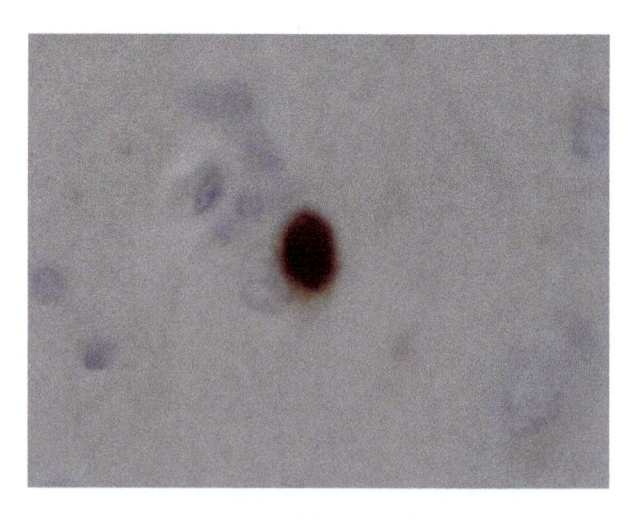

FIGURE 13.5 A temporal lobe Lewy body in DLB (staining for α-synuclein).
By kind permission of Dr Andrew King

Memory

Dementia often begins with forgetfulness for recent events; it's hard to lay down new memories (*anterograde amnesia*). This may start with uncharacteristic mistakes, e.g. muddling up appointments, mislaying items. With time, long-term memories are lost (*retrograde amnesia*), starting with more recent memories, then older, more established memories. People become disorientated for time (as it's always changing), *then* place, *then* (very late) person.

Language

Problems with speech and language include:

- *Receptive dysphasia*—difficulties *understanding* language.
- *Expressive dysphasia*—difficulties *producing* speech. Initial word-finding problems may progress to muddled, disjointed sentences.

Personality changes

Familiar traits may be lost or exaggerated, and new traits can appear. Carers often find this heartbreaking, watching the person they love become a stranger. For example, someone who was always easy-going and friendly may become bad-tempered and uninterested in others.

Subcortical symptoms

(See p. 133.) Deep brain structural damage can cause mental slowing (bradyphrenia), movement disorders (e.g. bradykinesia, chorea), depression, and executive dysfunction.

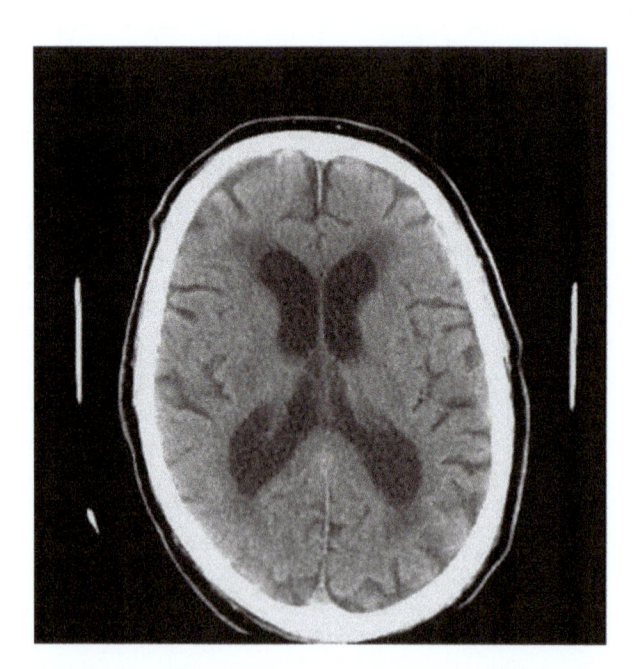

FIGURE 13.4 CT head showing VD: this non-contrast scan shows areas of lower density adjacent to the anterior and posterior horns of the lateral ventricles, due to chronic ischaemia.
By kind permission of Dr Mona Sriharan

Other functions

Parietal lobe involvement (common in AD) causes various problems, e.g.:

- *Agnosia*: difficulties *recognizing* things, e.g. familiar objects, faces (prosopagnosia).
- *Apraxia*: difficulties performing skilled tasks (e.g. drawing, dressing) despite normal sensory and motor function.
- *Dyscalculia*: problems using or understanding numbers.

Frontal lobe damage (see p. 137) can cause executive dysfunction, socially inappropriate behaviour, and personality change.

> 💡 When someone can't recognize their *own* face (*auto*prosopagnosia), they may see 'strangers' invading their home or staring in through their 'window' (mirror).

Mood symptoms

Anxiety or depression may occur early, especially while people understand that they have dementia.

Behavioural and psychological symptoms of dementia (BPSD)

BPSD symptoms usually occur later, and may make care at home difficult or risky, e.g.:

- *Behavioural*:
  - Restlessness, wandering.
  - Disturbed sleep/day–night reversal.
  - Shouting, screaming, swearing.
  - Inappropriate/sexually disinhibited behaviour.
  - Aggression.
- *Psychological*:
  - Delusions.
  - Hallucinations.
  - Depression, anxiety.

> 💡 People with dementia can become more confused, agitated, and frightened in the evening (*'sundowning'*). This may relate to tiredness, illusions in poor light, reduced need for sleep with age, or disrupted circadian rhythm ('internal body clock' thinking it's daytime at night).

Effect on life

Losing independence with ADLs (**Box 13.1**) can be extremely upsetting and place a heavy burden on carers. Additionally, dementia can make the world feel confusing, frightening, or overwhelming.

Dementia causes a wide range of risks (**Figure 13.6**), e.g.:

- *To self*:
  - Suicide/self-harm (especially early in illness, while aware of prognosis).
  - Self-neglect, e.g. poor oral intake/hygiene, forgetting medications, squalor.
  - Getting lost/wandering.
  - Accidents, e.g. leaving gas on (explosion), flooding, fires.
- *From others*:
  - Financial exploitation.
  - Neglect/abuse (emotional, physical, sexual).
- *To others*:
  - Aggression.
  - Sexual disinhibition.
  - Dangerous driving.

Clinical presentation: subtypes

See **Table 13.1**.

Alzheimer disease

AD shows a gradual decline. *Spatial navigation* problems (hippocampal involvement) may be an early sign, contributing to people getting lost. Clinicians sometimes talk about the *4As of Alzheimer* as key problem areas:

- **A**mnesia.
- **A**phasia.
- **A**gnosia.
- **A**praxia.

Depression or anxiety may present early on, with later flattened affect, social withdrawal, and personality changes.

Vascular dementia

Classically, there's *stepwise progression* (**Figure 13.7**): sudden deteriorations (representing new infarcts), which are stable until the next 'step' down. However, many smaller infarcts make 'steps' less obvious, causing a more gradual progression, and in some cases, a single, importantly located stroke suddenly causes dementia (*strategic infarct dementia*).

Symptoms tend to reflect the sites of lesions, so the presentation may be 'patchy' with sparing of certain cognitive abilities. A subcortical picture can develop where VD affects small, white matter blood vessels. Neurological signs may further support a VD diagnosis, e.g. hemiparesis, dysarthria.

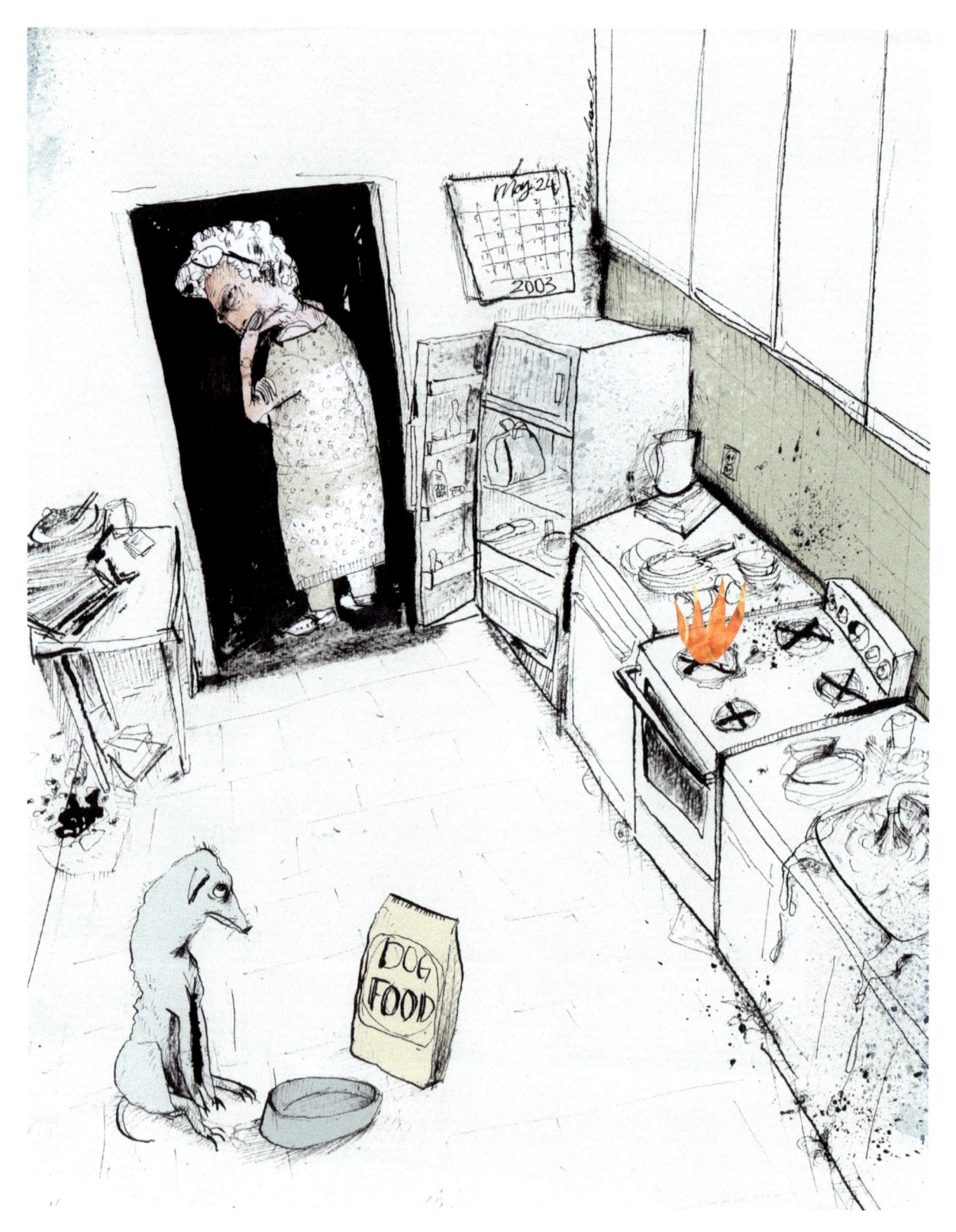

FIGURE 13.6 If undertaking a home visit, which risks would you identify from this woman's kitchen? How could you manage them?

Table 13.1 Summary of dementia subtypes

	AD	VD	DLB
Risk factors	Age Female Vascular risk factors Low IQ/education Head injury Previous depression *Late onset:* APOE ε4 allele *Early onset:* APP mutations, presenilin 1 and 2 mutations	Age Male Vascular risk factors	Age Male APOE ε4 allele
Pathology	Plaques and tangles Cortical atrophy Cholinergic pathway loss	Multiple cortical infarcts Arteriosclerosis	Lewy bodies
Onset	Insidious	Sudden	Variable
Course	Gradual decline	Stepwise decline	Gradual decline, but fluctuating symptoms
Main features	Amnesia Aphasia Agnosia Apraxia	Patchy cognitive impairment	Fluctuating cognition Visual hallucinations Parkinsonism
Other suggestive features	*Absence* of physical signs	Focal neurological deficits	Neuroleptic sensitivity Autonomic instability (e.g. syncope) Recurrent falls
Imaging	Cortical atrophy, especially medial temporal and parietal lobes	Multiple white matter lucencies, atrophy	Atrophy (less than AD), without features of other types

Lewy body dementia

Memory problems are often less prominent than in AD, at least at first. Two of the following symptoms should alert you to the possibility of DLB:

- Fluctuating cognition and alertness.
- Vivid visual hallucinations (often of people/animals).
- Parkinsonian signs (see p. 140).

DLB can be hard to diagnose, especially if parkinsonism presents late. Clues include recurrent falls, syncope, autonomic dysfunction (e.g. incontinence, constipation, postural hypotension), and REM sleep disorder (acting out dreams while asleep). REM sleep disorder may predate DLB by years.

DLB can resemble delirium due to fluctuating cognition and visual hallucinations. However, while delirium may require antipsychotics (neuroleptics), people with DLB must *not* be prescribed antipsychotics: up to 50% experience *neuroleptic sensitivity* (extreme and potentially fatal side effects).

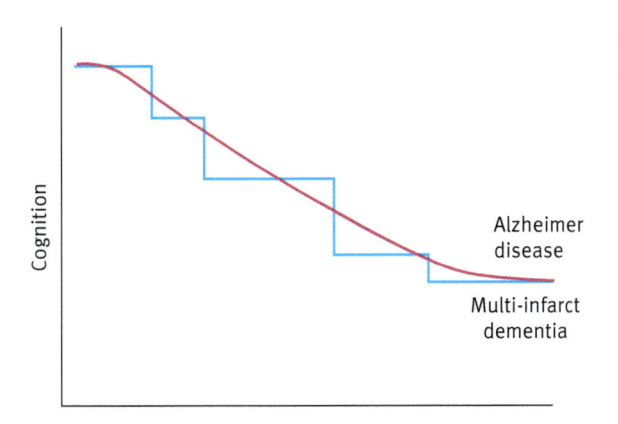

FIGURE 13.7 Cognitive decline: gradual (AD: red) and stepwise (VD: blue).

Differential diagnosis

A low cognitive test score doesn't diagnose dementia; there are many possible reasons (**Box 13.2**). The key

> **BOX 13.2** Causes of a low cognitive test score
>
> - Dementia.
> - Delirium.
> - Current mental disorder, e.g. depression, anxiety, psychosis.
> - Intellectual disability.
> - Limited education or literacy.
> - Sensory impairment.
> - Language or cultural barrier.
> - Feeling unwell, tired, irritable, or unmotivated.

differentials for dementia are mild cognitive impairment (MCI), delirium, pseudodementia, and 'reversible' causes.

- **MCI** (or 'mild neurocognitive disorder') is impairment on cognitive testing which doesn't cross the threshold for dementia. MCI affects 5–20% of people over 65 years, and 10–15% of people with MCI progress to dementia each year. *However*, some people never develop dementia, or simply need treatment of an underlying physical, psychiatric, or sensory problem.
- **Delirium** presents relatively *suddenly* with *fluctuating* confusion, poor attention, and various other symptoms (see p. 130). It's caused by physical ill health; treatment of this resolves the delirium.
- **Pseudodementia** (see p. 38). The *gradual decline* may resemble AD, but in pseudodementia, low mood usually *precedes* cognitive problems and there may be a history of previous depression. Depressed people classically lack motivation and give 'don't know' answers to questions.
- **Reversible causes of new cognitive impairment**, e.g.
  - Brain: subdural haematoma, space-occupying lesion, normal pressure hydrocephalus.
  - Endocrine: hypothyroidism, hypo-/hyperparathyroidism, Addison disease, Cushing syndrome.
  - Vitamin deficiency: B_{12}, folate, thiamine, niacin.

💡 People who develop delirium or pseudodementia are at increased risk of dementia. They should be followed up to optimize their physical and mental health and to monitor cognition.

Investigations

- **Cognitive testing**, e.g. M-ACE (see p. 144).
- **Collateral history**: particularly of duration and course of cognitive impairment, effect on life, risky behaviours.
- **Physical examination and observations** (RR, HR, BP, SpO_2, temperature).
- **Essential blood tests** (for explanations, see p. 130):
  - FBC, U&Es, LFTs, TFTs, vitamin B_{12}, folate, bone profile, CBG (HbA1c if known diabetes), HIV and syphilis testing.
  - Lipid profile (risk factor for AD/VD).
- **Additional tests as suggested by clinical presentation**, e.g. MSU, CXR, blood cultures, wound swabs, sputum/stool samples.
- **Neuroimaging** to exclude other cerebral pathology and help distinguish types of dementia (unless diagnosis is clear, clinically). Focal neurological signs and unusual presentations (e.g. new psychosis in older adults) always require brain scanning.
  - **MRI** is better than CT for early diagnosis and detecting subcortical vascular changes.
  - **SPECT or PET scan** if DLB suspected.
- **ECG** before starting anti-dementia medication.

Management

Although dementia can't be cured, management focuses on enhancing quality of life, independence, and dignity. MHOA teams work closely with carers, GPs, social services, and voluntary organizations to deliver multidisciplinary management. For prevention, see **Box 13.3**.

Biological interventions

Optimize physical health

To reduce confusion and potentially slow the progression of the disease, teams *treat or prevent*:

- *Sensory impairments*, e.g. with hearing aids, spectacles, magnifying glasses.

> **BOX 13.3** Dementia prevention: The Lancet Commission (2017)
>
> A third of *all* dementias could be prevented by modifying risk factors[2]:
>
> - Early life: poor education.
> - Midlife:
>   - Hearing loss.
>   - Hypertension.
>   - Obesity.
> - Late life:
>   - Smoking.
>   - Depression.
>   - Physical inactivity.
>   - Social isolation.
>   - Diabetes.
>
> Data from Livingston G., et al. (2017). Dementia prevention, intervention, and care. *The Lancet* **390**; 2673–734.

- *Causes of delirium* (see p. 129).
- *Pain*—BPSD may communicate pain; simple analgesia may help, e.g. paracetamol.
- *Vascular risk factors*—important in all dementias, but the mainstay of VD management, e.g. with antihypertensives, smoking cessation.

Differences in metabolism and elimination make older people more sensitive to medication side effects. All medications are reviewed, particularly for side effects which impair cognition:

- *Anticholinergic*, e.g. tricyclic antidepressants, urinary antispasmodics.
- *Sedative*, e.g. analgesics, antipsychotics, antihistamines.

Polypharmacy (multiple medications) causes extra drug interactions and side effects; medications are removed or reduced where possible.

Psychotropic medications

The golden rule when prescribing for older people is to use small doses and increase gently (*start low, go slow*).

- *Treat comorbid mental illness*, e.g. consider an antidepressant if depressed.
- *AChEIs*, e.g. donepezil, rivastigmine, are prescribed by specialists for mild to moderate AD or DLB. They stop acetylcholinesterase breaking down acetylcholine, increasing neurotransmitter levels in the synapse. This partially compensates for cholinergic loss, temporarily slowing disease progression or stabilizing symptoms.
- *NMDA receptor antagonists*, e.g. memantine can be used in moderate to severe AD, where acetylcholinesterase inhibitors are contraindicated.

BPSD are managed with behavioural and environmental strategies (see p. 133). Medication is reserved for BPSD causing *extreme distress or immediate risk* to the person or others (e.g. aggression). Antipsychotics or benzodiazepines are used short term and low dose, after carefully weighing benefits against risks (e.g. increased risk of stroke with antipsychotics, falls, confusion). Antipsychotics aren't used in DLB due to parkinsonian side effects, but AChEIs and memantine may help.

> 💡 Medication concordance is hard if you don't *remember* you need tablets, aren't sure if you've taken them, can't read instructions, or can't open bottles. Ask to *see* the person's medications—this may be very revealing!

Psychological interventions

Psychoeducation and *counselling* may help people come to terms with a new, early diagnosis of dementia. Other therapies include:

- *Reminiscence therapy*—encouraging someone to talk about their life, often using prompts from their past, e.g. music, photographs, objects.
- *Cognitive stimulation therapy*—activities that stimulate thinking, concentration, and memory, e.g. word association, categorization and number games; discussing the news.
- *Validation therapy*—validates the emotions behind the person's behaviour, e.g. if someone's looking for their (deceased) mother, carers would recognize and respond to their underlying need for reassurance.
- *Multisensory therapy*—as speech is lost in advanced dementia, touch, music, and other non-verbal stimuli can soothe or stimulate.

Behavioural approaches identify and modify triggers for challenging behaviour. For example, wandering may be triggered by disorientation, anxiety, boredom, hunger, or needing the toilet; it may resolve with reorientation, reassurance, or regular activities/food/toileting. This can be formalized with *ABC charts* (Antecedents, Behaviours, Consequences).

Social interventions

Planning

In early dementia, MHOA teams explore the person's wishes for the future, supporting them to formalize these, e.g. writing an advanced decision ('living will'); appointing a Lasting Power of Attorney (LPA) to manage financial/health decisions, should they lose capacity to make these. Driving is discussed early on: independence must be balanced against safety behind the wheel (see p. 147).

Home support

Teams support people to stay at home as long as possible: it's what most want *and* is therapeutic—people function better in familiar places, and tend to be more confused (at least briefly) when moved to hospitals or residential homes. Additionally, care is *means tested*—the State only pays for the poorest, or those with the greatest needs. This causes tremendous stress, as people may spend thousands of pounds (or even sell their home) to afford care. Social services assess care needs, and undertake means testing.

Practical interventions to help people stay at home include:

- *Dosette boxes/blister packs:* aid medication concordance.
- *Orientation aids:* clearly visible clocks, calendars, written reminders.
- *Environmental modifications*, e.g. remove patterned rugs (trigger visual illusions); change gas to

electric hobs (reduce fire risks from accidentally leaving gas on).
- *Helpcards*: essential information people carry in case of getting lost (e.g. their name, that they have memory problems, carer/GP contact details).
- *Care packages*: help at home, e.g. personal care, meal preparation, medication supervision.
- *Assistive technology*, e.g. sensors alert carers if someone leaves home overnight; tracker watches with panic alarms can help people who get lost or anxious while out and about.

Additionally, *day centres* can provide enjoyable daytime activities and social contact. *Day hospitals* may avoid admission to hospital by providing daily psychiatric care and rehabilitation for those with greater needs.

Care homes

When people *can't* live safely or comfortably at home, they need residential or nursing home care. EMI (elderly mentally infirm) care homes offer maximum support for people with the most complex or challenging needs, e.g. extreme BPSD. GPs and MHOA 'in-reach' support teams can optimize residential and nursing home care.

Carer support

Relatives often soldier on in very difficult circumstances; a *carer's assessment* is essential to identify and support *their* needs, e.g.

- *Emotional* support.
- *Education* about dementia and support services.
- *Training* to manage common problems and know where to seek help.
- *Respite care*, e.g. sitting services/temporary placements.

Voluntary sector organizations

Organizations like the Alzheimer's Society and Age UK offer essential services, including information, advice, advocacy, social groups, befriending, home care, and carer support.

Prognosis

Two-thirds of people with dementia live in their own or their carer's home. Five-year mortality of people diagnosed with dementia is 65% in men and 59% in women, but significantly higher in people who have been admitted to hospital for any cause. This is due to a combination of frailty, comorbid medical conditions, complications (e.g. poor swallow causing aspiration pneumonia), and the disease process itself.

> **!** **Elder abuse** (neglect, psychological, emotional, financial, physical, or sexual abuse) is associated with dementia. It's highest for women living alone with a carer on whom they're dependent for physical or mental health needs. Overwhelmed carers may need extra support: they're at greater risk of perpetrating abuse if they're isolated, unsupported, suffering mental health problems (e.g. depression, substance use), or experienced abuse themselves. Abuse also occurs in care homes or at-home care services: it's more likely with poor supervision and training of low-paid staff, working long hours, in isolation. *Safeguarding concerns* (e.g. bruising, malnutrition, behavioural changes) are documented in detail and reported to social services for investigation.

REALITY

General approach: tips, tricks, and cautionary tales

1. Basics

Home visits are vital to understand how someone's coping with their ADLs; if you can't visit, ask detailed questions about their home situation and seek permission to talk to close contacts.

2. Sensory problems

Before starting, check that the person can hear and see you: find their hearing aids/glasses and remove distractions, e.g. ask to turn off the television.

Don't shout! Many people lip-read to some extent, so don't cover your mouth. Speak clearly and *slightly* slowly, sitting nearer their 'better ear' if they have one. When speaking to carers, keep your face in view of the patient, to help them follow the conversation. Age-related hearing loss (*presbycusis*) affects high-pitched noises most, so using a slightly deeper voice may help. If you're still struggling to communicate, try writing down short questions.

3. Speech problems

People feel frustrated or embarrassed when they can't make themselves understood due to expressive dysphasia or dysarthria. Explain that their point of view is important to you, so you'd like them to speak slowly and may ask carers to help explain what they're saying. If they have dentures, ask them to use them, as these help with clarity. Repeat their key points to check that you've understood correctly.

4. Cognitive impairment considerations

Speak slowly, clearly, and simply. If you're not understood the first time, repeat yourself exactly, and don't be afraid to pause: people with dementia take time to process information and different phrasing can confuse them further. If this doesn't work, use simpler closed and clarifying questions:

> You: What did you do for a living?
> Molly: Huh?
> You: What did you do for a living?
> Molly: Huh?
> You: Did you work?
> Molly: Yes.
> You: What did you do?
> Molly: I was a biochemist.

Be encouraging. If they become upset about their memory, explore easier areas of their history (e.g. childhood/early adulthood memories).

5. Respect

Older people may prefer to be addressed formally, especially by a youthful stranger; they may be insulted if you assume you can use their first name. So start formally (e.g. Ms Patel) and *never* infantilize by calling an older person *Honey, Sweetie, Poppet, Love,* etc. This *may* be appropriate for a carer who knows the person well, but not for you as a medical student or junior doctor.

> 💡 Accept a cup of tea if offered. It builds rapport and tells you lots about functioning. If it's served cold with a sink's plug instead of a teabag, your host needs help around the house (or wants you to leave).

The interview

- • = Example question. * = Question linking to other parts of the history. C = Question best answered by carers.

General screening

- *Do you worry about your memory? Why?*
- *Have other people noticed problems? Such as?*
- *Do you find things confusing? Which things?*

- When did problems begin?
  * Did anything happen around then? *[Life events suggest depression; stroke/TIA suggests VD; physical illness suggests delirium]*
- C How did it progress? *[Screen: gradual/stepwise/sudden or fluctuating]*
- What are you most worried might be causing these problems?

Four As
Amnesia

- *How is your memory? [Screen: forgetting conversations, appointments, people's names; losing things, getting lost]*

Aphasia/dysphasia

- *Do you have any problems communicating?*
  - Do you struggle to find words? *[Expressive dysphasia]*
  - Can you make yourself understood easily? *[Expressive or receptive dysphasia]*
  - Can you always understand what other people are saying? *[Receptive dysphasia]*

Agnosia

- *Do you have difficulties recognizing objects?*
  - What about people's faces? *[Prosopagnosia]*

Apraxia

- *Do you struggle with everyday practical tasks?*
  - For example, tying shoelaces, fastening buttons, driving?
  - *Why? [Exclude motor/sensory impairment]*

Delirium/BPSD
Mood

- *Have you been feeling miserable? Sad?*
  * Which came first: forgetfulness or sadness? *[Pseudodementia]*

Psychosis

- *Have you seen or heard anything that other people don't notice?*
  - For example, hearing people talking? Seeing animals or (tiny) people?
- Is anyone against you? Is anyone trying to harm you?

Personality change

C *Do people think your/their personality has changed?*

Effect on life

ADLs

- *How do these problems affect you, day-to-day?*
- Are there things you can't do easily by yourself now? [Screen Box 13.1]
  * What makes it hard?
  * Have you got any coping strategies?
  * Who helps you?

Risk (Always check with carers too)

General

* *Has anything happened that's worried your family or friends?*

* What do you worry will happen if these problems continue?

Risk to self

* *Do you ever feel like life isn't worth living?*
* Have you ever walked off without knowing where you were, or become lost?
* Have you had any cooking accidents? What happened? [Screen for fires/leaving gas on, especially unlit]
* What did you eat and drink yesterday?
* Are you looking after yourself?

Risk to others

* Do you lose your temper with people? What happens?
  – Have you been violent?
* Have people said you've been too friendly or flirtatious?

---

1. Memory loss history (15 minutes)

Candidate's instructions

Thomas Locke is 66 and works in a sports shop. He's seeing the GP at the request of his manager, who's worried about his memory. You're a medical student at the practice. Please take a history of memory loss.

Patient's brief

Key characteristics

- I don't remember exact details and need to be asked directly about most symptoms to remember that they've been problematic.
- I feel frustrated and worried when I can't remember things.
- I sometimes struggle to find the right word.

History

My manager called me in for a chat, 2 weeks ago. He said I'd been making mistakes for a few months, like not setting the alarm each evening and forgetting to reorder stock. He wasn't angry but wanted to know if there was anything on my mind. When I couldn't think of anything, he said I should see the GP. I'm the best employee he's ever had and the firm doesn't want me to retire!

When I told my husband (Geoffrey), he admitted he'd been worried for about 6 months. He's noticed I go shopping and come home with random items, not the things I went for. He reminded me I keep losing my keys and locking myself out. We attended a party last week and Geoffrey said I was very repetitive.

I've started writing things down so I don't forget them, like the names of Saturday staff and a 'to do' list at work. I've even started taking notes on *EastEnders*, because I can't follow the storylines. I've only got lost once, a few weeks ago: Geoffrey and I split up to shop and agreed to meet at the car park but I couldn't find my way back and had to call him to find me.

I don't struggle with old friends' names, and can remember events from years ago as clearly as if they'd happened yesterday. I'm not depressed—life is good . . . as far as I can remember! I'm full of energy and really enjoy life, especially gardening. I look after myself, but Geoffrey's taken over the cooking and shopping because I make mistakes. He hasn't mentioned a change in my personality. Actually, keeping lists and writing things down means I'm more organized than I used to be, which is a good thing, right?

Other history
- My older brother, Jack, got Alzheimer's in his late fifties. He died in a nursing home at 63.

- Nobody in my family, including me, has had a mental illness.
- I have high blood pressure and take tablets for this.
- I don't smoke or use drugs. I drink 2 pints of beer a week.

Questions
What happens next?

Worries
I'm losing my memory, like Jack. I'll end up in a home.

💡 **Thomas may have dementia (most likely AD, given his family history), but it's important not to jump to conclusions. Acknowledge his anxiety but reassure him that there are many causes of memory problems, and most are reversible. The GP will want to talk to his husband, perform memory tests (e.g. M-ACE), and organize some tests (bloods, urinalysis, CT head, ECG). If needed, he can then be referred to a memory clinic for expert input, including medicines to help with memory.**

2. Cognitive impairment: collateral history (15 minutes)

Candidate's instructions
Naomi Johnson is a 21-year-old bank clerk who lives with her grandmother. She's brought her grandmother to the GP because she's worried about her memory. You're a medical student and will see Naomi while the GP examines her grandmother. Please take a collateral history of cognitive impairment.

Carer's brief
Key characteristics
- I'm worried about Gran and whether I can cope; I feel I'm letting her down.
- I'm tearful, tired, and need help.

History
Gran's always been a great cook and loved having the whole family for Christmas dinner every year. This year she couldn't get the timings right and all we had was roast potatoes. That wasn't like her, and she seemed really muddled, so I decided to move in to help out. Her memory was perfect until December (9 months ago); it seemed like a sudden change. She suddenly got a lot worse in March, but seems to have stayed at that level since.

I have to wash and dress her. It's not that she can't physically do it, but she can't organize herself and wouldn't remember it needed doing. I do all the cooking and shopping. She comes shopping with me but I keep a close eye on her because she gets lost easily, even though she's lived here her whole life. Gran sometimes confuses me with my mum and calls me Moira.

She's got too much energy, always pacing about. She hasn't tried to leave, but I've caught her 'cooking' in the middle of the night. Once, she put the instant coffee in the kettle with the water before she boiled it, which really worried me. We've got a gas stove and I worry she'll leave it on. She's wet herself a couple of times and it's really upset her. Sometimes she gets really scared and says she sees 'spirits' but I can't see anything. Otherwise, she seems fairly happy and enjoys pottering about the garden. She pulls the heads off the flowers before they've died now, but I know she's trying to be helpful.

Other history
- Gran's never had any mental health problems.
- She had two 'mini strokes' last autumn: one side went limp and her speech was slurred. She got better each time within a few hours.
- Gran's had high blood pressure and diabetes for years; she takes aspirin, a water tablet, and insulin injections.
- She's never smoked or drunk alcohol.
- My great-granny died of a heart attack.

Questions
Will social services help us? Does she have Alzheimer's?

Worries
She's home alone during the day, but I'll lose my job if I take more time off.

> 💡 Naomi's grandmother may have VD, but it's essential to rule out delirium and other reversible causes first. Social services should be contacted urgently to assess her for a package of care and provide Naomi with a carer's assessment. Naomi needs support in her own right; she shouldn't be expected to cope with this alone.

NEXT STEPS

Capacity and a dangerous discharge

You're an FY1 in elderly care medicine. Lily Watson, 78, is a retired librarian. She was admitted following her fourth fall at home in 6 months. She has a year's history of DLB and is reluctantly under the care of the MHOA team. Ms Watson has twice-daily carer visits and her niece, Laura, phones daily and visits monthly, despite living 50 miles away. Laura describes her aunt as 'fiercely independent' and says she's vowed she'll 'never go into a home'.

The ward physiotherapist is worried that Ms Watson won't be safe at home; she can't climb stairs and has trouble turning around. He tried to discuss this with her today, but she said she'd manage 'perfectly well' using the stairs to reach her bedroom and bathroom, then crossly packed her bags and demanded a taxi to take her home. You've been called to the ward.

- How will you assess and manage this situation?

Immediate containment

Attend as soon as possible, but while on the telephone, ask staff to let Ms Watson know that you're coming and how long you'll be. *Don't* call a taxi just yet! Courtesy and a cup of tea should suffice, but if Ms Watson makes active attempts to leave the ward, staff may keep her there until you arrive, if they believe that she lacks capacity to self-discharge against medical advice, under the MCA.

Preparation

Gather information from Ms Watson's notes, the MHOA team, and ward staff. With her permission, speak with her niece and any other close contacts. Focus on:

- Concerns about her ability to manage at home, especially risks, e.g. falls, leaving gas on, not eating, wandering, refusing carers' visits.
- Objective evidence of problems, before and during this admission, e.g. falls.
- Multidisciplinary team recommendations about increasing her care package and how soon these could be implemented (check with social worker).

Check whether she has a LPA or any advance directives regarding her medical care; these should be consulted and followed, if present.

Assessment

Assess Ms Watson:

- Look for evidence in your mental state examination of disorientation, poor memory or concentration, low mood, delusions, and hallucinations.
- Test her cognitive function, e.g. M-ACE ± frontal lobe testing (p. 143).
- Briefly assess mobility, e.g. walking, transfers, turning.

Check she understands the risks:

- Is she aware of the concerns?
- Does she foresee any problems?
- How will she manage at home?
- Will she need/accept help?
- Share the team's concerns, e.g. she can't climb stairs/ she falls because she forgets to use her walking frame.

Assess Ms Watson's capacity to make the decision to go home. To lack capacity, she must have:

- A disorder of brain or mind (e.g. DLB) *and*:
- Inability to do at least one of the following:
    - *Understand* the relevant information.
    - *Retain* the information long enough to . . .
    - *Weigh* the decision (pros and cons) to come to a conclusion, and . . .
    - *Communicate* her decision.

Management: has capacity

People can make *unwise* choices, if they have capacity to make the decision. Ms Watson can choose to go home, accepting a high risk of falls, provided she can understand, retain, and weigh these concerns, and communicate her decision.

Document your assessment clearly and discuss with your registrar/consultant. Inform Laura, and ensure urgent social services and MHOA follow up.

Management: lacks capacity

If you suspect a *reversible* problem affecting Ms Watson's capacity to make this decision, you must make every effort to address this before reassessing her capacity, e.g.:

- Deafness/non-English speaker: locate her hearing aid/book an interpreter.
- Delirium: treat the underlying cause in Ms Watson's best interests, using the MCA, and allow time for delirium to resolve.

Unfortunately, Ms Watson still wants to go home, adamant that she's been using the stairs safely all week, has never fallen, and will be safe at home without any help.

Document that she lacks capacity to make the decision about going home, detailing what she can't currently understand, retain, weigh, and/or communicate. It's in her best interests to be prevented from leaving the ward in the meantime. The MCA (or very occasionally, the MHA) will be needed as a legal framework; discuss this with a liaison psychiatrist.

Arrange a 'best interests meeting', involving Laura and the multidisciplinary team. Discuss the risks and benefits of discharge home, and Ms Watson's known wishes prior to losing capacity to make this decision. An independent mental capacity advocate (IMCA) can be arranged to help her represent her views. Although she may be at high risk of falls, this *doesn't* mean she *must* go into a care home. It may be possible to honour her wishes by minimizing the risks, e.g.:

- Arranging a limited *microenvironment* with a bed and commode on the ground floor of her home.
- Increasing her care package to four visits a day.
- Arranging a personal alarm so that she can call for help in case of falls.
- Leaving notes to remind her to use her Zimmer frame.
- Turning off the gas supply to her stove.
- MHOA team follow-up.

💡 Unfortunately, 3 months later, Ms Watson is readmitted after falling again and breaking her arm. Another best interests meeting is convened, and it's decided that her risk can no longer be managed safely at home. Although Laura's sad that her aunt now needs a residential home, she thinks the last 3 months were 'exactly what Aunt Lily would have wanted'.

Movie buff
Amour (2012).
Away From Her (2006).
Iris (2001).
Still Alice (2014).

Book shelf
Bayley, J. (1998) *Iris: A Memoir of Iris Murdoch*: a husband's poignant account of life before and after the acclaimed writer's dementia.

Boylan, C. (1999) *Beloved Stranger*: a beautifully written novel on the impact of late-onset affective disorders on children and partners.

Brown, M., Clegg, D. (Eds.) (2007). *Ancient Mysteries: Stories from the Trebus Project*: available from: www.trebusprojects.org/read/stories-from-the-archive. Remarkable narrative series by people living with dementia, bearing witness to 28 people's experiences and memories.

Everett, P.L. (2001) *Erasure*: coping with a parent's dementia, dignity, care, safety, ethnicity, identity, and individuality are poignantly explored in this readable novel.

Grant, L. (1998) *Remind Me Who I Am, Again*: a memoir exploring VD, loss, guilt, and bureaucratic intervention.

Ignatieff, M. (1993) *Scar Tissue*: AD from a son's perspective, examining the gulf between scientific explanation and personal experience.

Rule, J. (1987) *Memory Board*: a novel praised for its frank expression of sexuality and inclusion of older adults as central characters.

Notes

1. Genova, L. (2007) *Still Alice*. Bloomington, IN: iUniverse.
2. Livingston G., Sommerlad, A., Orgeta, V., et al. (2017) Dementia prevention, intervention, and care. *The Lancet*, **390**, 2673–734.

Journal club

Alzheimer's Disease International (2015) World Alzheimer Report 2015. The global impact of dementia: an analysis of prevalence, incidence, cost and trends. www.alz.co.uk/research/WorldAlzheimerReport2015.pdf

Alzheimer's Society (2014) Dementia UK update (2nd ed.). www.alzheimers.org.uk/sites/default/files/migrate/downloads/dementia_uk_update.pdf

Go to www.oup.com/uk/stringer2e for a wealth of additional resources, including an OCSE mark scheme, filmed scenarios, and self-assessment questions.

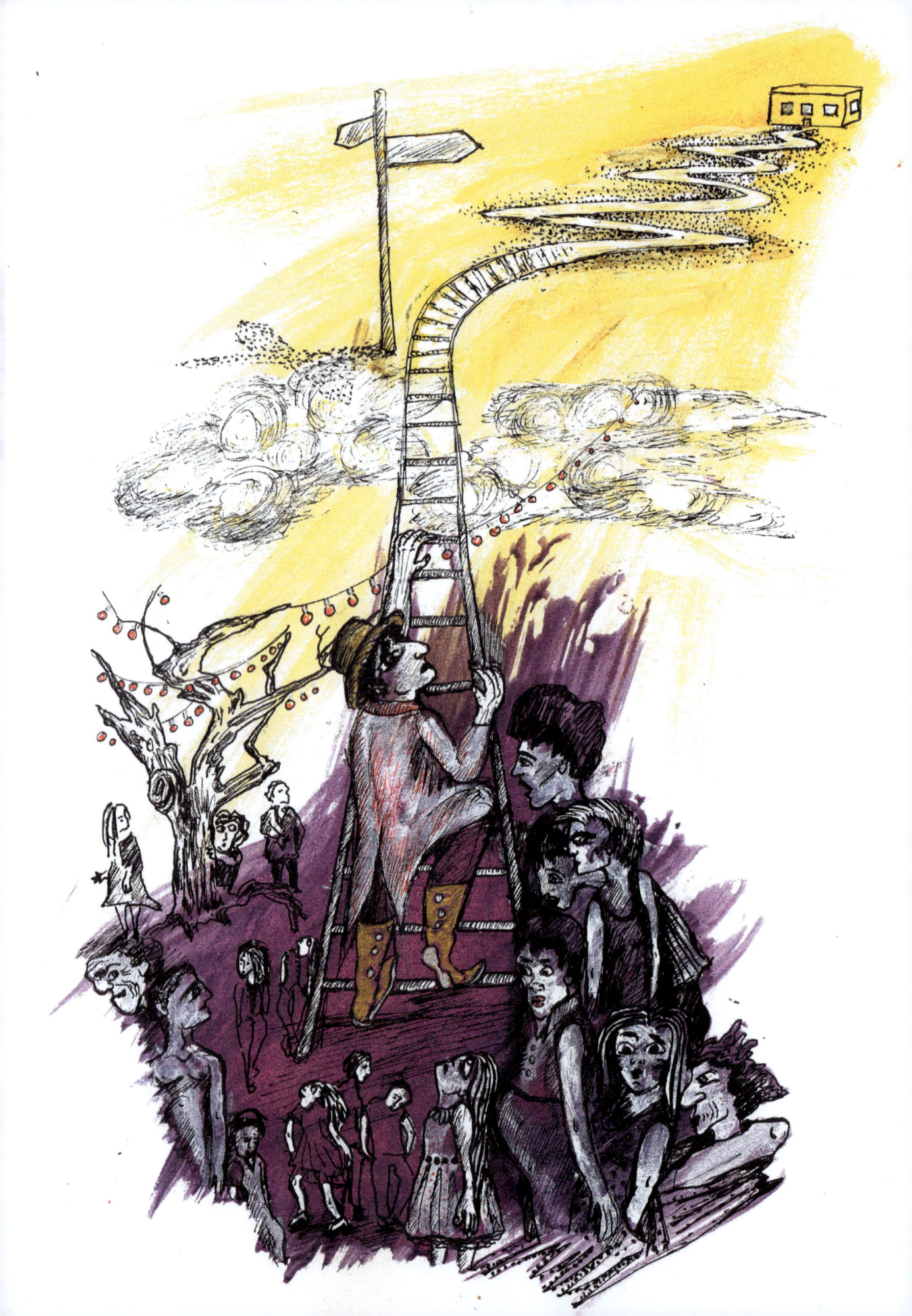

14 Anxiety Disorders

True or false?

Answers on p. 277

1. GABA receptor agonists reduce anxiety.
2. Negative reinforcement allows habituation to a fearful stimulus.
3. Social anxiety disorder is equally common in men and women.
4. Streptococcal throat infections are a risk factor for obsessive–compulsive disorder (OCD).
5. During a panic attack, paraesthesia may be experienced, secondary to hypocalcaemia.
6. Anxiety should reduce during the first few days on a selective serotonin reuptake inhibitor.
7. Systematic desensitization is useful in treating OCD.
8. Following a catastrophic event, formal psychological debriefing helps prevent post-traumatic stress disorder.
9. An anxious patient with tachypnoea should be helped to rebreathe CO_2 with the use of a paper bag.
10. A medical student confides that her GP prescribed beta-blockers for examination anxiety. You should report this to her clinical tutor if she refuses to do so.

Contents

Principles
Introduction
Epidemiology
Aetiology
- Genetics
- Childhood and life events

Main theories
- Neurotransmitter theories
- Neuroanatomical theories
- Psychological theories

Clinical presentation
- Generalized anxiety disorder
- Panic disorder
- Phobias
- Obsessive–compulsive disorder
- Body dysmorphic disorder
- Post-traumatic stress disorder

Differential diagnosis
Investigations
Management
- Biological interventions
- Psychological interventions
- Social interventions

Prognosis

Reality
General approach: tips, tricks, and cautionary tales
The interview
- OCD history
- Agoraphobia history

Next steps
An anxious colleague in need of help
- Differential diagnosis
- Immediate intervention
- Treatment

PRINCIPLES

'The thing that is in Room 101 is the worst thing in the world . . . The worst thing in the world', said O'Brien, 'varies from individual to individual. It may be burial alive, or death by fire, or by drowning, or by impalement, or fifty other deaths. There are cases where it is some quite trivial thing, not even fatal . . . In your case,' said O'Brien, 'the worst thing in the world happens to be rats.'

George Orwell, *Nineteen Eighty-Four*[1]

Introduction

Anxiety is a normal and necessary human emotion. Over the years, it's protected us from nonchalant extinction, inspired us to bungee jump, and given us the extra 'push' we needed to pass exams. Anxiety is vital, if a little uncomfortable at times.

In anxiety *disorders*, the normal anxiety response is exaggerated, and triggered by a trivial or non-existent threat. This chapter covers disorders in which anxiety is central: generalized anxiety disorder (GAD), panic disorder, phobias, obsessive–compulsive disorder (OCD), body dysmorphic disorder (BDD), and post-traumatic stress disorder (PTSD).

> 💡 In some cultures, there's no equivalent word for anxiety. People might describe their bodily experiences or a specific aspect of their anxiety, e.g. 'my heart is not at rest' (West Africa) or 'thinking too much' (Cambodia).

Epidemiology

Anxiety disorders are very common (**Table 14.1**). Most affect women roughly twice as commonly as men. The exceptions are social anxiety disorder, OCD, and BDD, where men and women are affected equally.

Aetiology

Genetics

Family and twin studies support a genetic contribution to anxiety disorders, conveyed by multiple genes of small effect. Risk is four to six times higher in relatives of affected people, and heritability is estimated at 30–50%. Relatives of people with a particular anxiety disorder are at increased risk of a *range* of anxiety disorders. This may reflect vulnerability conferred by certain personality traits such as introversion, harm avoidance, and neuroticism (see p. 261). A quarter of patients with OCD have premorbid anankastic personality traits. There's also a strong genetic overlap between anxiety disorders and depression.

Childhood and life events

Childhood adversity predisposes people to anxiety disorders. Life events can trigger anxiety disorders, especially

Table 14.1 Prevalence of anxiety disorders

Disorder	12-month prevalence[a]	Lifetime prevalence[b]
Any anxiety disorder (meeting criteria for 1 or more disorders)	18%	29%
Specific phobia	9%	13%
Social anxiety disorder	7%	12%
PTSD	4%	7%
GAD	3%	6%
Panic disorder	3%	5%
OCD	1%	2%
Agoraphobia (without panic disorder)	0.8%	1%
BDD	1.7%	2.4%

Data from: (a) Kessler, R.C., et al. (2005) Prevalence, severity, and comorbidity of twelvemonth DSM-IV disorders in the National Comorbidity Survey Replication (NCS-R). *Archives of General Psychiatry*, **62**, 617–27; (b) Kessler, R.C., Berglund, P.A., Demler, O., Jin, R., and Walters, E.E. (2005) Lifetime prevalence and age-of-onset distributions of DSM-IV disorders in the National Comorbidity Survey Replication (NCS-R). *Archives of General Psychiatry*, **62**, 593–602.

if they're experienced as threatening, e.g. someone's employer making redundancies.

By definition, PTSD is caused by *extreme* trauma: the risk of developing PTSD is associated with the degree of exposure, proximity, and human contribution to the traumatic event (e.g. torture is more strongly associated with PTSD than natural disasters). However, only about 10% of people who experience extreme trauma develop PTSD. Twin studies show that around a third of the variance in susceptibility is genetic. Risk factors include neuroticism, a personal or family history of psychiatric problems, childhood abuse, and poor early attachment. 'Survivor guilt' and continued exposure to the trauma or other stressors can perpetuate symptoms.

Main theories

Neurotransmitter theories

It's thought that the central neurotransmitters serotonin, noradrenaline, and gamma-aminobutyric acid (GABA) are dysregulated (underactive) in anxiety disorders. This is supported by the fact that drugs for anxiety target their action:

- Serotonin: selective serotonin reuptake inhibitors (SSRIs).
- Noradrenaline: tricyclic antidepressants (TCAs).
- GABA: benzodiazepines (GABA agonists).

Other substances may also play a role, such as the excitatory neurotransmitter glutamate, and a range of neuropeptides, e.g. cholecystokinin (CCK) and corticotropin-releasing factor (CRF) (influence stress and emotional circuitry).

Neuroanatomical theories

Functional hyperactivity of the amygdala (part of the limbic system with a key role in fear processing) is found in anxiety disorders. This is marked in PTSD, and associated with atrophy of the hippocampus, which plays a key role in short-term memory. This suggests that distorted processing and storage of traumatic memories could explain how they're involuntarily 'relived' rather than voluntarily 'remembered' in PTSD.

The basal ganglia and OCD are linked in several illnesses including Sydenham's chorea, encephalitis lethargica, and Tourette syndrome. Streptococcal throat infection may be followed by Sydenham's chorea; by OCD symptoms accompanied by anti-basal ganglia antibodies; and by PANDAS (paediatric autoimmune neuropsychiatric disorder associated with streptococcal infection)—in which OCD develops suddenly in children. Neuroimaging studies link OCD with deficient frontal lobe inhibition, possibly explaining why obsessions are so hard to suppress in OCD.

> **BOX 14.1** Little Albert and the rat
>
> Albert, an 11-month-old boy, played happily with a white rat until scientists made loud clanging noises whenever the rat appeared. Being very young, Albert was frightened of loud noises. However, through pairing the rat with noise, Albert became terrified of the *rat* (and anything resembling the rat, including white beards).
>
> Data from Watson, J.B. and Rayner, R. (1920) Conditioned emotional reactions. *Journal of Experimental Psychology*, **3**, 1–14.

Psychological theories

Classical conditioning: repeatedly pairing a neutral stimulus with a frightening one creates fear in response to the neutral stimulus alone (**Box 14.1**).

Negative reinforcement: behaviours which *relieve* anxiety (e.g. running away) are repeated. This prevents habituation (getting used to the stimulus and calming down), so anxiety is maintained after escaping a fearful stimulus.

Cognitive theories: worrying thoughts are repeated in an automatic way, which both induces and maintains the anxiety response.

Attachment theory: the quality of attachment between children and their parents affects their confidence as adults: insecurely attached children become anxious adults.

Clinical presentation

Anxiety presents with a range of physical and psychological symptoms (**Table 14.2**, **Figure 14.1**). The pattern, timing, and trigger(s) differ according to the particular anxiety disorder (**Table 14.3**). Avoidance and escape are common to most anxiety disorders, and people may develop safety-seeking behaviours (SSBs). SSBs are coping strategies, which *temporarily* reduce anxiety or seem to avert catastrophe (e.g. seeking reassurance).

Generalized anxiety disorder

In GAD, anxiety is *continuous and generalized* ('free-floating'). The person *worries about anything and everything*, e.g. work, health, relationships, past mistakes, imminent catastrophes. Physical symptoms (**Table 14.2**) are often prominent (e.g. tension headaches). Panic attacks occur in severe cases. To diagnose GAD, symptoms must be present for at least several months, although their intensity may fluctuate.

Panic disorder

Anxiety is intermittent and without an obvious trigger: it comes 'out of the blue'. A panic attack is a sudden attack

Table 14.2 Symptoms of anxiety

Symptom group	Examples
Psychological	Fears/worries
	Poor concentration
	Irritability
	Feelings of unreality (depersonalization, derealization)
	Insomnia
	Nightmares
Motor	Restlessness, fidgeting
	Feeling 'on edge'/unable to relax
Neuromuscular	Trembling/tremor
	Headache (e.g. tension headache: like a 'tight band')
	Muscle aches (especially neck and back)
	Feeling dizzy, light-headed, unsteady
	Tinnitus
Gastrointestinal	Dry mouth
	Difficulty swallowing/'lump in the throat'
	Nausea
	Indigestion/stomach pains
	'Butterflies' (churning stomach)
	Flatulence
	Frequent/loose motions
Cardiovascular	Chest discomfort
	Palpitations: feeling the heart 'pound' or 'miss beats'
Respiratory	Shortness of breath
	'Tight'/constricted chest
Genitourinary	Urinary frequency
	Erectile dysfunction
	Amenorrhoea

of extreme ('100%') anxiety, associated with physical symptoms, such as:

- Breathing difficulties.
- Choking sensations.
- Chest discomfort/tightness.
- Palpitations.
- Pins and needles/numbness (hands, feet, lips; see **Box 14.2**).
- Depersonalization/derealization.
- Tremor.

- Dizziness, fainting.
- Sweating.

People commonly think they're having a heart attack or stroke, or fear they'll die, 'lose control', or 'go mad'. These alarming thoughts exacerbate panic, until they gain reassurance or engage in SSBs (e.g. calling an ambulance, taking aspirin). Panic attacks are self-limiting, usually lasting less than 30 minutes, although they can *feel* never-ending.

For a diagnosis of panic *disorder*, there must be recurrent panic attacks (several within a month). Between episodes, the person is fairly anxiety free.

> The mischievous Greek god, Pan, supposedly leapt out and surprised travellers in the woods, causing attacks of extreme anxiety—hence, *panic*.

Phobias

In these disorders, *intermittent anxiety occurs in specific but ordinary circumstances.* People characteristically *avoid* or *escape* feared situations, only seeking treatment when this becomes disabling.

Specific phobias

Specific objects or situations trigger anxiety, e.g. spiders (arachnophobia). Phobias often develop in childhood, although sometimes begin later, usually after a frightening experience. The level of disability depends on how easily the person can avoid the thing they fear, e.g. a doctor with haemophobia (blood phobia) would be severely disabled. Phobias rarely resemble other diagnoses, but comorbid depression should be excluded.

> Blood, injury, and needle phobias cause strong vasovagal reactions, with bradycardia and hypotension. Although this has an evolutionary advantage (fainting into the 'recovery position' once injured), it complicates phlebotomy! Take blood with the person lying down, to avoid fainting and falls.

Social anxiety disorder (social phobia)

Onset is usually in late teenage years. *The core fear is of being scrutinized, judged, or criticized by others; they dread embarrassment or public humiliation.* People struggle with situations where the focus is (potentially) on them, e.g. dinner parties, board meetings, dating, public speaking. SSBs include self-medication with alcohol/drugs, which afford *psychological avoidance*. People may seek help for 'embarrassing' symptoms, which draw attention to their anxiety, e.g. blushing, trembling, sweating, stuttering. Note that they can usually tolerate crowds (unlike in agoraphobia), as the focus isn't on *them*.

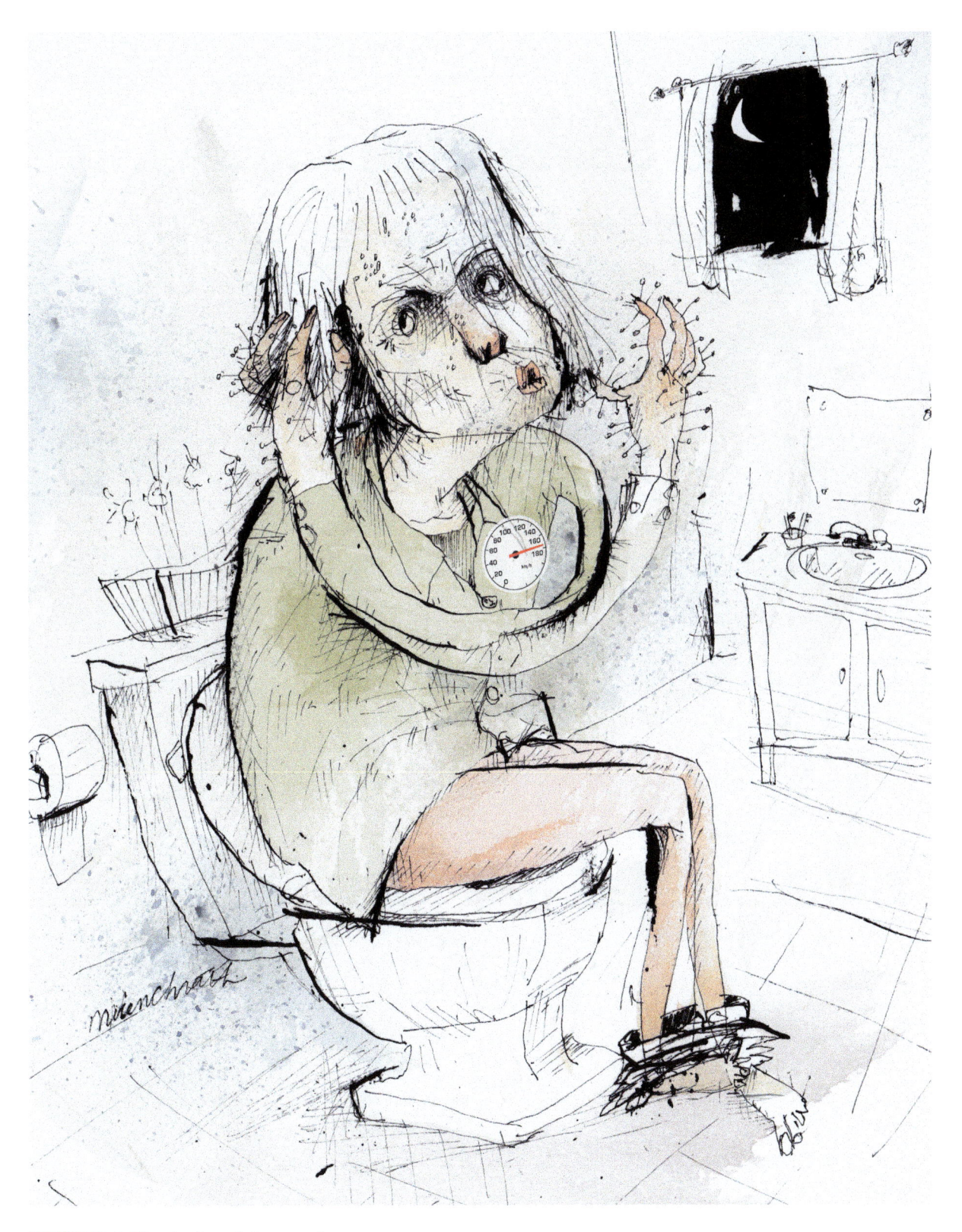

FIGURE 14.1 Physical anxiety symptoms

Agoraphobia

Onset is commonly in the twenties or mid-thirties and may be gradual or precipitated by a panic attack. The uniting fear is of being *unable to escape to a safe place* (usually home). Agoraphobia *includes fear of open spaces (e.g. parks) and situations that are confined or difficult to leave*, e.g.:

- Trains, planes, or buses.
- Lifts.

Table 14.3 Anxiety disorders overview

Diagnosis	Anxiety pattern Continuous	Anxiety pattern Episodic	Triggers/worries	Ask specifically about...
GAD	✓		Everything/many things, e.g. relationships, money, work, health, future	Chronic physical anxiety symptoms Apprehension
Panic disorder		✓	Nothing/don't know (panic attacks *just happen*)	Recurrent panic attacks Beliefs about what's happening, e.g. heart attack, stroke, dying?
Specific phobia		✓	Specific thing, e.g. cockroaches/vomit/spiders	Effect on life
Social anxiety disorder (social phobia)		✓	Judgement/scrutiny, humiliation, e.g. intimate gatherings, public speaking	'Visible anxiety,' e.g. sweating, blushing, trembling Self-scrutiny/judgement
Agoraphobia		✓	Feeling trapped, unable to escape to a safe place, e.g. crowds, public transport	Shrinking of the area considered 'safe' Panic attacks
OCD		✓	*Obsessions*: recurrent, unpleasant thoughts/images/impulses/doubts. Common themes: sex/violence/danger/contamination/illness/immorality/religion/order Triggers for obsessions, e.g. seeing dirt if worried about contamination	*Compulsions*: repetitive, stereotyped rituals (relieve anxiety caused by obsessions) Commonly: counting, cleaning, ordering, checking
BDD		✓	Excessive worry about appearance or a body part being ugly/abnormal Social scrutiny/reminders of appearance	Self-checking: mirror-checking, photos, measuring Covering, camouflaging, grooming Attempts to change appearance
PTSD	✓*	✓**	Extremely severe trauma (and reminders of this), e.g. rape, war, major fire **Re-experiencing*: flashbacks, nightmares, intrusive memories	*Hyperarousal Mood changes, e.g. irritability, numbness, depression

- Supermarkets and queues.
- Crowds.
- Sitting in the middle of the row in cinemas.

The overwhelming urge is to return home to safety. The prospect of leaving home generates anxiety, the severity increasing with distance from home or difficulty returning. Access to a dependable companion (or sometimes a car) can increase the person's geographical range and makes situations more bearable. Those worst affected become housebound, dependent on a small circle of family or friends. See p. 184 for a case study.

💡 **Agoraphobia literally means 'fear of the market place'.**

> **BOX 14.2** Panic attack biochemistry
>
> Hyperventilation (rapid, shallow breathing) blows off carbon dioxide (CO_2), lowering pCO_2 and raising pH (*respiratory alkalosis*). This lowers the level of (unbound) Ca^{2+} ions in the blood (hypocalcaemia), affecting nerve conduction and causing paraesthesia (tingling, numbness) in hands, feet, and around the mouth. In extreme cases, carpopedal spasm (involuntary contraction of hands and feet) occurs.

Obsessive–compulsive disorder

Obsessions are unwanted, unpleasant, and intrusive, repeatedly entering the mind despite attempts to resist them. They can be:

- *Thoughts*, e.g. 'I'm dirty!'
- *Images*, e.g. imagining your parents having sex.
- *Impulses*, e.g. the urge to shout 'bomb' in an airport.
- *Doubts*, e.g. 'Did I turn off the oven?'

Obsessions are *egodystonic* (conflict uncomfortably with the person's self-image) and are in no way enjoyable. Common themes include:

- *Contamination/illness*, e.g. catching HIV.
- *Sex*, e.g. fear of being a paedophile (when this feels repugnant, *not* enjoyable).
- *Harming self or others*, e.g. through violence, accidents, or mistakes.
- *Sacrilege/immorality*, e.g. urges to shout something blasphemous in a mosque.
- *Need for order or symmetry*, e.g. to feel 'right', be 'lucky', or prevent harm.

Although generally the sufferer recognizes that obsessions are *irrational or untrue,* they cause deep discomfort or anxiety, often because they bring a terrible feeling that *something bad might happen*. This anxiety is 'neutralized' with a *compulsion*.

Compulsions are repeated, stereotyped rituals that the person feels they must *do, to end the anxiety from an obsession.* They're neither pleasant nor inherently useful. They may be 'overt' (observable by others, e.g. cleaning, checking, counting aloud, ordering objects, hoarding) or 'covert' (e.g. mentally counting or repeating a phrase). The link between obsessions and compulsions may seem vaguely logical or completely unrelated. Compulsions are usually done in a very particular way, and if done 'incorrectly', the person may have to start all over again, taking hours, causing 'obsessional slowness', and severely affecting quality of life. Long term, resistance to both obsessions and compulsions may decrease or disappear.

So, a loving mother with OCD might have urges (obsessions) to throw her baby downstairs—it's the last thing she'd ever do, but makes her feel extremely anxious, *just in case* she succumbs. To reduce anxiety, she might touch the safety gate at the top of the stairs 100 times, or order the baby's clothes to make them symmetrical (compulsions). She might also have SSBs, e.g. only holding the baby if her partner is nearby. See p. 183 for a full case study.

> 💡 We all have intrusive thoughts that pop into our heads for no reason. We usually ignore them, e.g. while standing on a train platform: 'I could jump in front of that train!' People with OCD try to resist these thoughts, bringing them on more strongly. To experience this, *don't* think of purple penguins for 1 minute.

> 💡 *Thought–action fusion* is the idea that *thinking something is as bad as doing it* or that *thinking something makes it more likely to happen*. It's a type of *magical thinking*, common in OCD, and an extension of superstition. To experience it, think of the person you love most in the world. Picture them clearly in your mind. Now, write their name in the gap: 'I want _____ to die.' How do you feel? Can you do it? If not, why not? You know it's silly, but *what if it makes it happen*—right?

Body dysmorphic disorder

In BDD, people are *excessively worried about their appearance, believing that part of their body is ugly or abnormal,* often focusing on their face, head, or skin. The flaw is either imagined or extremely minor (e.g. slightly crooked nose), but they can't stop thinking about it. As in OCD, thoughts are recurrent, intrusive, and unpleasant, producing anxiety, which the person tries to decrease with repetitive actions. Insight into the irrationality of the belief varies. Behaviours include recurrent checking (via photos, mirrors, measuring, or touch); protracted and excessive grooming; or using make-up or clothing to camouflage or cover the area. They may try to 'correct' the perceived defect, e.g. taping back ears, cosmetic surgery, or desperate self-surgery (e.g. cutting their ears with scissors).

Post-traumatic stress disorder

PTSD was initially recognized in military psychiatry, where labels included 'shell shock', 'combat fatigue', and 'battle exhaustion'. *PTSD occurs after suffering or witnessing an exceptionally threatening or catastrophic traumatic event.* The trauma is often experienced as life-threatening, and should be likely to cause anyone extreme distress, e.g. natural disasters, war, serious

Clinical presentation **173**

assault, rape, torture, terrorism. There's no 'normal' way to react to such terrible events; everyone copes in their own way, and PTSD is only considered where symptoms are prolonged and disabling. PTSD usually begins within 6 months of the trauma, though there's often a delay before symptoms appear ('latency period'). Symptoms fall into the following groups:

Hyperarousal

- Unable to relax.
- Hypervigilance: constantly feeling on 'red alert'.
- Enhanced startle reflex (exaggerated reaction to unexpected stimuli).
- Insomnia.
- Poor concentration.
- Irritability.

Re-experiencing

- Flashbacks: vividly *reliving* the trauma (e.g. hearing, seeing, smelling the event, 'as if it's happening all over again').
- Nightmares.
- Intrusive memories: remembering the trauma without wanting to (NB: despite these, the person may not remember the entire trauma).

Avoidance

- Avoiding reminders of the event, including the setting, in case they trigger re-experiencing and anxiety.
- Trying not to *think* about the trauma.

Other changes

- Emotional detachment ('numbness').
- Reduced interest in activities.
- Powerful emotions including anger, depression, shame, and uncontrollable crying.

People may suffer comorbid depression or use drugs or alcohol to block out painful memories.

Complex PTSD is a severe and disabling condition, resulting from *inescapable, repeated or prolonged trauma*, e.g. childhood sexual abuse, slavery, torture. Extra, chronic symptoms include difficulties regulating emotion, pervasive negative views of self (worthless, shameful, guilty, a failure), and problems trusting people and maintaining close relationships.

> 💡 People may feel that they *should* have coped with a trauma, and are somehow 'weak' to suffer PTSD. Gently put them right—even the Marines get PTSD.

Differential diagnosis of anxiety disorders

Broadly speaking, the following differentials and comorbidities should be considered

- **Organic:** before diagnosing any anxiety disorder, consider physical causes for symptoms via history, examination, ± investigations (see **Table 14.4**).
  - **Substance misuse:** comorbid alcohol/drug use is common (especially in social phobia). Additionally, some intoxication or withdrawal states produce anxiety symptoms.
- **Psychosis:** can create anxiety, social withdrawal, or unusual thoughts.
- **Depression:** often comorbid; anxiety symptoms are common in depression, and depression can complicate anxiety disorders. *Generally, diagnose the disorder which came first and is most prominent, but don't be afraid to diagnose both*, if criteria are met.
  - *Mixed depressive and anxiety disorder:* low-level anxiety and depressive symptoms present equally together, neither justifying diagnosis alone.
- **Another anxiety disorder:** anxiety disorders can be hard to distinguish. *Diagnosis is based on the most important and disabling features, but remember that in real life, things aren't always clear cut, e.g. someone with OCD might also have agoraphobia symptoms.* Common mix-ups include:
  - *Panic disorder versus panic attacks:* panic disorder lacks triggers; panic attacks mark severity in another disorder with clear triggers.
  - *Panic disorder versus agoraphobia:* people often avoid or escape the places where they experience panic attacks, which can produce a broader picture of agoraphobia (agoraphobia is classified as *with or without panic disorder*).
  - *Social anxiety disorder versus agoraphobia:* both can cause social withdrawal. Ask which they'd dislike most: being in the middle of a large crowd (agoraphobia) or having to speak in a small group of strangers (social anxiety disorder).
  - *OCD versus agoraphobia:* time-consuming compulsions or contamination fears can make people housebound. Ask *why* they can't go out.
  - *OCD versus BDD:* repetitive rituals are common to both. Distorted body image suggests BDD.
  - *BDD versus social anxiety disorder:* fear of scrutiny is shared, but focused on physical appearance in BDD.
  - *PTSD versus acute stress reaction*—see **Box 14.3**.

> **BOX 14.3 Acute stress reaction**
>
> Most people would regard an acute stress reaction as an understandable 'state of shock' in response to traumatic events: the same events which can ultimately trigger PTSD. Acute stress reactions are characterized by:
>
> - Transience: start within minutes of the trauma and resolve spontaneously within hours to a few days.
> - Dazed/detached presentation.
> - Amnesia for the event; depersonalization/derealization.
> - Disorientation, agitation, irritability, panic, or aggression.
>
> People should be given medical treatment for any injuries, then emotional support and reassurance. Benzodiazepines can alleviate extreme short-term distress, but don't prevent later PTSD. *Formal*, immediate, psychological 'debriefing' (describing the trauma and your emotional response to an expert) may *increase* the likelihood of later PTSD, so is discouraged.

- **Personality disorder:** presents from late adolescence onwards and is pervasive across all situations, rather than having a more recent onset, relapsing–remitting course or specific triggers. Cluster C personality disorders, where there are traits of negative affectivity, anankastia, or detachment are key differentials for anxiety disorders.

Specific anxiety disorders have the following differential diagnoses

GAD

- Organic:
  - Hyperthyroidism causes continuous anxiety symptoms.
  - Dementia: anxiety may be an early presentation.
  - Intoxication, e.g. amphetamines, caffeine.
  - Withdrawal, e.g. from benzodiazepines, alcohol, opioids.
- Psychosis: free-floating anxiety may precede delusions and hallucinations, in the 'at-risk mental state' (see p. 81).
- Depression.
- Personality disorder.

Panic disorder

- Organic:
  - Asthma, angina, stroke/TIA can feature panic symptoms.
  - Rarely, phaeochromocytoma causes paroxysmal anxiety.
  - Intoxication, e.g. amphetamines, caffeine.
  - Withdrawal, e.g. from benzodiazepines, alcohol, opioids.
- Depression.
- Other anxiety disorders:
  - Panic *attacks* can arise in any anxiety disorder and indicate severity.
  - Agoraphobia *with* panic disorder.

Social anxiety disorder

- Organic: benign essential tremor (familial tremor *without* anxiety).
- Psychosis can cause social withdrawal due to persecutory delusions or negative symptoms.
- Depression: social withdrawal is secondary to fatigue or anhedonia, not fear.
- Agoraphobia.
- Personality disorder.
- Shyness: social discomfort not meeting criteria for personality disorder *or* social anxiety disorder.

Agoraphobia

- Organic: dementia (loss of function can make people housebound).
- Psychosis can cause social withdrawal due to persecutory delusions or negative symptoms.
- Depression: social withdrawal is secondary to fatigue or anhedonia, not fear.
- Other anxiety disorders:
  - Social anxiety disorder.
  - OCD.
- Personality disorder.

OCD

- Organic: movement disorders with repetitive, stereotyped movements resembling compulsions,
  - E.g. Tourette syndrome (see p. 250), Sydenham's chorea, Huntington disease, PANDAS.
- Psychosis: delusions are believed *absolutely* ± thoughts may feel alien (thought insertion) (see p. 82). People with OCD recognize their obsessions as being *irrational* on some level (even if only when they're calm); they also know the thoughts come from their *own* mind.
- Depression: obsessions can occur in depression, and 50% of OCD sufferers have depressive symptoms. If the episode meets criteria for depression, this diagnosis takes priority, unless there's a full pattern of comorbid OCD.

- Other anxiety disorders:
  - Agoraphobia.
  - BDD.
- Anankastic personality disorder (see p. 261): rigidity, inflexibility, liking of order. This shouldn't include obsessions and compulsions unless OCD is comorbid.
- ASD (see p. 247). In ASD, repetitive behaviours and need for routine/order are lifelong, with social and communication difficulties. However, ASD increases the risk of OCD.

BDD

- Organic: objectively severe physical deformity.
- Psychosis: persistent delusional disorder is diagnosed if beliefs reach delusional intensity, without other psychotic symptoms.
- Depression.
- Other anxiety disorder:
  - OCD.
  - Social anxiety disorder.

PTSD

- *Psychosis:* flashbacks can resemble hallucinations, but should *relive* past experiences. The sense of threat in PTSD may be severe, but relates entirely to the trauma (not to delusional themes).
- Depression: trauma commonly triggers depression or adjustment disorder (**Box 14.4**), and people with PTSD often experience depressed mood. PTSD is diagnosed when re-experiencing phenomena and avoidance are present.

> **BOX 14.4 Adjustment disorders**
>
> Life events, such as going to university, moving house, or ending a relationship, require adaptation to cope with new situations, tasks, roles, and responsibilities. It's normal to experience fleeting symptoms of anxiety, low mood, irritability, or sleeplessness. In *adjustment disorders*, the person's reaction is greater than expected for the situation, but *not* severe enough to diagnose an anxiety or depressive disorder:
> - Symptoms start within 1 month of the stressor and resolve within 6 months.
> - Support, reassurance, and problem-solving often suffice.

- Other anxiety disorder:
  - Acute stress reaction.
  - Adjustment disorder.

💡 Anyone would seem to have GAD if they drank 20 espressos each day. Check consumption via drinks, chocolate, caffeine tablets, and cold and 'flu preparations—especially in occupations requiring sustained alertness, e.g. night shift staff, lorry drivers.

Investigations

- History, physical examination, ± investigations to exclude organic causes (**Table 14.4**).
- Anxiety rating scales quantify severity or provide baseline 'scores' against which to measure treatment

Table 14.4 Organic causes of anxiety: anxiety pattern and investigations

Problem	Continuous	Episodic	Investigations
Hyperthyroidism	✓		TFTs
Caffeine	✓	✓	History
Alcohol	✓	✓	History + LFTs including GGT, FBC including MCV
Recreational drugs		✓	History ± UDS
Arrhythmia		✓	12-lead ECG/24-hour ECG
Hypoglycaemia		✓	CBG (while symptomatic)
Phaeochromocytoma		✓	BP, 24-hour urine for vanillylmandelic acid (VMA)

response, e.g. Beck Anxiety Inventory (BAI), Hospital Anxiety and Depression Scale (HADS).
- Collateral history.

Management

New or mild anxiety disorders may improve with simple forms of help (**Box 14.5**).

Biological interventions

Antidepressants

See p. 40. Antidepressants are effective antianxiety medications, but therapeutic doses may be higher than for depression, and the response can take longer (6–8 weeks). Before prescribing, let people know that anxiety can *increase* briefly when starting antidepressants, or upon missing or suddenly stopping them. Ideally, also offer CBT.

- *SSRIs* are usually first line, e.g. sertraline.
- *SNRIs* are increasingly used in PTSD, GAD and panic disorder, e.g. venlafaxine
- *TCAs* can help in panic disorder, e.g. imipramine. Avoid if suicidal, as TCAs are toxic in overdose.

An SSRI *or* clomipramine are effective in OCD, and a low-dose second-generation antipsychotic can be added for resistant symptoms.

Anxiolytics

Pregabalin is an antiepileptic licensed for neuropathic pain and GAD. It reduces excitatory neurotransmitter secretion, by acting on calcium channels.

> **BOX 14.5** Management of new or mild anxiety presentations
>
> - **Psychoeducation and support:** explain and normalize the physiological effects of anxiety; provide information, advice, and emotional support.
> - A **problem-solving** approach can identify and address stressors.
> - **Self-help** material, including CBT-based books, websites, podcasts, and apps can help. The person should be encouraged to access their natural support networks, especially if they've been avoiding their friends, family, and faith groups.
> - **Relaxation techniques, breathing exercises, mindfulness** (see p. 44): taught in person or using electronic resources. They're based on *reciprocal inhibition*: it's not possible to panic *and* relax at the same time, so relaxation can combat panic. These must be mastered while calm, as it's impossible to use them for the first time when panicking!

Benzodiazepines (e.g. diazepam) are very effective anxiolytics, but tolerance builds rapidly and people quickly become dependent. They can be a useful *short-term* anxiety treatment (e.g. while waiting for SSRIs to take effect) but *use mustn't exceed 2–4 weeks*. Benzodiazepines enhance GABA transmission in the brain by interacting with the GABA-A receptor. Side effects include amnesia, ataxia, and respiratory depression, especially in older adults and those with pre-existing respiratory disease.

Beta-blockers (e.g. atenolol, propranolol)

These are sometimes used to treat uncomfortable adrenergic symptoms (especially in social phobia), e.g. tremor and palpitations. Caution is required, as contraindications include asthma, heart block, and heart failure.

> 💡 Remember to treat comorbid depression and substance use disorders.

> 💡 Specific phobias rarely need medication, as they're usually intermittent problems.

Psychological interventions

Cognitive behavioural therapy

People with anxiety disorders often think, feel, and behave as if they're in imminent danger when they're not; CBT changes behaviours and thoughts that maintain anxiety. In the UK, it's often provided initially via the Improving Access to Psychological Therapies (IAPT) service. Therapy starts with psychoeducation about the physiology of anxiety and techniques for managing arousal, such as controlled breathing and relaxation exercises.

CBT uses *exposure therapy* when avoidance and escape are central to the presentation (**Figure 14.2**).

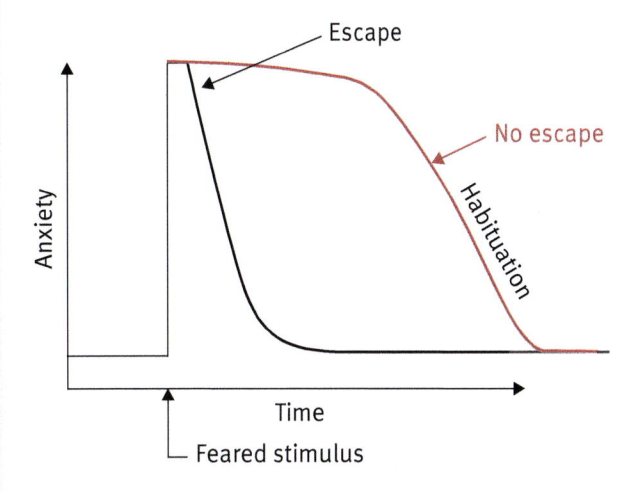

FIGURE 14.2 Response to feared stimulus: fear and escape versus habituation

People avoid or escape the things they fear, sometimes through SSBs or substance use disorders (e.g. drinking for 'Dutch courage'). This reduces anxiety and makes them feel better (negative reinforcement, see p. 169) but means they never learn the truth: that anxiety decreases (*habituates*) as they get used to the feared stimulus. In the absence of actual harm, the body only stays *extremely* anxious for a short time (usually 30–45 minutes). Repeated exposure to the same stimulus produces lower and lower anxiety levels, and faster habituation, until there's no fear response at all (*extinction*).

We'll illustrate this with an editorial phobia: cockroaches. The editor wants to 'cope' if a cockroach enters her clinic (*not* by squashing it; this apparently releases millions of eggs, creating an infestation). Given that no reasonable person would hold a live cockroach, the therapist suggests they work towards catching the cockroach in a jar to remove it.

A gradual approach is used: *systematic desensitization*. The therapist helps the editor construct a 'hierarchy' of feared situations, from the least to the most frightening (**Table 14.5**).

Starting with the easiest task (looking at a cockroach photograph), the editor *stays* in the situation until her anxiety habituates, and she learns she doesn't need to run away. She works upwards, tackling each step repeatedly during sessions or as homework, until she reaches her goal (level 9, as 10 isn't necessary). In a matter of weeks, she's fearlessly removing cockroaches from her own and other people's offices.

> **Flooding** isn't used anymore. This was where people were plunged into their worst fear (level 10) until they habituated. Though effective, most people were too terrified to try it!

Later sessions explore thoughts with a *cognitive approach*. For example, in **GAD**, the main feature is worry (**Figure 14.3**).

The therapist discusses automatic assumptions (e.g. 'My daughter will be abducted if I don't drive her to school!') and tests the person's anxious predictions through behavioural experiments, e.g. letting the daughter walk to school with friends. The outcome (repeated non-abduction) helps disprove the worry and informs more realistic thoughts, e.g. 'She'll call if she *needs* me'.

The therapist also identifies *thinking errors*. For example, *catastrophizing* (jumping to the worst possible conclusion), e.g. 'I feel ill. It's cancer! I'll die!' The therapist would challenge this and help the person look for evidence that proves or disproves it.

These techniques gradually help people reassess the true level of threat, notice when their anxiety is making them think illogically, and relax their SSBs (e.g. decreasing calls to school). Over time, more adaptive coping strategies are developed to replace the avoidance, escape, and SSBs, which had reinforced the anxiety.

CBT can treat all anxiety disorders, but the focus and techniques are adapted to each disorder.

Panic disorder: people often misinterpret physical anxiety symptoms as a medical catastrophe (e.g. stroke),

Table 14.5 Anxiety hierarchy

Anxiety level[a]	Activity
10	Hold a live cockroach with bare hands
9	Catch a cockroach in a jar
8	Hold a dead cockroach
7	Watch *the therapist* hold a dead cockroach ('*modelling*')
6	Hold a jar containing a *live* cockroach
5	*Hold* a jar containing a dead cockroach
4	Look at a jar containing a dead cockroach
3	Look at a picture of a cockroach

Evil cockroach (courtesy of Dr Richard Lin)

[a] 10 = maximum anxiety, 0 = no anxiety.

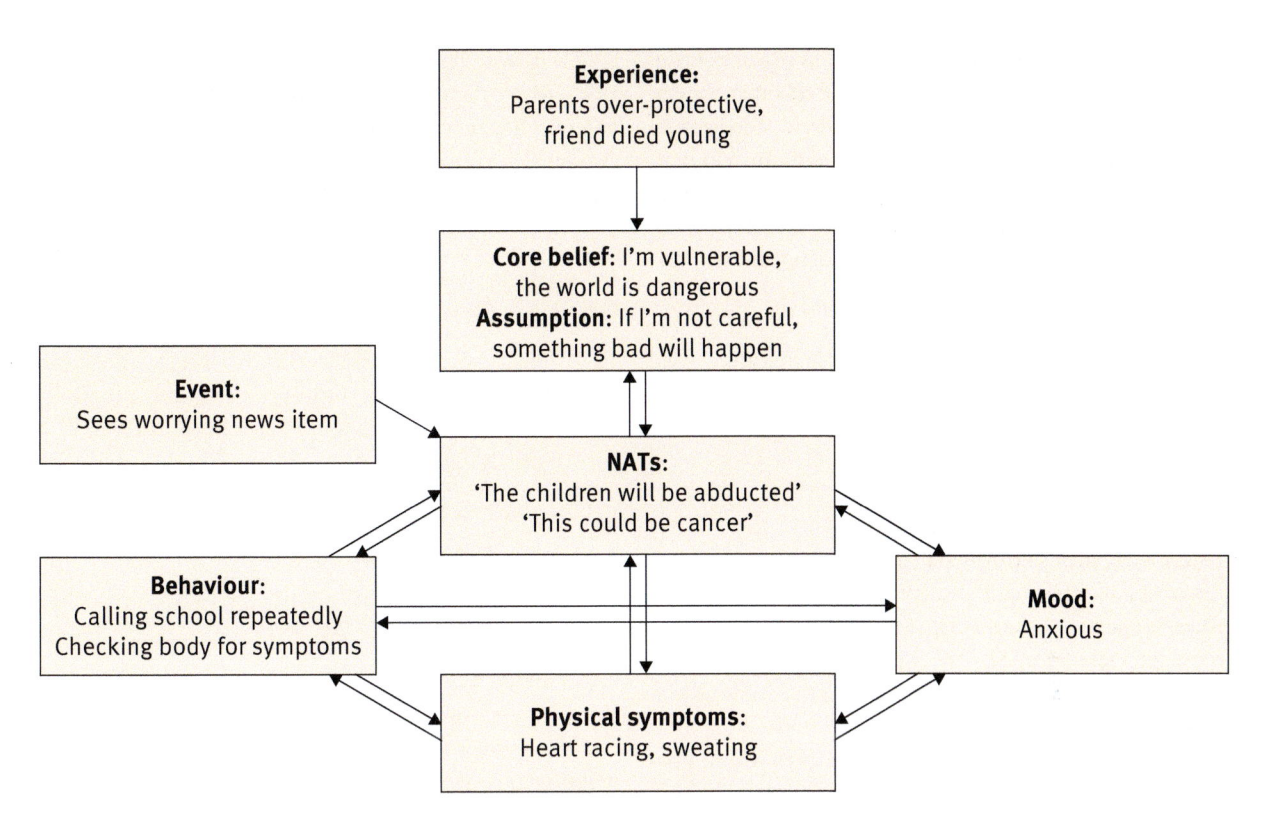

FIGURE 14.3 Example CBT formulation for GAD. An event triggers negative automatic thoughts (NATs), setting up a vicious cycle of worry

escalating their panic. They adopt SSBs (e.g. calling an ambulance), and conclude that their behaviour prevented the catastrophe, as nothing bad happened. The SSBs take the place of escape in **Figure 14.3**. CBT educates the person about the true meaning of their symptoms ('panic, not perish'). It helps them test whether their behaviours really keep them safe, and whether their beliefs are true, or misinterpretations.

Social anxiety disorder: SSBs and excessive self-monitoring to avoid embarrassment actually make things worse, e.g. if someone focuses attention on their own performance, they can't listen or respond properly to others, and seem socially awkward. Therapy involves stopping SSBs during social situations, to challenge assumptions. Video feedback and role-play can help.

Agoraphobia: exposure tasks might tackle gradually leaving the house, starting by stepping outside the door, before walking up the road, then going to a small, local shop, before progressing to a big supermarket. During each experiment, the person stays in the situation until their anxiety resolves. The first attempt at a task might be with a companion (e.g. spouse); once successful, it's repeated alone.

OCD: *exposure and response prevention*. CBT deliberately exposes the person to situations which trigger obsessions, then supports them *not* to use compulsions (response prevention). Remember, compulsions 'neutralize' anxiety, similar to escape in other disorders. For example, someone with contamination OCD will touch something dirty (e.g. toilet seat), triggering obsessions, e.g. 'I've caught AIDS!' Instead of immediately scrubbing their hands (compulsion), they're supported to tolerate the anxiety until it habituates. A hierarchy of feared situations is used, as in exposure therapy.

BDD: therapy supports the person to challenge their thoughts about their appearance and its importance, and to reduce time spent on SSBs (e.g. mirror-checking). Behavioural experiments may include testing what others think of their appearance, and exposing them to social situations without performing SSBs, such as going out without wearing make-up.

PTSD: *trauma-focused* CBT is used. Trauma can shatter belief systems, resulting in new beliefs, e.g. 'The world is unsafe and unpredictable'/'I'm weak and vulnerable'. These are examined and challenged through discussion and behavioural experiments. *Exposure therapy* supports the person to work through their memories, rather than avoiding them, e.g. by recording a detailed narrative of the traumatic event and listening to it repeatedly; going to the place where the trauma happened.

Eye movement desensitization and reprocessing (EMDR)

In this PTSD-specific therapy, the original trauma is deliberately re-experienced by the person narrating or imagining everything that happened in as much detail as possible. They simultaneously fix their eyes on the therapist's finger as it quickly passes from side to side in front of them. Eye movements can be replaced by any alternating left–right stimulus, e.g. tapping left then right hands. Strange as it seems, this can treat PTSD, possibly by aiding memory processing in addition to exposure work.

Mindfulness

See p. 44. This meditative approach is increasingly used in anxiety disorders (especially OCD). People are taught to 'notice' thoughts, rather than trying to avoid them or ruminate on them.

Social interventions

Psychoeducation through self-help literature and online resources is often highly effective in reducing anxiety. Carer education is essential, as friends and family are often recruited in SSBs, or may facilitate escape and avoidance, believing they're protecting the anxious person from harm or distress.

It's important to address social stressors where possible, as these often perpetuate problems, e.g. writing letters in support of housing, signposting to Citizen's Advice or benefits advisors. Where employment or parenting skills are affected by anxiety, it's helpful to liaise with employers or social workers, to help the person explain their problem, suggest short-term adjustments and longer-term hopes for a return to full function. For example, someone with severe social anxiety disorder would struggle with direct customer contact, but could temporarily undertake administrative work until CBT enables them to face their fears.

Third-sector organizations provide essential information, advice, and telephone support for sufferers and carers. They may facilitate peer support through groups or online forums, and try to raise public awareness and reduce stigma.

Prognosis

Early diagnosis and treatment are essential, as the shorter the duration of symptoms, the better the prognosis. Anxiety disorders are often chronic. Overall, a rule of thirds applies:

- One-third recovers completely.
- One-third improves partially.
- One-third fares poorly, suffering considerable disability and poor quality of life.

OCD tends to run a chronic course, with symptoms worsening at times of stress. Without treatment, it's often disabling and commonly comorbid with depression. The majority of people with PTSD recover, although some suffer for many years; chronicity and complex PTSD can lead to enduring personality change. Symptoms can relapse around anniversaries associated with the trauma.

❗ **Overall, people with anxiety disorders are at greater risk of self-harm and suicide; other risks may relate to the response to anxiety, e.g. fears of contamination in OCD may lead to restriction of eating. Despite their fears, people with obsessional thoughts about violence or sexually inappropriate behaviour are *not* at increased risk of acting on them.**

REALITY

General approach: tips, tricks, and cautionary tales

1. Ooze calm

If *you* seem nervous, you'll panic an anxious person. Take a deep breath. Relax. Smile.

2. Read body language

Remember: even *discussing* anxiety can make people nervous. Observe signs of anxiety, e.g. crossing arms and legs, trembling, fidgeting. Don't automatically change the subject if they become tense; they may need time, encouragement, or reassurance before continuing. Ask how you can help them to feel more comfortable.

3. Trust me, I'm (nearly) a doctor

Anxious people (especially those with GAD) may have *pressure of speech* and be hard to interrupt. Let them talk for a while, then gently interrupt, e.g.:

> **Ahmed:** ... and then it all happened again, and I ...
> **You:** Sorry, Ahmed? You've told me so much, so quickly. Are you worried we'll miss something important unless you get it all out at once?

> **Ahmed:** A bit!
>
> **You:** I know all the essential areas we need to cover to help you. Could you trust me to ask the right questions? I may interrupt you to bring you back on track if needed. How does that sound?

This can decrease anxiety *and* give you permission to lead the interview.

4. Never dismiss fears

Students rarely *laugh* at fearful patients, but there are more subtle ways of being dismissive. For example, by immediately suggesting solutions, you can make someone feel that *you* see their problem as silly or easily overcome. Empathize first, solve later.

People sometimes dismiss their *own* fears out of embarrassment—don't join them in putting themselves down. Instead, legitimize their concerns, e.g.:

> **Neil:** I'm sorry. It's stupid. Cats terrify me!
>
> **You:** Don't apologize; everyone's scared of something. Most people just aren't brave enough to admit it.

Embarrassment stops people seeking help, so your acceptance and encouragement may facilitate their recovery.

5. Tough topics

Topics provoking fear, guilt, or shame can be extremely difficult to discuss—especially if they've been kept secret until now. Make the interview feel safe, unrushed, kind, and non-judgemental; explain confidentiality if needed.

You don't need *every* detail—only enough to understand the problem, so that you can empathize and identify the best way to help. Don't interrogate the person, or panic if your progress is slow. Instead, see information as *their* property: they'll choose whether to share it or not. Paradoxically, giving permission to say nothing sometimes makes people more willing to say what they're thinking, e.g.:

- You don't have to tell me anything. But if you *want* to tell me what happened, I'm listening.
- It's clearly hard to talk about. If you feel able, try and tell me *a little* of what happened. Take all the time you need.
- This is difficult to talk about. Are you OK to go on, or would you like to take a break?

Don't unpack a trauma without allowing enough time to conclude the discussion in a supportive and contained way. *Make time* to empathize, normalize their response, and to provide a way forward, even if that's simply offering a follow-up meeting, perhaps with a relative or friend for support.

6. Don't panic

If someone has a panic attack in front of you, *stay calm*. Be kind but firm: ask them to sit still, and explain that it's a panic attack and, although frightening, won't hurt them, and will pass in a few minutes. Explain that they need to slow their breathing (e.g. breathing in through their nose, *slowly* counting to three, then out, counting to three through their mouth). Successfully 'surviving' a panic attack (without using SSBs) demonstrates that it *isn't* a medical emergency. Reflect on this with the person afterwards, if possible.

The interview

• = Example question. ∗ = Question linking to other parts of the history.

Symptoms of anxiety

Physical

> • *How does your body feel when you're nervous?*
> ∗ What do you think is happening when you get these feelings?

Psychological

> • *What worries you?*
> • What's the *worst* thing you worry might happen?
> • Is it hard to concentrate?
> • Can you relax?
> • Have you felt as if you weren't real? *[Depersonalization]*
> • Has the world felt unreal? *[Derealization]*

💡 If someone *presents* with physical symptoms (and organic causes have been excluded), don't jump to diagnose 'anxiety', as this can feel dismissive. Use their words in place of 'anxiety' (e.g. 'horrible feeling'/'breathing problems'). You can then start to consider the role of anxiety by asking what they're *thinking* during these episodes.

Diagnosis

You can often diagnose anxiety disorders by checking two features (**Table 14.3**):

Episodic or continuous

> • *Do you feel anxious* all *the time or just* some *of the time?*

Trigger

- *What triggers your anxiety?*
- What do you worry about (or fear) the most?

💡 If someone can avoid all triggers of their anxiety disorder, they might experience little or no anxiety now. Ask about past situations.

Coping

Avoidance

- *Are there things you avoid because they'll make you too anxious?*
- Are there places you can't go because it feels too frightening?
- ∗ Have you missed out on anything important because of it?

Escape

- *Have you ever felt so bad that you've had to leave a situation?*
- ∗ How has this affected you?

SSBs/other strategies

- *Are there other things you do to feel better/calmer?*
- Do you seek reassurance that you'll be OK?
- ∗ Some people use alcohol or drugs to cope with anxiety. Do you?
- ∗ Does it ever get so bad that life doesn't feel worth living?

Specific disorders

GAD

- *Are you constantly overwhelmed by worry?*
  - Tell me your top three worries.
- What were you like *before* you started feeling anxious all the time? *[Lifelong anxiety suggests negative affectivity personality traits]*
- Do you get lots of aches, pains, or physical symptoms?
- ∗ How do you see the future? *[Apprehension]*

Panic attacks/disorder

- *Take me through what happens when you have one of these episodes.*
- Do you notice . . . ? *[Screen: pins and needles, can't breathe, palpitations]*
- How long does this last? How does it end? How often does it happen?
- What do you think is happening? *[Screen: physical illness, dying, 'going mad', losing control]*
- What thoughts go through your head when this happens?
- ∗ Are there places you can't go now? *[Agoraphobia?]*

Social anxiety disorder

- *Which social situations are the hardest?* *[Screen: meeting new people, dating, speaking/eating in public, interviews]*
- Do you become *visibly* anxious? How? *[Screen: tremble, blush, sweat, stutter, wobbly legs]*
- What do you most fear will happen in front of people? *[Screen: embarrassment/looking foolish/failure]*
- What do you worry others will think of you?

Agoraphobia

- *Where have you stopped going?* *[Screen: public transport, supermarkets/shopping centres, crowds, cramped spaces]*
  - If you *must* go there, how do you cope?
- How did this start? Do you ever have panic attacks?
- Which places still feel safe?
- Do you rely on someone to help you?

OCD

Obsessions

- *Do worrying thoughts or ideas bother you? Tell me about them.*
- Do you worry about . . .
  - . . . doing something wrong?
  - . . . germs or dirtiness?
  - . . . sex, violence, or causing harm?
  - . . . religious ideas?
  - . . . things not being symmetrical/perfect?
- How do these thoughts make you feel?
- Do you try to block them out? Does that work?
- Are they your own thoughts? *[Exclude thought insertion]*
- When you're *calm*, how true/logical do these thoughts seem? *[Exclude delusion]*
- ∗ How do you make the anxiety/discomfort go away?

Compulsions

- *Some people have rituals or tasks they must do in a very particular way. Do you?*
- ∗ Does it take you a long time to complete everyday tasks? Why?

- Do you . . .
  - . . . clean or wash a lot?
  - . . . count or check things?
  - . . . have to put things in order or get them *just right*?
  - . . . have to *think* things in a certain way?
- Does [*ritual*] make you feel calmer for a while?
- What happens if you don't do [*ritual*] perfectly? *[Repeat?]*
- ∗ How often do you do [*ritual*]? How much time does it take in a day?
  - Do you wish you could do it less?

💡 OCD can make people ashamed and guarded. Try, 'Some people worry about things they find shocking or embarrassing. They might worry they've done or could do something bad. They feel awful, as these are things they'd never *want* to do. Do you ever have worries like that?'

BDD

- *Do you worry about your appearance?*
- Which part(s) of your body don't you like? Why?
- How do you think other people view it?
- Are there things you have to do because you dislike your appearance?
  - Do you keep checking it? *[Mirrors/measures/photos]* How often?
  - Do you do anything to hide or disguise it?
  - How much time does this take, in total, in a day?
- ∗ Have you tried to physically change it in any way? *[Surgery/self-mutilation]*

PTSD
Trauma

- *Did something (terrible) happen? Take your time. Tell me what you can.*
  - At the time, what did you think would happen to you/them?
  - ∗ What's happened since? *[Screen: disability, legal proceedings, ongoing threats]*

Hyperarousal

- *Have you felt constantly on edge or jumpy?*
  - Does it feel like you're almost *waiting* for something bad to happen again?
  - ∗ How's your sleep?
  - ∗ How do you feel, mostly? *[Screen: detached/numb/depressed/irritable]*

Re-experiencing

- *Do you ever feel like it's happening all over again?*
  - Do you get flashbacks? What are they like?
  - ∗ What triggers them?
  - Have you had bad dreams or nightmares?
  - Is it hard to block out horrible memories of what happened?
  - Do you find yourself thinking about it, even though you don't want to?

Avoidance

- *Are there things you can't face since this happened?*
  - Have you been back to the place where it happened?
  - ∗ What happens if you can't avoid these things? *[Flashbacks?]*

💡 If someone *presents* with re-experiencing (flashbacks, nightmares, intrusive thoughts/memories), try, 'Does it remind you of something that happened to you before?'

1. OCD history (15 minutes)

Candidate's instructions
Jeremy Blaker is a 27-year-old bus driver. He's attended the GP surgery because his manager is concerned about his fitness to drive. You're a medical student at the surgery. The GP has asked you to take a psychiatric history.

Patient's brief
Key characteristics
- I'm fairly calm but feel anxious and embarrassed when explaining my thoughts.
- If the student makes me feel silly/ashamed, I'll close down.

The interview   183

History

My manager's received complaints about my bus running late. At first he said not to worry, but the complaints kept coming and he's losing patience.

About a year ago, I suddenly thought: 'I'll crash the bus and everyone will die.' I couldn't get it out of my head. What kind of a person thinks *that*? I got so distracted I went through a red light. I pulled over and tried to clear my head by counting everyone on the bus. When I finished, I felt calm enough to drive again.

Since then, the thought comes more often (ten times a day), and however hard I try to block it, it comes back. It makes me feel terrible: sick, sweaty, my hands shake, my heart pounds. I can cope until the next bus stop, when I have to count everyone again. It feels like counting puts everything right and keeps my passengers safe, making me calmer. If I think I've miscounted, I have to recount until I'm *sure*—that's why I'm running late.

Last week I had a full bus and couldn't get the count right, so I couldn't leave the bus stop. People were shouting, getting off and on; it was too confusing. I couldn't drive unless I was sure it was safe, so I turned the engine off, took the keys out and sat down at the bus shelter. My passengers had to get off and another driver came out and drove me back to the depot. When I tried to explain it to my manager, he said I shouldn't work again until I'd seen the GP.

Deep down, I know it's ridiculous. I don't *believe* that knowing the number of passengers will stop me crashing! I just can't stop thinking, 'What if? What if I *do* crash and everyone dies?' I can't take the risk of *not* counting, just in case. I can't tell my friends about this. They'd think I was crazy. I've always been the calm, practical one, not someone too superstitious to drive. I've stopped driving my car recently, because similar thoughts started happening there: 'I'll run someone over.' Fortunately, the thoughts only happen while I'm driving, so otherwise I'm fine.

Other history

- I'm not depressed or suicidal. My energy's good, but I worry too much to enjoy work.
- I'm physically fit. I had my tonsils removed after many bouts of tonsillitis.
- I don't drink heavily or do drugs—it'd be dangerous in my job.
- Nobody in my family (including me) has ever suffered mental illness.
- Just before this started, I moved house—I guess that was a bit stressful.

Question
Am I going mad?

Worry
I'll lose my job.

Jeremy's OCD is disabling, but likely to respond well to CBT ± an SSRI. Although his obsessions might distract him slightly, he's likely to be an extremely conscientious driver. Ideally, the GP/CBT therapist will support Jeremy to *stay* at work (exposure, not avoidance) and educate his manager. With the manager's support, behavioural experiments will be easier and more effective.

2. Agoraphobia history (15 minutes)

Candidate's instructions
Ms Grace Teaney is a 55-year-old solicitor. Her son, Robert, has asked the GP to visit as Ms Teaney is housebound. You're a medical student accompanying the GP. Take a history with a view to making a diagnosis.

Patient's brief
Key characteristics
- I'm eloquent, personable, and try to make light of matters.
- I'm embarrassed to need a house call; Robert insisted.
- I'm calm, but feel anxious when describing panicky episodes.

History

Everything started about 9 months ago when I took the lift to my office on the 18th floor and it became stuck. I wasn't a great fan of enclosed spaces, but I thought I could cope, and calmly pressed the alarm button. Nothing happened. I called out a little 'Hello?' but nobody answered. I banged on the doors and shouted, to no avail. I realized I was trapped, and panicked: the air seemed to be running out, my throat closed up and my heart beat hard and fast, as if it would jump right out of my chest. Then my hands tingled and I thought I'd had a stroke. Just then, the engineer's voice came through the speaker, the lift shunted up, and the doors opened. I practically fell out. I was dizzy, crying, and sweaty. Everything felt unreal, as if people were talking to me through water or thick glass. I was in such a state that I took the day off. I told myself it was a one-off event, but found that even *thinking* about lifts made me panicky, so I took the stairs from then on. Eighteen flights: quite the workout!

Things didn't stop there. First, it was the trains. Going through tunnels felt a bit like being in the lift all over again. One morning it was so bad, I got off a stop early and walked 3 miles to work. I haven't been on a train since. Buses became problematic a few weeks later. With the fear that it might happen again, my world shrank down to this house. I didn't plan to, but there was always a reason to stay home: holding dinner parties for friends to visit *me*, giving Robert managerial experience by leaving him in charge at work. Eventually, I realized I was trapped.

The further from home I am, the more frightened I feel. For over 6 months, I've only been to the local mini-market with Robert. I trust him, and he understands that I might need to run off. I really can't cope with queues, so he queues while I wait in the car, which feels safe. I've told colleagues my back's playing up, so I work from home using Skype, and e-mailing or sending work in via Robert.

Though I keep up the facade of coping and being the boss, I feel vulnerable, miserable, and lonely. The work Robert brings home is starting to feel overwhelming, and I don't enjoy it as I used to; it's becoming hard to concentrate on it. I wish I could get out and see my friends. It's pathetic that I can't leave home without pep talks and handholding.

Other history

- I've never seen a psychiatrist. Nobody in my family has had similar problems, though my father struggled with 'nerves'.
- I'm not a big drinker but have the occasional cognac. I've never smoked.
- I have high blood pressure, controlled with tablets.

Question

I want help, but I've heard it means facing my fears. Could it harm me?

Worry

These 'incidents' are mini strokes.

💡 Ms Teaney's agoraphobia is severely disabling, but the short duration suggests a good prognosis; this should respond to treatment. Normalize her experiences and explain how CBT works. Emphasize that it won't harm her, and that exposure to her fears will be in *small, manageable steps*, decided between her, her therapist, and (if wanted) Robert. If depression is present, it may resolve as agoraphobia is treated, or require treatment in its own right; an SSRI is a good choice for both diagnoses.

NEXT STEPS

An anxious colleague in need of help

You're a surgical FY2. Toby is a medical student on your firm. You know he recently failed a mock OSCE, which knocked his confidence, and note that he's bright but shy, and tends to blush and stutter whenever questions are directed at him. He confided in you that he finds the group teaching intimidating, and is terrified of making a fool of himself in front of your consultant, Ms Brand. You suggested he ask his GP for a CBT referral to treat his anxiety. He seemed appreciative, but hasn't attended teaching for the last 2 weeks. Ms Brand threatened to fail Toby if he missed the end-of-term case presentation.

Toby attends the presentation and seems calm but vague, performing poorly, despite excellent slides. You catch him afterwards, and ask whether he started CBT. Toby explains he didn't need therapy, as 'a little diazepam' (10mg) 'took the edge off' his anxiety.

- What's your immediate response?
- What treatment will Toby need?

Differential diagnosis
Includes social anxiety disorder, GAD, personality difficulties—negative affectivity, ASD, depression, substance misuse.

Immediate intervention
Don't let Toby onto the wards, where he may place patients at risk. Find somewhere private to talk and find out whether the diazepam was prescribed—if not, he acted unprofessionally and possibly unlawfully, and you may need to involve the General Medical Council (GMC). Support him to explain the situation to Ms Brand or his clinical tutor *in order to gain help* (this isn't about punishment). If he refuses, it's your professional responsibility to discuss matters with a senior doctor.

This may sound extreme, but it's a serious situation: if Toby needs diazepam *now*, his substance misuse will probably escalate with future stress, posing risks to him and his patients. This won't be comfortable for either of you, but Toby needs your support.

Treatment
Toby may well have social anxiety disorder. Check he's registered with a GP, and whether he's already receiving support. His GP may refer to a CMHT or treat problems in primary care. Toby needs a full psychiatric assessment, physical examination, and appropriate investigations. Social anxiety disorder would be managed primarily by psychological treatments (e.g. CBT), although SSRIs and beta-blockers may also help. Benzodiazepines should be avoided because of the risk of dependence. A broader substance misuse problem will need input from an addictions specialist, and may require referral to the GMC if it's affecting Toby's fitness to practise.

Organizations that help UK doctors and medical students with mental health problems or provide information include:

- **Doctors' Support Network:** www.dsn.org.uk
- **British Medical Association:**
  - *Counselling*: www.bma.org.uk/advice/work-life-support/your-wellbeing
  - *Doctors for doctors scheme*: www.bma.org.uk/doctorsfordoctors
- **Sick Doctors Trust:** www.sick-doctors-trust.co.uk
- **British Doctors' and Dentists' Group:** www.bddg.org
- **Practitioner Health Programme:** php.nhs.uk/
- **General Medical Council:** www.gmcuk.org/concerns/doctors_health_concerns.asp

💡 Mental health and substance misuse problems are more common in doctors than the general population, yet we often ignore them or avoid seeking treatment. We're *allowed* to be unwell, but professionalism requires that we recognize our problems and seek the same help we'd recommend to our patients.

Movie buff
Apocalypse Now (1979) and *The Deer Hunter* (1979): two classics focusing on the traumatic experiences of American soldiers in the Vietnam War. Vivid portrayals of the traumatized soldiers in conflict and civilian life afterwards.

As Good As It Gets (1997): lead actors Helen Hunt and Jack Nicholson both won Oscars in this romantic comedy which has some great, strong characters. Nicholson plays a highly disagreeable, cynical novelist with OCD; his condition is challenged as he is forced out of his comfort zone.

The Aviator (2004): featuring a wealth of Hollywood stars, this is a biographical film of Howard Hughes—movie director, aviation pioneer, and wealthy airline owner. Hughes appears to become increasingly eccentric and socially withdrawn due to severe OCD.

Two Days, One Night (2014): Sandra is off work with depression and anxiety. Her colleagues vote for a bonus, rather than Sandra returning to work. She has one weekend to change their minds. This film confronts us with the interrelationship of anxiety, social problems, and stigma in the twenty-first century.

Book shelf
Barker, P. (1991) *Regeneration*: this renowned trilogy is themed around First World War trauma and shell-shock, using real-life characters, including famed war poets Siegfried Sassoon and Wilfred Owen, to explore attitudes towards hysteria in men and treatment methods, such as the then-new use of talking therapy.

Haddon, M. (2006) *A Spot of Bother*: touching and amusing novel focusing on a middle-aged retired man who becomes acutely anxious after finding a lesion on his leg which he believes to be cancerous.

Wilensky, A. (1999) *Passing for Normal*: this autobiography examines OCD in the context of Tourette syndrome. Wilensky's positive portrayal explores heredity, medication, behavioural therapy, and support groups. Her symptoms are thoroughly explored: hoarding, tics, compulsions, skin-picking, and self-medication with alcohol and cannabis.

Note

1. Orwell, G. (1949) *Nineteen Eighty-Four*. London: Penguin, 1987.

Journal club

Baldwin, D.S., Anderson, I.M., Nutt, D.J., et al. (2014) Evidence-based pharmacological treatment of anxiety disorders, post-traumatic stress disorder and obsessive-compulsive disorder: a revision of the 2005 guidelines from the British Association for Psychopharmacology. *Journal of Psychopharmacology*, **28**, 403–39.

Bandelow, B., Michaelis, S. (2015) Epidemiology of anxiety disorders in the 21st century. *Dialogues in Clinical Neuroscience*, **17**, 327–35.

Heyman, I. (2006) Obsessive–compulsive disorder. *British Medical Journal*, **333**, 424–9.

Lancaster, C.L., Teeters, J.B., Gros, D.F., et al. (2016) Posttraumatic stress disorder: overview of evidence-based assessment and treatment. *Journal of Clinical Medicine*, **5**, E105.

Resources

Combat Stress—for Veterans with PTSD and other mental health conditions: www.combatstress.org.uk/

No Panic—for panic disorder: www.nopanic.org.uk/

OCD Action: www.ocdaction.org.uk/

OCD UK: www.ocduk.org

Go to www.oup.com/uk/stringer2e for a wealth of additional resources, including an OCSE mark scheme, filmed scenarios, and self-assessment questions.

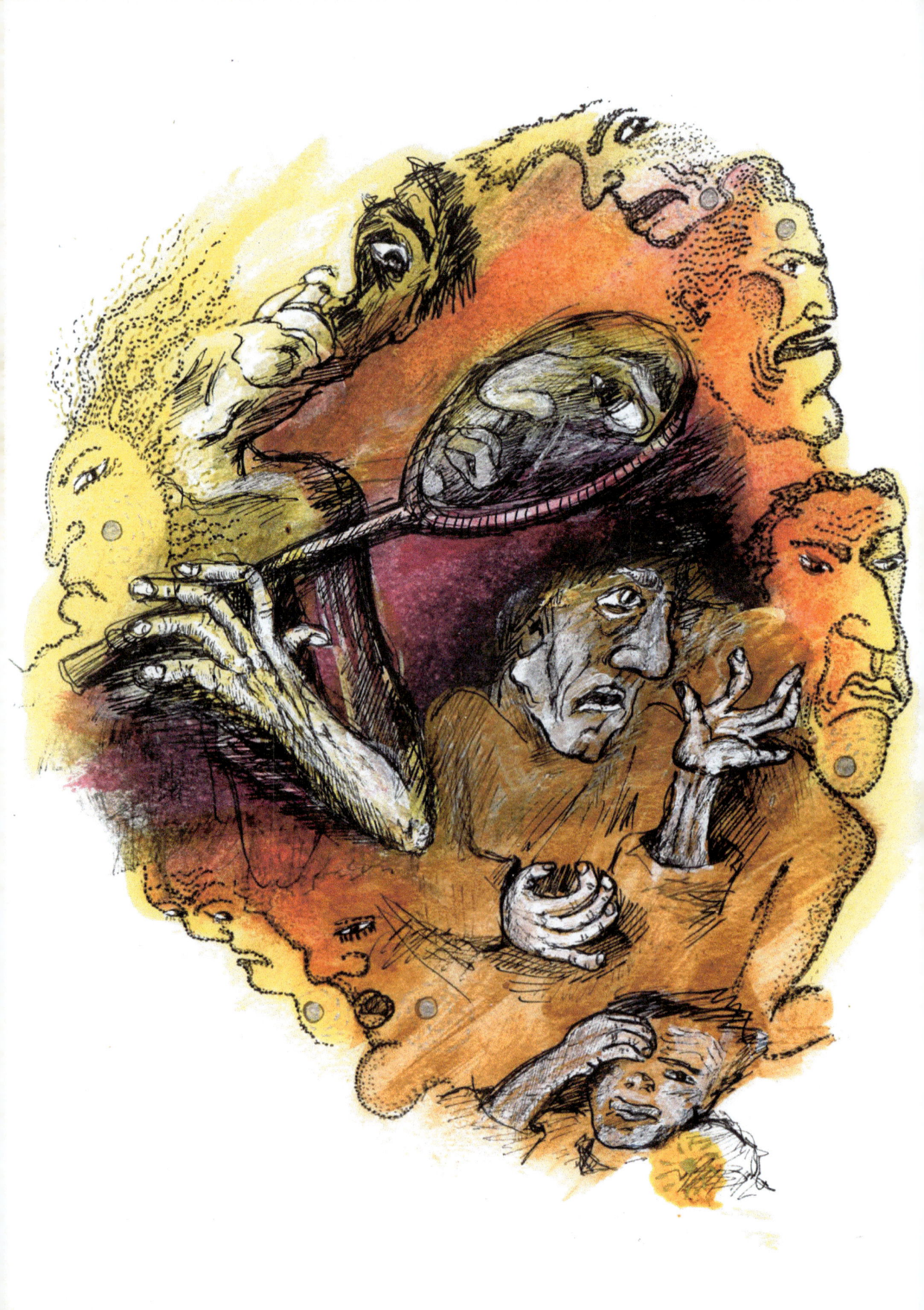

15 Medically Unexplained Symptoms

True or false?

Answers on p. 277

1. Cognitive models propose that a person with medically unexplained symptoms (MUS) typically reduces their anxiety by taking their own pulse.
2. People with chronic fatigue syndrome should be encouraged to exercise vigorously to break the cycle of fatigue.
3. In bodily distress disorder, symptoms are repeatedly focused on one particular part of the body.
4. Relative lack of concern despite worrying symptoms is highly suggestive of dissociative neurological symptom disorder.
5. In psychogenic amnesia, the main symptom is retrograde memory loss.
6. Factitious disorder is the intentional production of physical or psychological symptoms to receive medical attention.
7. Iatrogenic harm is one of the greatest risks to the health of people with MUS.
8. The reattribution model consists of contemplation, pre-attribution, reattribution, and maintenance.
9. People with MUS have better outcomes when seen by multiple GPs, as it gives reassurance.
10. A person with irritable bowel syndrome should be referred for investigation if they develop rectal bleeding, despite the potential to reinforce their anxiety.

Contents

Principles
Introduction
Epidemiology
Aetiology
- Psychodynamic models
- Cognitive models
- Biological models
- Psychosocial

Clinical presentation
- Bodily distress disorder
- Hypochondriasis
- Dissociative neurological symptom disorder
- Factitious disorder

Differential diagnosis
Management
Prognosis

Reality
General approach: tips, tricks, and cautionary tales

The interview
- Fatigue history

Next steps
Suspected malignancy after MUS
- Issues
- Your response
- Other measures
- Effects on current treatment

PRINCIPLES

[O]ften when I have been consulted in a Case, and found it to be what is commonly call'd Nervous, I have been in the utmost Difficulty, when desir'd to name the Distemper, for fear of affronting them … If I call'd the case 'Glandular with nervous Symptoms', they concluded that I thought them pox'd, or had the King's Evil. If I said it was Vapours, Hysterick or Hypochondriackal Disorders, they thought that I call'd them Mad or Fantastickal … I was in a Hazard of a Drubbing for seeming to impeach their Courage … I myself was thought a Fool, a weak and ignorant Coxcomb, and perhaps dismiss'd in Scorn.

Dr George Cheyne, *The English Malady*[1]

Even if medical tests cannot explain your pain or tiredness or disability, it does not lessen your suffering. The pain of medically unexplained illness is every bit as real as any other and, if anything, is multiplied by the lack of understanding.

Suzanne Sullivan[2]

Introduction

Although it can be convenient in medicine to treat the mind and body as distinct entities ('dualism'), the relationship between the two is complex, and separating them is not always helpful. *Somatization*—in which psychological stress manifests as physical symptoms—is a common experience; it's also known that established physical conditions (e.g. eczema, asthma) may be exacerbated by stress. Nevertheless, when somatization becomes a constant pattern, causing distress or affecting functioning, it may be considered a disorder.

People with medically unexplained symptoms (MUS) are distressed and preoccupied by symptoms not fully explained by an organic cause; and will typically seek repeated medical attention for these symptoms. Terminology is varied, but MUS can be described as 'functional' (as opposed to structural) illness, somatoform disorder (formerly called Briquet syndrome), or disorder of bodily distress (ICD-11). Most people with MUS are managed in general practice or medical outpatient clinics; a minority require psychiatric referral. Conflict (as described in the earlier quote from Dr Cheyne), can arise when a patient and their doctor disagree about the origin of their symptoms. Without clear understanding and communication, MUS can lead to frustration, excessive investigations, and chronic disability.

Epidemiology

MUS are extremely common, and people with MUS are seen by *every* medical professional. About 20–25% of people attending their general practice report MUS, and rates can be higher among medical outpatients. They are more common in women than in men: for disorder of bodily distress the prevalence is up to 2% in women and 0.2% in men. There is a strong association with less time in formal education. It's particularly common for MUS to be present *alongside* an organic condition.

Aetiology

Psychodynamic models

Traditional psychoanalytical models suggested that unconscious (often sexual) conflict was 'converted' into physical symptoms; thus providing primary gain (reduction in anxiety), and secondary gain (care and attention from others). Sometimes the form of the symptom was regarded as a re-enactment of traumatic childhood experiences. More recent psychodynamic theories have focused on early childhood experiences, including trauma, loss, and insecure attachment, leading to later difficulties, e.g. dependency on caregivers/doctors. Related theories suggest that in non-psychologically minded people, or those who are 'alexithymic' (find it hard to identify their own emotions), physical symptoms may be more comfortable than facing underlying distress. Cultural and family attitudes to disease also play a role—and illness behaviour models may be learned and carried into adulthood, e.g. when a child experiences prolonged illness themselves or in a parent or sibling.

Cognitive models

An individual's interpretation of normal physiology can create anxiety and perpetuate MUS. Someone concerned about palpitations might misinterpret normal physiological experiences, such as a rapid heartbeat while anxious, as a sign of a heart attack. Selective attention to the problem leads to acute awareness of palpitations whenever they occur. Behaviours such as repeated checking (e.g. of pulse rate) maintain anxiety in the long term; reassurance reinforces the importance of these safety behaviours while preventing the person from learning that symptoms are benign.

Biological models

Repeated experience of physical sensations may lead to 'sensitization', causing an enhanced response to future sensations. Similarly, the brain cytokine system (which coordinates immune response to threat) may become sensitized and less quick to 'shut down' after a period of threat. Abnormalities in autonomic function, proprioception, and the cortisol response have all been suggested as relevant to MUS. Genetic factors, though not clearly identified, are likely to play some part.

Psychosocial

MUS may be precipitated by stressful life events.

Clinical presentation

Bodily distress disorder

Typically the person experiences multiple symptoms, affecting any body system, and persisting over time. Symptoms are difficult to treat and prone to evolve, resulting in distress, numerous clinical consultations, and fruitless investigations. The disorder is often associated with disruption in social/family relationships, work, and daily activities. Symptoms may cluster within specific body systems, leading specialists to identify well-recognized syndromes:

- *Rheumatology*—fibromyalgia (widespread pain, touch sensitivity, fatigue, headache, 'brain fog'), chronic fatigue syndrome (CFS) (**Box 15.1**).

> **BOX 15.1** Chronic fatigue syndrome
>
> - CFS is also known as myalgic encephalomyelitis (ME).
> - May follow viral infection (e.g. glandular fever), but also arises spontaneously; no clear aetiology—including infection—has been identified.
> - Main symptom is extreme fatigue; people are typically exhausted by mild exertion. Leads to alternating pattern of activity and debilitating fatigue, or complete exercise avoidance.
> - Other symptoms common, e.g. poor concentration, myalgia, sore throat, depression.
> - Some evidence for benefit of *graded exercise* (scheduled, gradually increasing activity) rather than rest or unplanned overactivity.
> - CBT improves fatigue and physical functioning.

- *Pain clinics*—headache, pelvic pain, lower back pain.
- *Gastroenterology*—irritable bowel syndrome (abdominal pain, bloating, diarrhoea/constipation), non-ulcer dyspepsia.
- *Otolaryngology*—dizziness, tinnitus.
- *Cardiology*—non-cardiac chest pain, palpitations.
- *Military medicine*—shell shock (historically), Gulf War syndrome.

Some people may have clear associated psychosocial stressors but deny their relevance, perhaps because they fear their physical symptoms will be dismissed as being 'all in the mind'. A person's expectations of illness may inform their symptoms, leading to uncharacteristic patterns, e.g. pain which is constant and severe throughout the day, without the usual relieving and exacerbating factors.

Hypochondriasis

This is an extreme form of health anxiety. Rather than being distressed by the *experience* of multiple unexplained symptoms, the person fears that they are suffering a specific serious illness (e.g. cancer) despite reassurance/investigations to the contrary. Usually the focus is upon one particular system or symptom, e.g. palpitations (must mean serious heart disease), abdominal pain (must mean bowel cancer). Insight may be good, poor, or absent.

Dissociative neurological symptom disorder ('functional neurological symptom disorder', 'conversion' disorder)

Considered a subset of MUS, here the person develops a specific neurological symptom not consistent with a recognized neurological disease. The presentation is often acute and dramatic, and may follow a conflict or stress (which may not always be obvious—to you or the person). The disorder is regarded as an involuntary loss of normal integration of neurological functions; the older term 'conversion' comes from the traditional Freudian view that internal psychological conflict is unconsciously 'converted' into a physical symptom. Presentations include:

- Paralysis, sensory loss, movement disorder.
- Blindness.
- Aphonia (inability to produce speech).
- Seizures ('non-epileptic seizures' or—unhelpfully—'pseudo-seizures').
- Amnesia ('psychogenic amnesia')—the loss of all personal memories including one's own identity.
- Fugue—temporary loss of retrograde and anterograde memory, accompanied by wandering far from home.
- Stupor.
- Dissociative identity ('multiple personality') disorder—rare.

Although recognized neurological signs can be present, again the person's own concept of illness may inform the presentation: sudden anaesthesia might follow a distribution that doesn't reflect dermatomes or other sensory loss patterns; a seizure may not follow the usual tonic–clonic pattern. These anomalies can be helpful in identifying conversion disorder; but do not mean that people are 'faking' symptoms!

People with conversion disorder were traditionally thought to show 'la belle indifference'—a relative lack of concern despite obviously worrying symptoms. Recent studies suggest this sign may be equally as common in those with a confirmed organic disorder!

Factitious disorder

In contrast to the previously mentioned conditions, the person *deliberately* produces, feigns, or exaggerates physical symptoms to receive medical treatment. Examples include contaminating urine samples, creating skin lesions, or feigning amnesia. The motive is psychological, e.g. to obtain sympathy or attention, to re-enact a child–parent relationship through a doctor, or to test authority. When severe, it is known as *Munchausen syndrome*, and when imposed on another (e.g. a parent tampering with their child's laboratory samples), as *Munchausen-by-proxy*.

Malingering

As in factitious disorder the person deliberately feigns physical symptoms; however, the motive is for external rather than psychological reward, e.g. to avoid military service, gain insurance or compensation, or obtain drugs.

Differential diagnosis for MUS

- Organic: rule out any possible physical cause. When symptoms are multiple and variable, a multisystem organic pathology may be responsible, e.g. sarcoidosis, occult malignancy, chronic infection (e.g. tuberculosis, HIV).
- Psychiatric conditions:
  – Anxiety and depression can cause and exacerbate symptoms (e.g. depression lowers the pain threshold) and are commonly comorbid with both medical illness and MUS.
  – Personality disorder may underlie factitious disorder; and may be comorbid with all MUS (particularly clusters B and C; see p. 258).
  – Psychosis may present with somatic hallucinations and hypochondriacal delusions.

The Hospital Anxiety and Depression Scale (HADS) focuses on the *cognitive* symptoms of anxiety and depression, helping to diagnose these disorders when physical symptoms (e.g. fatigue) are present.

Management

1. Therapeutic assessment: engagement is crucial, so take a full history and perform an appropriate physical examination.
2. Explain and reassure: many people will be reassured by knowing that their symptoms are not serious, but common and familiar. The reattribution model (**Box 15.2**) can help.
3. Don't over-investigate: unnecessary specialist referrals and physical medications reinforce physical illness beliefs and may increase anxiety. Clinicians face a dilemma in deciding when to stop investigating; however, try to ensure no more than *reasonable* investigation of possible organic causes, and review old notes and tests to prevent duplication.

> **BOX 15.2** The reattribution model
>
> Feeling understood, changing the agenda, and making the link constitute Goldberg's reattribution model.[3]
>
> 1. **Feeling understood**
>
> 2. **Changing the agenda**
>
> Your patient's agenda is physical. Your task is to bridge the gap to include a psychological *and* physical understanding. Feed back your (normal) examination/investigation findings while recognizing the reality of their symptoms, e.g.
>
> > **You:** Your examination was normal, though your neck muscles are very tight. These headaches have been causing you a lot of pain, haven't they?
> >
> > **Kirsty:** Yeah—they're driving me mad.
> >
> > **You:** Constant headaches are miserable! People can get headaches like this when under pressure. Other signs of being under pressure can include feeling shaky and tearful—a bit like you've been feeling since starting your new job. Do you think it's possible that this might be having an effect on your headaches?
> >
> > **Kirsty:** I guess . . .
>
> This reframes your patient's symptoms in the context of life events and other symptoms identified during your assessment.
>
> 3. **Making the link**
>
> Make an explicit link between symptoms and your patient's emotional state, normalizing their experience. One way to is to draw a CBT-style diagram with them, e.g.
>
> Intense worry
> 'I have a brain tumour!' → Increased muscle tension → Tension headache
>
> This opens the way for a shared understanding of the reality of symptoms, while recognizing psychosocial contributing factors.
>
> Data from Goldberg, D., Gask, L. and O'Dowd, T. (1989) The treatment of somatization: teaching techniques of reattribution. *Journal of Psychosomatic Research*, **33**(6), 689–695.

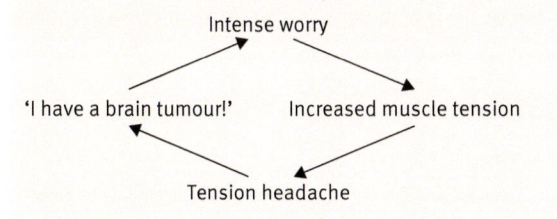

4. Emotional support: encourage the person to discuss emotional difficulties; involve their social network and support them to deal with stresses.

5. Encourage normal functioning: people with MUS may avoid normal activities, but they are crucial to recovery and preventing disability. Avoid reinforcement of symptoms or disability (e.g. providing a wheelchair in dissociative neurological disorder when someone can walk).

6. Treat comorbid illness, particularly anxiety or depression.

7. CBT: discussion, diaries, and behavioural experiments help the person to identify and modify unhelpful cognitions, reducing avoidance and reassurance-seeking behaviours.

8. Graded exercise has some benefit in certain disorders, e.g. CFS, fibromyalgia. Physiotherapy may help in dissociative neurological disorder.

> 💡 The strength of patients' beliefs may encourage you to order excessive investigations. Always ask yourself if you would normally investigate these symptoms this way.

Prognosis

Shorter duration of MUS and milder symptoms have a better prognosis. Over a quarter of people with MUS attending primary care and two-thirds of people with functional neurological symptoms remain symptomatic after a year. Rates of completed suicide (but not mortality by other causes) in people with CFS are significantly higher than in the general population. Chronic presentations fluctuate and can be exacerbated by stress.

> ❗ **In the absence of an underlying organic cause, the greatest risk to people with MUS may be iatrogenic harm. Demands by the person and their family, frustration, and defensive medical practice may encourage doctors to request unnecessary, invasive investigations or even recommend speculative treatments. These prolong symptoms, defer diagnosis, and carry their own risks of harm.**

REALITY

General approach: tips, tricks, and cautionary tales

1. Conflict and teamwork

Conflict between the person with MUS and staff doesn't solve anything, and can compromise engagement, worsening prognosis. Sufferers often feel frustrated and hopeless: they *know* that something's wrong, but their test results are normal, they may feel that nobody believes them, and worry that they'll never get better. Staff often feel helpless and exasperated, thinking there's nothing wrong, not understanding why the person keeps attending their service. This can lead to negative labelling, e.g. 'heart-sink' or 'fat-folder' patients.

To enhance staff–patient teamwork, remember two key points:

- There *is* something wrong.
- The person has *unsolved*, rather than *unsolvable* problems.

In other words, the person's help seeking is legitimate *and* there is hope. The challenge now is to use your medical and psychiatric knowledge to help them to move forward.

2. Empathize and validate

Symptoms are *real*; an itch is itchy, whether due to stress or scabies. You don't need to know the cause to empathize. People with MUS have often been deprived of empathy, almost as though professionals think it'll make things worse. It won't; it helps.

Explore their problems, then empathize and validate their experience as being *real* and disabling, upsetting, painful, or frightening. Validating symptoms doesn't mean you're validating a physical cause.

3. Negatives are positive

Before ordering tests, explain the meaning of a normal or negative result—you can both feel reassured that a frightening physical illness *isn't* causing their symptoms. Explain that you'll still take their symptoms seriously if test results show no abnormalities; this isn't the end of their management plan.

4. Focus on the impact

Once you or other doctors have ruled out organic causes, you need to *stop* trying to 'get to the bottom of it'. Instead of focusing on the cause or diagnosis, focus on the *impact* of these symptoms on the person, as it leads on to what you can *do* to help. The BATHE[4] method provides a useful approach to asking about MUS and is of course relevant to taking a history in any specialty of medicine. Empathic exploration of the context of symptoms, and how people feel about them and cope with them, can help build a shared understanding of the problems.

5. Believe in yourself

People may expect or demand specialist referrals, while you worry that you're missing something or feel that your expertise is being challenged. If you're sure that you have excluded organic causes, don't join your patient in their anxiety. The exception to this rule is if symptoms change or show alarming new features, e.g. rectal bleeding in someone with presumed IBS.

6. Boundaries

Offer regular, scheduled appointments. One member of the team should see this person; ten people will say ten slightly different things—leading to ten different plans!

The interview

• = Example question. * = Question linking to other parts of the history.

MUS history

Symptoms

- *Tell me more about the problems you've been having.*
- Have you noticed any pattern to your symptoms?
- Check specifically for medications (including over-the-counter or internet-bought analgesics, benzodiazepines).
- Explore psychosocial context/triggers.

Illness behaviours

- *Are your symptoms the same every day?*
  – [Yes]
    - What can you do on a good day?
    - What's a bad day like?

- Does anything determine whether you have a good or a bad day??
  - *[No]*
    - Take me through what you do in a typical day.
- What steps have you already taken to try to reduce symptoms?
  - Have you sought any help so far? What's been suggested? *[Check if the person has seen more than one specialist about the same symptom]*
- What can't you do anymore?
  - What stops you?/What would happen if you did this?
- Are there things you have to *avoid* doing?
  - (For example, weight-bearing/particular movements/work.)
- Are there things you have to do to prevent further harm/keep yourself safe?
- Do you ever push yourself to do things despite your symptoms? What happens? *[Check for overburdening]*
- How do you relax?

Illness beliefs

- **What's your biggest worry about what's happening?**
- What do you worry might happen if you did *[activity]* despite *[symptoms]*?
  - Cause damage?
  - Worsen symptoms in the short-term?
- Have you read anything worrying? *[Online articles, fora]*
- Do you know anyone who's had similar problems?
  - What happened? *[Screen: severe illness/medical mismanagement, missed diagnosis]*

Other history
Effect on life

- **What do you miss doing most?**
- How's it affecting your work/studies/relationship/social life/family/hobbies?
- How do your family/friends/colleagues/partner help/react? *[Screen: support, (excessive) concern, criticism (reinforcing sick role?)]*

Emotional consequences

- How do your symptoms leave you feeling? *[Screen: depression, anxiety (pervasive versus just when symptoms present, severity]*

Risk

- **Do you ever feel so bad, you think of harming yourself? Ending your life?**
- Have your symptoms caused any other problems? *[Screen: medication dependence, complications from excess investigations (e.g. adhesions from exploratory surgery, infections from long-term catheter), privately funded tests]*

Fatigue history (15 minutes)

Candidate's instructions
Emily Joseph is an 18-year-old A-Level student who saw her GP twice this month, feeling tired all the time. Her mother, who attended both appointments, was concerned about glandular fever and brought printouts of online articles. The GP asked Ms Joseph to book a double appointment for follow-up, without her mother. Please take a history with a view to making a differential diagnosis.

Patient's brief

History
I'm subdued and slightly irritated about telling my story all over again; haven't you read my notes? I'm feeling exhausted and stressed because I had to defer my five A-Level exams and take a gap year because of the tiredness. It all started last summer when I was training for a marathon. I was running in Richmond Park every day and eating really healthily, buying supplements online, and studying hard: I want to be a vet. Then all of a sudden I came down with 'flu but *it never got better*. Mum advised bed rest but I had to run the marathon (I'd raised all that sponsorship!), so I did. It wasn't my personal best time and after that, I never got back to my old self. I read about a model who had Lyme disease and then I realized Richmond Park is full of ticks! I can't recall any bites or rashes, but it must be that.

> *Key characteristics*
> - I'm exhausted but preoccupied with getting a medical diagnosis.
> - When pressed, my family and I have high expectations that I excel.
> - I'm unsympathetic to a psychological model of fatigue: we're an army family. We value strength and resilience.
> - I'm still taking supplements I bought online, for when I can run again.
> - My periods are regular but *so* heavy. That doesn't help.
>
> *Other history*
> - I'm at the low end of a healthy BMI, but I'm anxious about weight gain now that I can't run.
> - I had the MMR vaccinations separately when I was five, after the army base GP insisted that I had to have them all.
> - I have three brothers and they're all in the army now. Everyone's quite protective of me: I'm the 'baby' of the family.
>
> *Question*
>
> I *can't* defer my A-Levels again. How will I ever have the energy?
>
> *Worry*
>
> I've read a lot online about Lyme disease. I'm considering sending samples by post to get the antibody tests. If you can't help me, should I see a specialist in America?

💡 **Ms Joseph may have CFS, but it's important to rule out differential diagnoses. These include anorexia nervosa, anaemia secondary to menorrhagia, viral and bacterial infections, endocrine pathologies (e.g. hypothyroidism, diabetes mellitus), and adverse effects from treatments purchased online. If CFS is diagnosed, a programme of graded exercise with or without CBT is likely to be beneficial. Skilful communication and psychoeducation for her and her mother will be key to engaging them in treatment and reassuring them that further investigations and seeing multiple specialists is likely to be counterproductive.**

NEXT STEPS

Suspected malignancy after MUS

You are a CT1 in a general surgical outpatient clinic, seeing Ms Vanessa Ouade, a 52-year-old woman who has two large volumes of hospital notes. Her GP has referred her due to a year's history of irregular bowel habit. She has been seen and investigated by several specialty clinics in the past. Ms Ouade tells you: 'My GP said it was my IBS playing up again, I had to fight to get a referral.'

The history reveals abdominal pain, loss of appetite, fatigue, bloating, and 5kg weight loss. In recent years, Ms Ouade's sister and their mother have been diagnosed with breast cancer, but breast examination identifies no abnormalities. You organize further urgent tests and she asks you anxiously if she has cancer, too. You explain that with her symptoms and family history, it will be important to rule out ovarian as well as intestinal problems. Ms Ouade tearfully asks, 'Should I have seen you sooner?'

- How will you answer her question?

Issues
- Managing the immediate situation.
- Management of a person with previous MUS.

Your response

This is an uncomfortable situation, but Ms Ouade asks a reasonable question. It's important that she understands the facts: she has worrying symptoms of weight loss, abdominal pain and altered bowel habit, and a family history which could implicate a genetic predisposition, but you do not know the diagnosis yet. Remain professional: neither leap to dismiss her concerns, nor criticize the GP, however tempting this may be. Focus on the here and now: Ms Ouade is in the right place and her investigations will be prioritized. If cancer is detected, this is a common and treatable condition. Ms Ouade may feel that her symptoms were not taken seriously enough, soon enough: this can happen when people present to their doctor with MUS. If she is unhappy, inform her of the complaints procedure and reassure her that complaints will not affect her care. Remember that this is an anxiety-provoking experience, and offer to call a family member, to be present and take her home.

Other measures

Document Ms Ouade's symptoms in her own words, including any concerns. Clearly detail the advice and explanations you have provided; your notes may be read if she makes a complaint. After the clinic, inform your consultant of the situation.

Effects on current treatment

Ms Ouade may have had a long history of unsatisfactory consultations already; her confidence and trust in doctors may be low, especially if a chance to diagnose ovarian cancer earlier was missed. This increases the complexity of her medical case: she may need extra time to explain her diagnosis and management, and vent her feelings.

Movie buff
I Remember Me (2001): film-maker Kim Snyder's documentary, inspired by her own experience of CFS, explores several 'epidemics' and asks what it's like to have an illness which is poorly understood.

Memento (2000): this psychological thriller tells the story of a man who suffers anterograde amnesia following trauma. It explores themes of confusion, time fragmentation, and paranoia associated with the condition.

The Falling (2014): starring a young Maisie Williams, the story of a mysterious fainting epidemic which breaks out at a strict girls' boarding school, following a tragedy.

Book shelf
Cardinal, M. (1975) *The Words to Say It*: this account of acute anxiety and depression, manifesting through medically unexplained vaginal bleeding, autobiographically describes the experience of treatment with Freudian psychoanalysis.

Haddon, M. (2006) *A Spot of Bother*: Haddon's novel tells the story of George Hall, who, after a period of acute stress, becomes convinced that a skin lesion is malignant.

Sacks, O. (1984) *A Leg to Stand On*: after an accident, neurologist Oliver Sacks found that during the anticipated routine recuperation, his leg no longer felt part of his body. Writing about the experience was his only relief.

Strouse, J. (1981) *Alice James: A Biography*: the less well-known sister of novelist Henry and psychologist William James was severely affected by 'neurasthenia' (today, CFS). Its development over her short life is traced in this compelling biography.

Sullivan, S. (2015) *It's All in Your Head: True Stories of Imaginary Illness*: disregard the title, because these words should never be uttered! Title aside, consultant neurologist O'Sullivan's sensitive book presents case studies of people with MUS, from paralysis, seizures and blindness to chronic fatigue and pain.

Footlights
Still Ill (2016): a play by the Kandinsky theatre company about conversion disorder. Written in collaboration with neuropsychiatrists it was well received by critics and patient groups. It explores the search for meaning following diagnosis and how it feels to be told that 'there's nothing wrong with you'.

Notes

1. Cheyne, G. (1733) *The English Malady: or A Treatise of Nervous Diseases of all Kinds.* London: G. Strahan.
2. Sullivan, S. (2015) *It's All in Your Head: True Stories of Imaginary Illness.* London: Chatto & Windus.
3. Goldberg, D., Gask, L., O'Dowd, T. (1989) The treatment of somatization: teaching techniques of reattribution. *Journal of Psychosomatic Research*, **33**, 689–95.
4. Lieberman, J.A., Stuart, M.R. (1999) The BATHE method: incorporating counselling and psychotherapy into the everyday management of patients. *Journal of Clinical Psychiatry*, **1**, 35–8.

Journal club

Carson, A.J., Brown, R., David, A.S., et al. (2012) Functional (conversion) neurological symptoms: research since the millennium. *Journal of Neurology, Neurosurgery & Psychiatry*, **83**, 842–50.

Fink, P., Rosendal, M., Toft, T. (2002) Assessment and treatment of functional disorders in general practice: the extended reattribution and management model—an advanced educational program for nonpsychiatric doctors. *Psychosomatics*, **43**, 93–131.

Hatcher, S., Arroll, B. (2008) Assessment and management of medically unexplained symptoms. *BMJ*, **336**, 1124–8.

Nimnuan, C., Hotopf, N., Wessely, S. (2001) Medically unexplained symptoms: epidemiological studies in seven specialities. *Journal of Psychosomatic Research*, **51**, 361–7.

Salkovskis, P.M. (1996) The cognitive approach to anxiety: threat beliefs, safety-seeking behaviour and the special case of health anxiety and obsessions. In: *Frontiers of Cognitive Therapy* (ed. P.M. Salkovskis), pp. 48–74. New York: Guilford Press.

Wessely, S., Nimnuan, C., Sharpe, M. (1999) Functional somatic syndromes: one or many? *The Lancet*, **354**, 936–9.

Resources

www.neurosymptoms.org/: written by neurologist Dr Jon Stone, a wealth of resources on dissociative neurological symptom disorder.

Go to www.oup.com/uk/stringer2e for a wealth of additional resources, including an OCSE mark scheme, filmed scenarios, and self-assessment questions.

16 Eating Disorders

True or false?

Answers on p. 277

1. Five per cent of people with eating disorders are male.
2. Perfectionism and low self-esteem are associated with anorexia nervosa but not bulimia nervosa.
3. Anorexia nervosa causes pancytopenia.
4. Russell sign indicates malnutrition.
5. ECG findings in eating disorders include tachycardia and shortened QTc.
6. Refeeding syndrome is characterized by low potassium, magnesium, and phosphate.
7. Failure to complete the SUSS (sit up–squat–stand) test suggests that inpatient treatment may be needed.
8. Eating disorders are culture-bound syndromes.
9. Selective serotonin reuptake inhibitors can reduce bingeing and purging in bulimia nervosa.
10. Family therapy is effective for eating disorders.

Contents

Principles
Introduction
Epidemiology
Aetiology
- Genetics
- Neurobiological factors
- Psychological and family theories
- Sociocultural
- Psychiatric comorbidity

Clinical presentation
- Anorexia nervosa
- Bulimia nervosa
- Physical complications
- Differential diagnosis

Investigations
Management
- Anorexia nervosa
- Bulimia nervosa

Prognosis

Reality
General approach: tips, tricks, and cautionary tales
The interview
- Eating disorder history

Next steps
An underweight woman with fertility problems
- Further information
- Enhancing motivation and understanding
- Management
- Weight gain

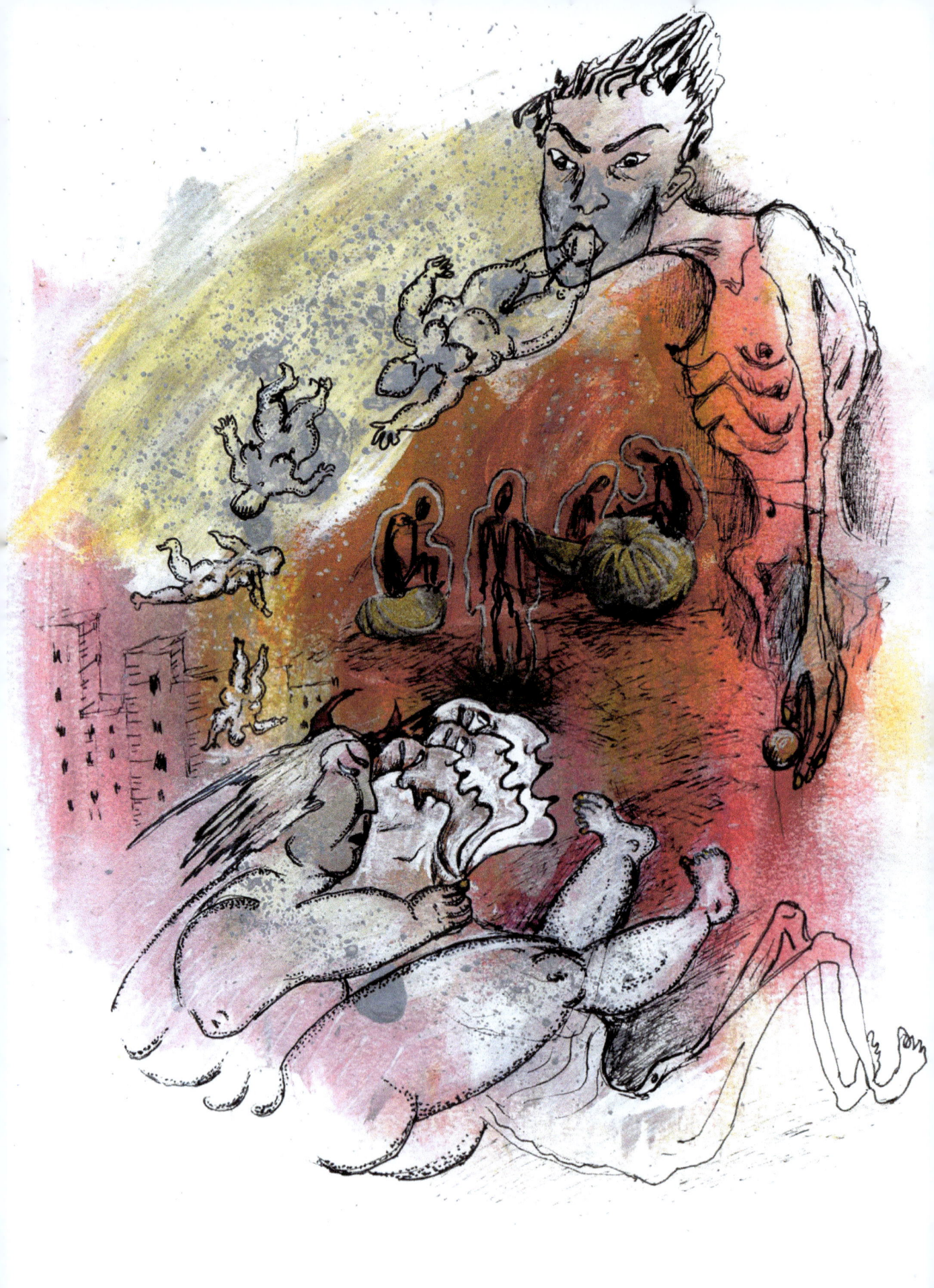

PRINCIPLES

This is a belief that you deserve slow torture, violent death. Without being entirely aware of it, I had settled on starvation as my torture of choice. When people think about killing themselves, they usually think about killing themselves with the least amount of pain, the briefest period of suffering. This is different.

Marya Hornbacher, *Wasted: A Memoir of Anorexia and Bulimia*[1]

Introduction

For most of us, food is functional (providing energy, abating a rumbling stomach) or enjoyable (delicious or a reason to socialize). We may have been on a diet or tried to change our body through exercise without it completely taking over our lives or endangering our health. While concern about body image is increasingly common in the general population, in people with eating disorders, food, weight, and body image become *all*-consuming. Eating disorders are suspected where the following behaviours aren't explained by physical health problems, developmental stage, food scarcity, or culturally sanctioned practices.

- **Anorexia nervosa** (AN): a persistent pattern of reduced energy intake (restricted eating), purging behaviours (e.g. self-induced vomiting, laxative or enema misuse), and/or increased energy expenditure (e.g. excessive exercise) associated with significantly low bodyweight for height, age, and development, usually associated with fear of gaining weight.
- **Bulimia nervosa** (BN): frequent, recurrent episodes of binge eating (e.g. once per week or more over at least 1 month), followed by repeated, inappropriate purging (to compensate for the binge). A *binge eating episode* is a confined period in which the person feels noticeably unable to control or stop eating. The person's bodyweight is normal for height, age, and developmental stage.
- **Binge eating disorder** (BED): the pattern of binge eating seen in BN, often accompanied by feelings of guilt or disgust, but without compensatory purging; this can cause obesity.
- **Avoidant/restrictive food intake disorder** (ARFID): insufficient quantity or variety of food intake to meet energy or nutritional requirements, in the absence of bodyweight or shape concerns.

Epidemiology

Although eating disorders mostly affect women, the incidence is rising in men; the current female-to-male ratio is 8:1. Onset is usually in mid to late adolescence, although symptoms can start in childhood and later adulthood. The lifetime prevalence of eating disorders in England is 0.6% (AN), 1.0% (BN), and 3.2% (BED). BN may be underdiagnosed because people aren't visibly underweight. Eating disorders are commoner in 'Westernized' societies, where there's pressure to conform to thin body ideals (typified by profoundly underweight celebrities); incidence in low- and middle-income countries is increasing in line with globalization. People from black and ethnic minority groups are at lower risk than white populations.

Aetiology

Genetics

Family and twin studies suggest a significant genetic contribution to eating disorders (via single nucleotide polymorphisms (SNPs): multiple genes of small effect); heritability estimates range from 30% to 80%. Relatives of people with BN also have higher rates of obesity, depression, and substance misuse.

Neurobiological factors

Brain imaging findings are inconsistent and possibly confounded by the effects of malnutrition. However, functional imaging suggests abnormal connectivity between reward centres (e.g. the striatum) and executive control (prefrontal cortex). Other studies suggest imbalances between dopaminergic (reward) and serotonergic systems.

Psychological and family theories

People with eating disorders more commonly have a history of obstetric complications, sleeping and feeding difficulties, and childhood abuse. Research into *allostatic load* seeks to understand the relationship between adaptation to stress (e.g. early emotional adversity) and its effects on the body. Personality traits (perfectionism, neuroticism, and low self-esteem) are risk factors for both AN and BN. One theory proposes that initial weight loss enhances someone's sense of achievement and autonomy, reinforcing perfectionist traits. When life feels out of control, the comfort associated with controlling *something* (weight) may also reinforce AN.

Parental overprotection and family 'enmeshment' are associated with AN. Enmeshment describes excessively close relationships, where unclear boundaries compromise independence. One theory views AN as a means of avoiding the stress of separation from family support or becoming an independent sexual being; AN maintains dependence on family *and* a peripubertal physique. BN is associated with disturbed family dynamics, parental weight concern, and high parental expectation.

Sociocultural

Societal pressure to be thin is an important factor in eating disorders and socially encouraged dieting may trigger eating disorders in genetically susceptible individuals. High-risk groups include people in occupations focused on weight or body image, including models, athletes, and dancers.

Psychiatric comorbidity

Eating disorders are commonly comorbid with other mental health disorders. Up to 75% of people report a history of depression; anxiety disorders, obsessive–compulsive disorder (OCD), body dysmorphic disorder (BDD), substance use disorders, and personality disorder (particularly anankastia and borderline pattern) are also more common. People with BN often have a history of obesity and up to 50% previously suffered AN (the reverse pattern is less common).

> 💡 Some features of eating disorders result from starvation itself. Healthy men subjected to semi-starvation develop preoccupation with food, unusual food preparation rituals, and binge eating with feelings of self-disgust.

Clinical presentation

The key similarities and differences between AN and BN are summarized in **Table 16.1**.

Table 16.1 Symptoms of AN and BN

Symptom	AN	BN
BMI	<18.5kg/m²	>18.5kg/m²
Deliberate weight loss	✓	✓
Bingeing	✗	✓
Purging	✓	✓
Body image distortion	✓	✓
Endocrine dysfunction	Common	Uncommon

Anorexia nervosa

See **Figure 16.1**.

- **Body mass index (BMI) <18.5kg/m²** (or <5th percentile BMI-for-age in children and adolescents). This is divided into AN with 'significantly low' bodyweight (BMI >14kg/m²) and AN with 'dangerously low' bodyweight (BMI <14kg/m²) or <0.3 percentile BMI-for-age.
- **Deliberate weight loss.** Methods may include:
  - Dietary restriction, reducing calorie intake and avoiding foods considered fattening (e.g. fat, complex carbohydrates, whole food groups).
  - Purging.
  - Excessive exercise.
  - Medication misuse, e.g. appetite suppressants, thyroxine, diuretics, stimulants such as cocaine. People with type 1 diabetes may omit insulin doses to prevent fat deposition.
- **Distorted body image:** people are preoccupied with their body shape; they see themselves as normal or overweight and dread gaining weight.
- **Endocrine dysfunction:** the impact of starvation on the hypothalamic–pituitary–gonadal axis may cause amenorrhoea in women and impotence in men. Libido is lost in both sexes. If AN begins before puberty, menarche and breast development are delayed or arrested.

Weight loss sets up a vicious circle, as starvation exacerbates preoccupation with food, e.g. baking or cooking elaborate meals for others. People with AN may conceal their symptoms, e.g. chewing but spitting food into a cup, talking about meals that they haven't eaten.

> 💡 BMI isn't particularly accurate in children and adolescents, so BMI-for-age is used instead.

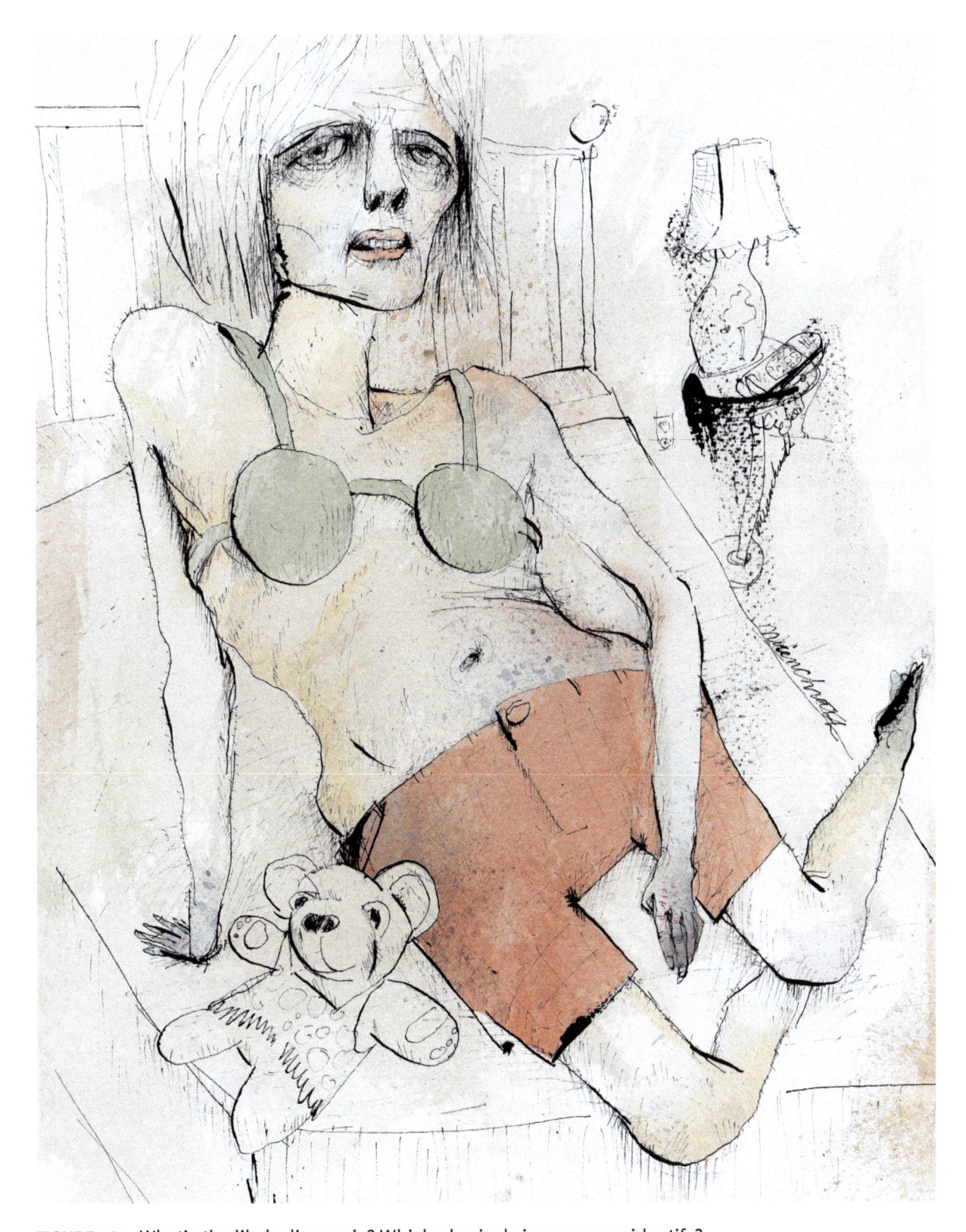

FIGURE 16.1 What's the likely diagnosis? Which physical signs can you identify?

Bulimia nervosa

- **Binge eating:** recurrent episodes of (usually secretive) overeating. People experience irresistible cravings for food and lose control, eating large amounts with a sense of urgency and compulsion. They may consume thousands of calories, often eating 'forbidden' foods, e.g. 20 doughnuts. Binges may be triggered by stress.

Clinical presentation **203**

- **Purging:** bingeing causes feelings of shame and guilt, triggering desperate measures to undo the 'damage', e.g. vomiting, laxatives.
- **Deliberate weight loss:** between binges, the person usually tries to control their weight through diet, exercise, etc.
- **Body image distortion:** people with BN feel fat, are preoccupied with their shape and weight, and often hate their body.
- **BMI >18.5kg/m²** unlike AN, people with BN have normal or slightly increased bodyweight, with normal endocrine functioning (regular periods).

🛑 Some people with eating disorders access harmful 'Ana' (AN) and 'Mia' (BN) websites, encouraging each other to lose weight, posting selfies, and sharing (often dangerous) weight loss methods. They normalize disordered eating and can make it harder for people to recover.

🛑 'Diabulimia' is an informal term for the omission of insulin by people with diabetes, to lose weight. Despite its name, people may present with BN *or* AN. Complications include blindness (diabetic retinopathy), diabetic ketoacidosis, and renal failure.

Physical complications

Table 16.2 summarizes the physical complications of eating disorders. Starvation-related problems are commoner in AN, while purging-related problems tend to affect people with BN. However, since purging and starvation occur in both conditions, all complications should be considered during assessments of AN or BN.

💡 Hypotension presents as lightheadedness on standing.

💡 Delayed gastric emptying makes people with AN feel bloated after eating small amounts.

💡 Lanugo hair is the body's attempt to keep warm following body fat loss.

🛑 In BN, electrolytes are closely monitored. Vomiting and laxative misuse cause hypokalaemia and hyponatraemia (causing arrhythmias and convulsions, respectively).

Differential diagnosis

Unintentional weight loss and difficulty eating enough always require a thorough history, physical examination, and MSE. People without eating disorders usually have a realistic understanding of their weight and want to regain lost weight. When the person denies deliberate weight loss, differential diagnoses for AN and BN include:

- *Organic causes*, e.g. malignancy, chronic infection (e.g. TB, HIV), gastrointestinal pathology (e.g. coeliac disease, Crohn disease, oesophageal stricture), endocrine dysfunction (e.g. diabetes mellitus, Addison disease, hyperthyroidism).
- *Affective disorders*: weight loss *can* be severe in depression and mania but only in the context of other affective symptoms (e.g. altered mood, energy, enjoyment).
- *Anxiety disorders*: OCD may cause food avoidance (e.g. due to contamination fears) or lengthy rituals which obstruct regular meals. In BDD, people believe that part of their body is abnormal or ugly (e.g. that their nose is grossly misshapen)—beliefs focused primarily on weight, 'fat', or size suggest a primary eating disorder.
- *Psychosis*: food restriction may result from persecutory delusions (e.g. poisoning) or grandiose delusions (e.g. no *need* to eat).
- *Autism spectrum disorder* is associated with rigid eating habits and preferred foods.
- *Other specified feeding or eating disorder (OSFED)* is sometimes used for atypical eating disorder presentations (e.g. AN-like *except* their BMI is still >18.5kg/m² or BN-like, but very infrequent binge/purging).

Differential diagnoses for BED include:

- *Depression*: overeating may occur, without distorted body image or compensatory behaviours.
- *Organic and genetic conditions*, e.g. brain tumours, Kluver–Bucy syndrome (hyperphagia and hypersexuality), Prader–Willi syndrome.

💡 Depression and OCD are relatively common comorbid disorders and can complicate diagnosis and management.

Investigations

1. Physical observations, including CBG, lying/standing BP (look for postural BP drop).
2. Height, weight, and BMI.
3. Sit up–squat–stand (SUSS) test: impaired in severe AN due to proximal myopathy. Ask the person to sit up from lying flat, then to rise from a squatting position—both without using their hands.

Table 16.2 Physical complications of eating disorders

	Starvation	Purging
General	<ul><li>Emaciation</li><li>Dehydration</li><li>Short stature</li><li>Lethargy</li><li>Cold intolerance</li><li>Blue/cold peripheries</li><li>Hypothermia</li><li>Infections (from reduced immunity)</li><li>Dry skin, brittle hair/nails</li><li>Fine, downy (lanugo) body hair</li><li>Peripheral oedema (low albumin)</li><li>Hypercholesterolaemia</li><li>Hypercarotenaemia (yellowish skin)</li></ul>	<ul><li>Dehydration</li><li>*Russell's sign* (knuckle calluses/cuts from self-induced vomiting)</li><li>Swollen parotid glands (puffy face)</li><li>Eroded dental enamel</li><li>Dental caries</li><li>Hypercholesterolaemia</li><li>Hypercarotenaemia</li></ul>
Haematological	<ul><li>Anaemia</li><li>Leucopenia</li><li>Thrombocytopenia</li><li>Pancytopenia (severe AN causes bone marrow hypoplasia)</li></ul>	
Cardiovascular	<ul><li>Bradycardia</li><li>Hypotension</li><li>Mitral valve dysfunction</li><li>Cardiac failure (e.g. oedema)</li><li>Syncope</li><li>Sudden death</li></ul>	<ul><li>Arrhythmia (hypokalaemia)</li><li>Sudden death</li></ul>
Gastrointestinal	<ul><li>Constipation</li><li>Abdominal pain</li><li>Gastro-oesophageal reflux</li><li>Delayed gastric emptying</li><li>Gastroduodenal ulcers</li><li>Malnutrition: deficiency diseases</li><li>Nutritional hepatitis (↓albumin; ↑bilirubin, lactate dehydrogenase, alkaline phosphatase)</li></ul>	<ul><li>Abdominal pain</li><li>Oesophageal tears</li><li>Gastric rupture</li><li>*Melanosis coli* (mucosal pigmentation from laxative misuse, seen on colonoscopy)</li></ul>
Endocrine	<ul><li>Delayed/arrested puberty</li><li>Amenorrhoea</li><li>Erectile dysfunction, loss of morning erections</li><li>Low libido</li><li>Infertility (ovarian/testicular atrophy)</li><li>Hypothyroidism</li></ul>	
Musculoskeletal	<ul><li>Osteoporosis and fractures</li><li>Muscle wasting, especially proximal myopathy</li></ul>	
Neurological	<ul><li>Peripheral neuropathy</li><li>Cognitive deficits</li><li>Delirium</li><li>Coma</li><li>Cerebral volume loss</li></ul>	<ul><li>Convulsions (hyponatraemia)</li><li>Peripheral neuropathy</li><li>Delirium</li></ul>

4. Blood tests (**Tables 16.3 and 16.4**):
   - FBC, U&Es, LFTs including albumin.
   - Bone profile, creatine kinase, glucose, TFTs.
5. ECG: bradycardia, arrhythmias, and prolonged QTc.
6. Others as indicated, e.g. dual-energy X-ray absorptiometry (DXA) scan in AN (osteoporosis); pregnancy test in *any* women with amenorrhoea.

> ❗ *Any* renal impairment increases a person's risk of electrolyte dysfunction when rehydrating or refeeding—take it seriously!

Management

The initial interview requires time and skill: engaging the person is crucial. GPs may manage people with mild or low-risk presentations but refer complex or high-risk presentations to specialist eating disorder services. Comorbid diagnoses (e.g. depression, anxiety disorders, substance use, personality disorder) require treatment in parallel.

Anorexia nervosa

Biological interventions

Nutritional management is essential to prevent and treat life-threatening complications. Specialist dieticians recommend meal plans, supplements, and help the team to determine a target weight range, with realistic weekly weight gain.

People with the greatest physical health complications need nutritional stabilization on a medical ward, applying MARSIPAN guidelines (**Table 16.4**). Otherwise, high-risk management is undertaken in specialist eating

Table 16.3 Biomarker changes in eating disorders

	Abnormality		Cause	
	Low	High	Starvation	Bingeing/purging
FBC	✓		✓ (WCC, Hb, platelets)	✓ (WCC)
U&Es	✓		✓ (Urea)	✓ (K^+, Na^+)
Chloride	✓			✓
Albumin	✓		✓	
Glucose	✓		✓	✓
TFTs (T_3)	✓		✓	
FSH, LH, oestrogen, progesterone	✓		✓	
Phosphate	✓		✓	✓
Calcium	✓		✓	✓
Magnesium	✓		✓	✓
LFTs (ALP, bilirubin)		✓	✓	
Creatine kinase		✓	✓	
Amylase		✓		✓
Cortisol		✓	✓	
Growth hormone		✓	✓	
Cholesterol		✓	✓	✓

Table 16.4 Adapted MARSIPAN (Management of Really Sick Patients with Anorexia Nervosa) guidelines: investigation results suggesting high complications risk

Investigation	Result
BMI (kg/m²)	• Lower risk: 15–17.5 • Moderate: 13–15 • High risk: <13 • Rapid weight loss (>1kg/week)
Physical examination	• Hypotension (especially if postural drop) • Bradycardia (<40bpm) • Core temperature <35°C • ↓muscle power (SUSS) • Purpuric rash
Blood tests	• ↓Na⁺ (<130mmol/L) • ↓K⁺ (<3.0mmol/L) • ↑transaminases • Hypoglycaemia (<3mmol/L) • ↑urea/creatinine
ECG	• Bradycardia • ↑QTc interval (>450ms) • Non-specific T-wave changes • ECG changes associated with hypokalaemia

NB: although MARSIPAN guidelines relate to severe AN, they also apply to people with BN or rapid weight loss.

Adapted with permission from The Royal Colleges of Psychiatrists, Physicians and Pathologists. *MARSIPAN: Management of Really Sick Patients with Anorexia Nervosa*, 2nd ed. College Report CR189. Copyright © 2014 The Royal College of Psychiatrists.

disorder units. Daytime hospital care is sometimes possible if risks are moderate and most people receive long-term management as outpatients.

Many people struggle to accept help: despite high risks of mortality and morbidity, AN narrows the person's focus. The illness can become their world, providing comfort, so relinquishing control over eating can feel terrifying. This is particularly true at very low bodyweight, when the person's thinking becomes rigid, limiting their ability to consider pros and cons of treatment. In life-threatening situations where the person refuses treatment or lacks capacity to accept treatment for AN, compulsory admission and refeeding (by nasogastric tube) is sometimes needed under the MHA.

> **Refeeding syndrome** is a potentially fatal complication of feeding extremely malnourished people. The switch from fat (in starvation) to carbohydrate (when feeding) metabolism increases insulin secretion, causing electrolytes (e.g. potassium, phosphate, and magnesium) to move rapidly from blood into intracellular stores, risking life-threatening arrhythmias from sudden electrolyte depletion.

> **Be alert to treatment sabotage.** People with AN may try to convince staff they're gaining weight, e.g. before being weighed, filling their pockets, or water loading (drinking excess water, sometimes causing hyponatraemia). They may covertly continue weight loss, e.g. purging, secretly or subtly exercising.

Psychological interventions

- *Motivational interviewing* (see p. 119) engages people who lack insight, feel ambivalent about AN, or view it positively.
- *Family therapy* involves the whole household. Several families may attend multifamily therapy, to share problems and solutions.
- *Eating disorder-focused cognitive behavioural therapy* (CBT-ED) addresses control, low self-esteem, and perfectionism. The person learns to monitor their dietary intake, and associated thoughts and feelings in daily diaries.
- *Focal psychodynamic therapy* (FPT) develops self-awareness, interpersonal skills, and self-esteem, through the relationship with the therapist. This suits people with later onset or chronic AN, or who've already tried CBT-ED.

Social interventions

- Families are usually involved early and offered information about the illness, as well as healthy eating and nutrition.
- Charities (e.g. BEAT) provide information and support for people with AN, their families, healthcare professionals, and the general public.
- People with severe AN often need help to maintain or re-enter education or employment. They may need support to shop, prepare meals, maintain portion sizes, and eat outside their home as part of recovery. This can be tackled through specialist occupational therapist-led inpatient or outpatient group activities.

Bulimia nervosa

Most management is provided in the community.

Biological interventions

Medical complications are managed accordingly. SSRI antidepressants (e.g. fluoxetine) can reduce bingeing and purging by enhancing impulse control.

Psychological interventions

- *BN-focused guided self-help programmes* provide psychoeducation and CBT. They encourage exploration of thoughts and feelings which trigger binges.
- *Adapted CBT-ED* may be offered if this is ineffective.
- *BN-focused family therapy* can help children and young adults living at home.
- *Longer-term psychotherapy* may be required to address underlying or comorbid difficulties contributing to BN.

Social interventions

In addition to interventions used for AN, dental care is required to manage complications of frequent vomiting.

> **!** MSE and risk assessment are as important as physical healthcare, due to elevated suicide risk.

> **💡** Relatives may share perfectionist traits with their loved one, making their caring role even more stressful.

Prognosis

The standardized mortality ratio (of observed deaths in people with that diagnosis compared to that expected in the general population) of AN is 5.86, among the highest for all psychiatric disorders; 20% of deaths are by suicide. Fifty per cent of people with AN are asymptomatic after 10 years. The remaining 40% have continued symptoms; conversion of AN to BN is common. Very low weight, later onset, longer duration, and comorbid BN symptoms are poor prognostic factors for AN. After 10 years, 70% of people with BN have recovered and 1% have died. Severe bingeing or purging, low body weight, and comorbid depression are poor prognostic factors for BN.

REALITY

General approach: tips, tricks, and cautionary tales

Much of this section applies to people who are under- *or* overweight.

1. Food/weight *isn't* the problem

You wouldn't tell someone choking on a peanut to *breathe more*—you'd deal with the peanut. Likewise, telling someone with an eating disorder to simply *eat more* or *less* misses the point: eating and weight changes are observable signs of deeper problems, like low self-esteem. Try to understand how the person feels about themselves, and what other things are worrying or stressing them. Exploring their priorities first can engage the person, making eating and weight difficulties easier to tackle.

2. Take concerns seriously

If someone thinks their eating is a problem, it *is* a problem—whatever their weight. Respect their courage for telling you, listen to their concerns, and take them seriously. Never judge by appearances:

- 'Normal' BMI can hide severe distress and life-threatening electrolyte imbalances.
- Although many people with AN are young, white females, don't overlook men, older people, and members of ethnic minorities.

Likewise, listen to carers' concerns: they know the person better than you (or your clinic scales).

3. Don't bully

People with eating disorders are usually extremely self-critical, like they're walking around with a bully in their head: '*You're not good enough/thin enough . . . You don't deserve food . . . Nobody wants you . . . You're disgusting . . .*' Online forums show that people with eating disorders often feel bullied or insulted by health professionals. Avoid:

- Giving frightening lectures about the dangers of their weight/behaviour.
- Sighing in response to weight gain or loss.
- Inadvertent humour about weight.
- Describing weight or BMI as '*bad*' or '*good*' (emphasizes their sense that weight makes *them* bad or good).
- Using negative words to describe someone who is:
  - Overweight, e.g. *fat, greedy, lazy, weak-willed*.
  - Underweight, e.g. *stick-thin, vain, attention-seeking, immature*.

Making someone feel worse *won't* motivate them to get better—it'll just fuel their self-hatred, worsening their problems.

4. Be on their side

Be the antidote to their spiteful inner bully, with compassion, support, and sensitive positivity. Weight problems often feel overwhelming. Show that you believe they can change, without setting them up for failure. Explain that sustainable change takes time: it's hard work and they may struggle, come to a standstill, or even go backwards at times. This is a normal part of learning how to do things differently, *not* a sign of failure.

Provide information about the dangers of extreme weight change methods in small, relevant chunks. Then use health *benefits* to reinforce successes, e.g. 'You've lowered your risk of osteoporosis.' Avoid making praise contingent on weight change. Rather, pay attention to the *process*, e.g.:

- 'You've worked so hard this week.'
- 'This was a challenging week. What made it difficult?'

Additionally, *validate*. Let the person know what you value about them, sticking to personality rather than physical traits, e.g. their sense of humour, honesty, courage. Don't overdo it: the person may find it hard to hear praise. Just validate when you notice something and really mean it.

5. Family matters

An eating disorder can feel like a war fought between the person, their loved ones, and the healthcare team. Don't expect to win every battle, or to solve entrenched problems overnight. Families often feel stressed and helpless. They may become overprotective, authoritarian, or critical, unintentionally reinforcing disordered eating. Encourage carers to stay calm, warm, and compassionate, and to access support for themselves. When arguments arise, facilitate discussions and keep everyone working together, rather than taking sides.

The interview

• = Example question. * = Question linking to other parts of the history.

Weight

Current

- *How do you feel about your weight?*
- Are you currently trying to lose weight?
- * How?

Progress

- *How's your weight changed? Since when?*

Ideal

- *What's your target weight? Why?*
- How will you know when to stop?

Deliberate weight loss methods

Rather than focusing on every dietary detail, explore the *overall* pattern and its social and emotional impact.

Dietary restriction

- *Tell me about your daily diet.*
- Can you take me through an average day?
- Are there rules to guide what you eat? *[Screen: calorie limit/avoided foods]*
- Do you ever skip meals? Do you ever fast?
- Have you ever pretended to eat more than you actually did? How?
- Does it sometimes feel like food dominates your life?
- * Do you ever lose control? What happens?

Exercise

- *What exercise do you do? [Check method, duration, frequency]*

Vomiting/laxatives

- *Some people make themselves vomit to lose weight. Have you done that?*
- Have you ever used laxatives?
- How often?
- * What triggers this?

Medications

- *Have you used any pills, medicines or drugs to lose weight?*

Bingeing

- *Do you ever lose control or binge? What happens?*
- How often? What do you eat?
- How do you feel? *[Screen: before/during/after]*
- * What do you do after a binge?
- * Do you do anything secretly to lose weight?

Body image distortion

Self-view

- *What do you think about your body?*
- * How does it make you feel?
- Which areas do you focus on? Why?
- How does this compare to what other people think about you?
- How do you keep track of changes? *[Screen: weigh/measure/photo]*

Fear of fatness/weight gain

- *Are you scared of gaining weight?*
- What would be the *worst* thing about that?

Hypothalamic–pituitary–gonadal axis disturbance

Amenorrhoea

- *How are your periods?* [Screen: menarche/regularity/last period]

Libido

- *Weight can affect sex drive. Have you noticed any changes?*
- Do you have any problems reaching orgasm?
- [Men] Do you still get erections?

Risk

Physical complications

- *How's your health at the moment?*

- Dieting can cause physical changes. Have you noticed any problems? [Screen: palpitations/dizziness on standing/weakness/cold sensitivity/constipation/rashes/periods/libido]

Self-harm

- *Have you ever harmed or hurt yourself?*
- Do you ever feel like life isn't worth living?

Psychosocial screen

- *What do your friends/family think about your weight?* [Screen: criticism/bullying/concern/support]
- How do you find eating with others?
- * How do weight and food affect other areas of your life?
- Do you talk to people online about your weight? What do they say?
- Who's your role model, weight-wise?

Eating disorder history (15 minutes)

Candidate's instructions

You're a final year medical student holding a GP surgery clinic. Alice Sangowa is an 18-year-old student; her mother booked an appointment after finding her vomiting. The practice nurse reports a BMI of 23.5kg/m² (height 171cm; weight 69kg). Take a history, sufficient to present Alice to your GP supervisor.

Patient's brief

Key characteristics

- I wear baggy clothes, fidget, and chew gum.
- I'm annoyed and initially snappy and guarded.
- I'm ashamed but open up if the student is kind.

History

I was sick! So? It's literally none of Mum's business! Or yours! I was bullied all through school for being fat; I had no friends and got trolled on Instagram. Mum and Dad were too busy getting divorced, so I coped through comfort eating, but got to 90kg and looked disgusting. A year ago, I joined a slimming club and reached my target weight of 70kg, about 3 months ago. The bullying stopped and people started saying I looked good.

I wanted to lose more but the club wouldn't help, so I kept going by myself. I avoid fat and sugar and eat 1500 calories a day, e.g. porridge for breakfast; chicken salad for lunch; pasta and fruit for dinner. I weigh myself daily and plan to be 53kg (size 8) for university in 6 months' time (I'm currently size 12). I've been asked out, but don't want to date anyone yet; I'd hate them to see my fat belly and thighs. It's frustrating, I'm not losing much weight now...

I'm always hungry and thinking about food. Sometimes, I get desperate. About five times a week, I get this growing feeling I *need* to binge, especially if I'm upset about something. Once everyone's gone to bed, I sneak out to the local shop and buy chocolate, biscuits, ice cream, bread, chocolate spread. I rush home and eat the lot, as fast as I can. Sometimes I can't even remember tasting it... Then I feel guilty and fat and have to vomit and take laxatives. The next day, I stick extra hard to my diet and run five (rather than my usual three) miles to burn off the extra calories.

Other history
- My sister had anorexia but 'recovered'. She's *enormous* now.
- I feel bloated and sometimes get weird, fluttery feelings in my chest. My periods are regular.
- I don't drink, smoke, use drugs or diet pills. I hadn't heard of thyroxine (I'll Google that later).
- I'm not depressed or suicidal. I sometimes cut myself when feeling guilty.
- My friends are mostly online. They think I'm fine, I just need to diet harder...
- I'm predicted straight A grades and have a place at Bristol to study medicine.

Question
What will you tell Mum?

Worry
You want to make me fat.

💡 Alice meets criteria for BN (prominent, regular binge–purge cycles, distorted body image and deliberate weight loss but BMI >18.5kg/m²). The GP should empathize and explain that her 'fluttery feelings' may be due to vomiting and laxatives and could represent heart complications; they should encourage her to accept urgent blood tests and an ECG. Once this has been managed, she may agree to work with a dietician and CBT therapist or specialist eating disorder team to safely manage her weight and regain a sense of control.

NEXT STEPS

An underweight woman with fertility problems

You're an FY2 in general practice. Rebecca Fox is a 32-year-old lawyer who attends to discuss referral for *in vitro* fertilization (IVF). She and her husband, Sean, haven't conceived after three years of trying. IVF guidelines require a BMI of 19–30kg/m² but Rebecca's BMI is 17.5kg/m². She admits to irregular periods, but irritably protests that she 'eats normally'.

- What further information is needed?
- How could you motivate Rebecca to accept help?
- What's your management plan?
- A week later, she's gained 5kg. Why?

Further information
Rebecca has a low BMI and irregular periods, but these *don't* mean she has an eating disorder. She'll be offended if you assume this, especially as she attended to talk about IVF. Start with safer ground: explore her general health and menstrual history, then explain that weight affects periods and fertility, so you'll need to ask about it.

Check whether her weight's changed recently. Was any loss deliberate? How does she view her current weight and body shape? Would she like to change them? Explore body image distortion and fears of weight gain or 'fatness'. Elicit deliberate weight loss methods, including dietary restriction, exercise, vomiting, laxatives, and medications. Screen for substance misuse, depression, and suicidal ideation.

Your physical examination should exclude organic causes of weight loss and identify signs associated with high mortality, e.g. hypothermia, bradycardia/arrhythmias, postural hypotension, rashes. A SUSS test is relevant, though likely to be normal at this BMI. Arrange blood tests (see p. 206) and an ECG.

Rebecca's risk dictates the urgency of referral. Unless her weight loss has been extremely rapid or she has electrolyte abnormalities or evidence of physical decompensation, she's unlikely to be at immediate risk of sudden death at this BMI. However, always assess suicide risk.

Enhancing motivation and understanding
Whether Rebecca has AN, BN, or another diagnosis, one appointment won't resolve it. Build rapport and explore her hopes of having children; this can be

powerfully motivating. Check her understanding of how weight affects fertility. Explain that she can't access IVF at her current weight, because it compromises her fertility (both natural conception and in a 'test-tube'). If her BMI enters the healthy range, her periods are likely to normalize, improving her fertility; either she won't need IVF or will be eligible for referral.

Management

Encourage Rebecca to explain (or let you explain) the situation to Sean. Even if she won't divulge all details, she may tell him she needs to gain weight to move forwards. This may let you involve Sean. It may be possible to manage Rebecca in primary care, perhaps using a weight gain plan with the support of an experienced dietician and referral for psychological therapy to explore underlying stressors. Specialist psychologist input for eating disorders is available via referral to a CMHT and is increasingly important, the more severe her symptoms. If worried or unsure about immediate risks, discuss Rebecca's case with an eating disorder specialist psychiatrist or the medical team on-call. She might require emergency psychiatric assessment or (in severe cases) admission for electrolyte correction, safe refeeding, or management of suicide risk.

Weight gain

Small weight variations *matter* when the person's BMI is low; this is a massive gain in 1 week. It's possible that Rebecca's desperately eaten to gain weight and meet referral criteria but more likely to be an erroneous result or an attempt to simulate weight gain (e.g. water loading, filling her pockets with weights). Avoid accusations! Use the same, calibrated scales; weigh her in normal indoor clothes, without shoes or coats, with empty pockets, and suggest she empties her bladder beforehand (especially if wriggly or restless).

💡 **Many illnesses cause weight loss with secondary subfertility, e.g. cancer, coeliac disease, hyperthyroidism. Don't miss organic causes!**

Movie buff
Black Swan (2010).
Malos Hábitos [*Bad Habits*] (2007).
Sharing the Secret (2000).
To the Bone (2017).

Book shelf
Hornbacher, M. (1998) *Wasted*: an autobiographical account of AN, including frank description of feigning apparent recovery.
Lamb, W. (1992) *She's Come Undone*: women's prison creative writing workshops bring out the story of how BED can develop following a traumatic experience.
Lee, C. (2004) *To Die For: The True Story of a Broken Childhood*: a carer's account.
Mantell, H. (1995) *An Experiment in Love*: this novel explores how eating disorders can manifest in high-pressure group situations, including social constructions of femininity and control.

Note

1. Hornbacher, M. (1999) *Wasted*. London: Flamingo.

Journal club

Royal College of Psychiatrists (RCPsych) (2014) *MARSIPAN: Management of Really Sick Patients with Anorexia Nervosa* (2nd ed.) (College Report CR189). London: RCPsych. www.rcpsych.ac.uk/docs/default-source/improving-care/better-mh-policy/college-reports/college-report-cr189.pdf?sfvrsn=6c2e7ada_2

Schmidt, U., Treasure, J., Alexander, J. (2015) *Getting Better Bite by Bite: A Survival Kit for Sufferers of Bulimia Nervosa and Binge Eating Disorders* (2nd ed.). Abingdon: Routledge.

Treasure, J., Alexander, J. (2013) *Anorexia Nervosa: A Recovery Guide for Sufferers, Families and Friends* (2nd ed.). Abingdon: Routledge.

Go to www.oup.com/uk/stringer2e for a wealth of additional resources, including an OCSE mark scheme, filmed scenarios, and self-assessment questions.

17 Conditions Related to Sexual Health

True or false?

Answers on p. 277

1. Sensate focus therapy initially bans sexual intercourse.
2. Compulsive sexual behaviour disorder is commoner in men than women.
3. Beta-blockers can treat male erectile dysfunction.
4. Morning erections indicate a psychological cause for male erectile dysfunction.
5. Transgender people are at increased risk of suicide and self-harm.
6. Sexual pain-penetration disorder can affect women who've never been sexually active.
7. Paraphilic disorders are treated with exposure therapy.
8. All transgender people undergo psychiatric assessment before receiving gender reassignment surgery.
9. Antidepressants may improve male early ejaculation.
10. A 36-year-old woman discloses previous rape at a routine smear test. If she doesn't want to report it, the clinician should inform the police.

Contents

Principles
Introduction
Sexual dysfunctions and sexual pain disorders
- Sexual desire problems
- Sexual arousal dysfunctions
- Orgasmic dysfunctions
- Ejaculatory dysfunctions
- Sexual pain disorders

Paraphilic disorders
Gender incongruence
Prognosis

Reality
General approach: tips, tricks, and cautionary tales
Psychosexual history

Next steps
Psychosexual problems in primary care
- Immediate management
- Diagnosis and explanation
- Further support and management

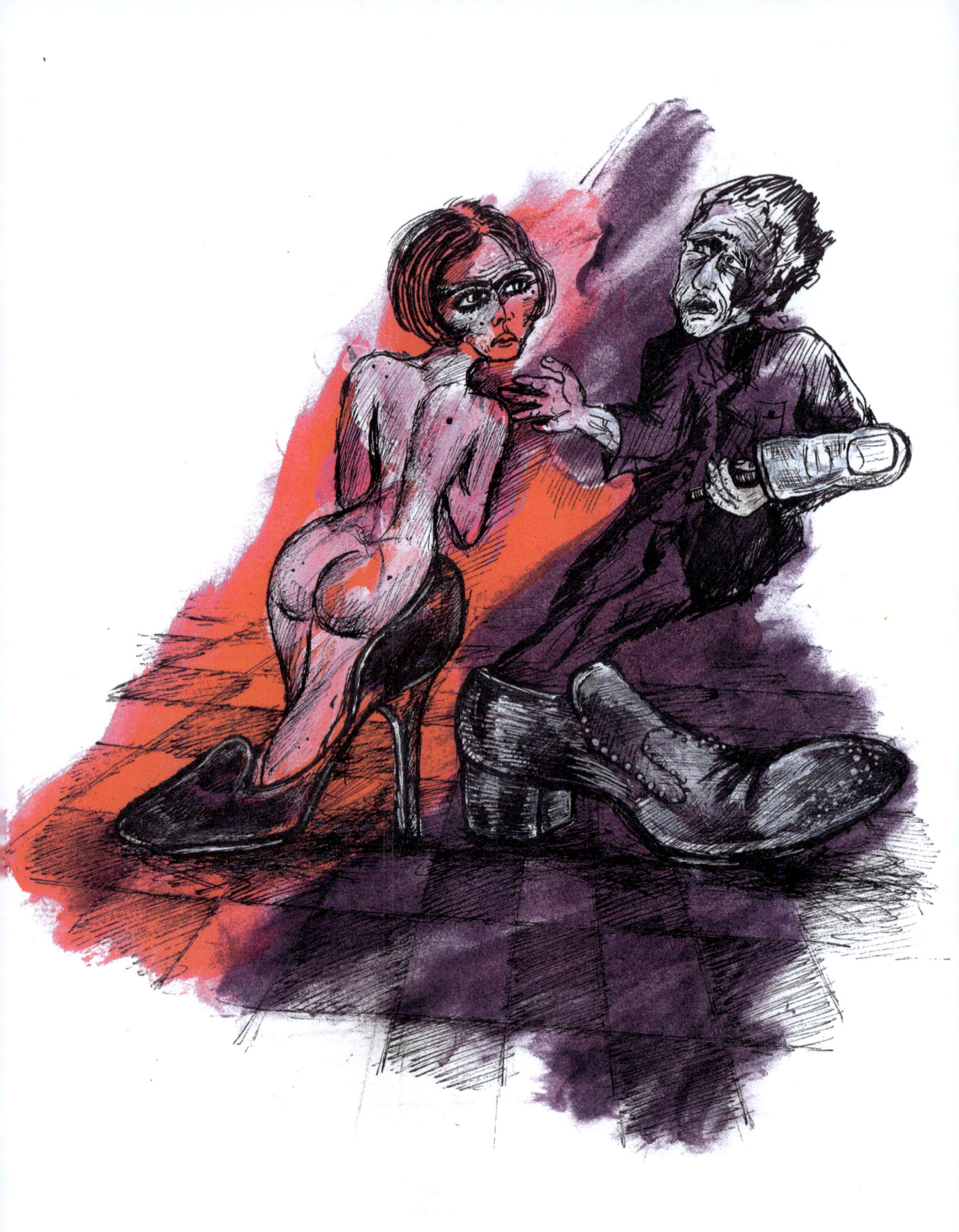

PRINCIPLES

The world is not to be divided into sheep and goats. Not all things are black nor all things white. It is a fundamental of taxonomy that nature rarely deals with discrete categories. Only the human mind invents categories and tries to force facts into separated pigeon-holes. The living world is a continuum in each and every one of its aspects. The sooner we learn this concerning human sexual behaviour, the sooner we shall reach a sound understanding of the realities of sex.

A.C. Kinsey et al., *Sexuality in the Human Male*[1]

Introduction

This chapter covers sexual dysfunctions, sexual pain disorders, paraphilic disorders, and gender incongruence. People won't always report symptoms or problems, due to shame and social taboos. By simply being relaxed and knowledgeable when discussing psychosexual matters, you can have a life-changing effect on the person.

Sexual dysfunctions and sexual pain disorders

Sexual dysfunctions include problems with sexual desire (libido), arousal, orgasm, and ejaculation, causing distress and/or affecting relationships (**Table 17.1**). Sexual pain disorders include sexual pain-penetration disorder (SPPD) and dyspareunia. Symptoms may be:

- *Lifelong* (normal function is never experienced) or a*cquired* (normal function is lost).
- *Generalized* (normal function is absent or diminished in all circumstances, including masturbation) or *situational* (normal function is absent or diminished in some circumstances, with some partners, or in response to some stimuli, but not others).

The following diagnoses are only considered where symptoms have been present episodically or persistently for at least several months, despite desire for sexual activity and sufficient stimulation, and where they cause the person significant distress. Despite under-reporting, studies suggest that 40% of adults experience such symptoms. Women most often seek help for hypoactive sexual desire dysfunction and men for erectile dysfunction (ED).

Table 17.1 Common sexual dysfunctions and pain disorders

Problem	Female	Male
Sexual desire	Hypoactive sexual desire dysfunction Compulsive sexual behaviour disorder	Hypoactive sexual desire dysfunction Compulsive sexual behaviour disorder
Arousal	Female sexual arousal dysfunction	Erectile dysfunction ('impotence')
Orgasm	Anorgasmia	Anorgasmia
Ejaculation	N/A	Early ejaculation Delayed ejaculation Retrograde ejaculation (organic)
Pain	Sexual pain-penetration disorder Dyspareunia (organic)	Dyspareunia

Sexual desire problems

Hypoactive sexual desire dysfunction (HSDD)

HSDD is the absence or significant reduction of sexual desire, evidenced by lack of spontaneous sexual thoughts and fantasies, desire in response to erotic cues and stimulation, or inability to sustain interest in sexual activity after starting.

Commoner in women, lifelong HSDD is often idiopathic but can follow childhood sexual abuse. Acquired

HSDD may be associated with physical illness or injury and its treatment; depression, anxiety, medication, or substance use; relationship problems; cultural factors; lack of knowledge or experience; menopause or childbirth in women; or low testosterone in men. The person may avoid intimacy, fearing it'll progress to sex; this can leave partners feeling rejected.

Once physical causes have been addressed, management is psychological. Tailored sexual education and *sensate focus therapy* are used (**Box 17.1**). Open communication is encouraged between partners, and *sex timetabling* may help couples to find a compromise if their libidos differ significantly.

> 💡 Some people have little or no libido but are happy with this. They may identify as asexual; without significant distress, this may be a normal variant of libido.

Compulsive sexual behaviour disorder (CSBD)

CSBD is a persistent pattern of uncontrolled intense, repetitive sexual urges resulting in repetitive sexual behaviour over at least 6 months, causing pronounced distress or functional impairment. It can have features of salience, rapid reinstatement after withdrawal, and continuance despite harm which are seen in harmful and dependent substance use, too. It more commonly affects men and can damage relationships. Psychiatric (e.g. mania, substance use) and organic causes (e.g. frontal lobe syndrome, testosterone or oestrogen use, dopaminergic medication in Parkinson disease) must be investigated before considering psychological treatments incorporating CBT.

Sexual arousal dysfunctions

Female sexual arousal dysfunction (FSAD)

The absence or marked reduction of a woman's response to sexual stimulation, evidenced by absent/markedly reduced genital responses (e.g. vulvovaginal lubrication), non-genital responses (e.g. increased heart rate), and feelings (excitement and pleasure). Its aetiology can be organic (e.g. menopausal atrophic vaginitis, infection) or psychological (e.g. anxiety). Treatments include lubricating gels, hormone replacement therapy, and psychological therapies.

Erectile dysfunction (ED)

ED is the inability/very reduced ability to sustain a sufficiently hard or lasting erection for intercourse to occur. Causes may be (**Table 17.2**):

Organic

- Vascular, e.g. diabetes, arteriosclerosis.
- Neurological, e.g. multiple sclerosis, autonomic neuropathy, surgical or traumatic nerve injury.
- Iatrogenic, e.g. antidepressants, antipsychotics, antihypertensives, beta-blockers, diuretics.
- Substance use, especially excessive alcohol ('brewer's droop').
- Pituitary failure, testicular underdevelopment (e.g. Klinefelter syndrome, mumps virus).
- Peyronie disease (penile fibrosis).
- Priapism (prolonged erection causing scarring if not treated promptly).

Psychosocial

- Performance anxiety.
- Depression.
- Relationship problems.
- Cultural factors.
- Lack of knowledge/experience.

In 'performance anxiety', there is fear of sexual 'failure', sometimes triggered by a past perceived failure

Table 17.2 Factors suggestive of organic versus psychosocial origins of ED

	Organic	Psychosocial
Age	Older	Younger
Onset	Gradual	Sudden
Some erections?	No	Yes (e.g. morning erections, masturbation)
Risk factors	Smoking, obesity, hypertension, chronic alcohol excess	Anxiety/alcohol before/during sex
Other diagnoses?	Physical, e.g. vascular history	Psychiatric, e.g. depression

---

BOX 17.1 Stages of sensate focus therapy

- *Intercourse* is initially banned.
- *Non-genital caressing* focuses on pleasure and relaxation.
- *Genital touching* focuses on arousal and subsequently, orgasm.
- *Intercourse* often occurs naturally, with time.

(e.g. when drunk). This creates a 'vicious circle': worry inhibits erections, causing more worry.

> 💡 Doctors often unintentionally cause ED through medication side effects; people experiencing ED often avoid raising it. *Ask!*

Investigations

- Physical examination, including genitalia (usually normal).
- Testosterone and sex hormones (low testosterone or hyperprolactinaemia indicate organic aetiology).
- CBG ± HbA1c (if diabetes is known/suspected).
- LFTs, including GGT (if alcohol use disorder is reported/suspected).

Management

Modifiable risk factors (e.g. smoking, weight, alcohol use, diabetes, hypertension) are addressed and medications changed to minimize sexual side effects, where possible. Psychological treatment (sensate focus therapy or CBT) can address psychosocial causes. Physical causes respond best to:

- Phosphodiesterase-5 inhibitors, e.g. sildenafil (e.g. Viagra®).
- Self-administered intracavernosal prostaglandin injections before intercourse (but can be painful).
- Vacuum pumps: a plastic dome and pump placed over the penis create a vacuum, producing an erection maintained by a tight ring placed around the base of the penis.

Orgasmic dysfunctions

Anorgasmia

Absent, very delayed, or infrequent orgasm experiences or particularly diminished orgasmic sensations in women. Causes include neurodegenerative conditions, medications (including antidepressants), alcohol use, depression, relationship factors, cultural factors, lack of knowledge/experience, previous abuse, or lack of connection with partner. Although some women can achieve orgasm solely through vaginal penetration, many need direct clitoral stimulation. Education, self-exploration, masturbation, and sensate focus therapy (**Box 17.1**) can help, although some people never achieve orgasm.

Ejaculatory dysfunctions

Male early ejaculation

Ejaculation occurs before or in a short time after vaginal penetration or other stimulation, with little/no perceived control. The cause is usually unclear, but it's commoner in young men, sometimes has a strong genetic contribution, or may be caused by medication (e.g. antiparkinsonian medications) or prostatitis; it usually improves with experience. Orgasm can be postponed by the *stop–start technique* (squeezing the glans penis) or SSRIs, although these can cause other sexual side effects.

Male delayed ejaculation

Inability to achieve ejaculation or excessive or increased delay to ejaculation can be caused by physical (e.g. antidepressants) or psychological factors (e.g. anxiety). Treatment includes psychological therapies, advice on varying sexual techniques, and medication review.

Sexual pain disorders

Sexual pain-penetration disorder

SPPD (older name: vaginismus) features at least one of:

- Significant difficulty attaining penetration, due in part to involuntary tightening of pelvic floor muscles.
- Marked pelvic pain during penetration.
- Fear of vulvovaginal or pelvic pain before, during, or after intercourse.

Symptoms can't be fully explained by an organic condition, mental health disorder, inadequate lubrication, or age-related changes. Sexual anxiety, previous sexual assault, or abuse *sometimes* contribute. Treatment involves education, relaxation, self-exploration, and pelvic floor exercises. Women can insert vaginal 'trainers' (plastic, tampon-like objects) of increasing sizes to get used to penetration.

Dyspareunia

Recurrent genital pain before, during, or after intercourse with an identifiable organic cause, such as:

- *Women*—infection, episiotomy, endometriosis, tumour, vaginal dryness.
- *Men*—urethritis, prostatitis.

Vulvodynia

Although not a sexual pain disorder, medically unexplained chronic pain, burning, or rawness of vulval skin can impact sexual health. *Vestibulodynia* causes localized redness and tenderness, in response to touch; it usually presents in younger women and is associated with secondary dyspareunia. *Dysaesthetic vulvodynia* causes spontaneous, diffuse pain independent of touch, usually seen in postmenopausal women who aren't sexually active. Treatments include minimizing irritation (e.g. cotton underwear, fragrance-free products, cooling), gentle sexual positions, anaesthetic gels, and stress reduction.

Paraphilic disorders

Persistent, intense patterns of atypical sexual arousal are evidenced by sexual thoughts, fantasies, urges, or behaviours focused on individuals whose age or status makes them unwilling or unable to consent. Paraphilic disorders are only diagnosed if the person has acted on their desires or are very distressed by them; they affect men more than women. Sexual arousal is triggered by atypical stimuli:

- **Paedophilic disorder:** prepubertal children.
- **Coercive sexual sadism disorder:** inflicting physical/psychological suffering on a non-consenting person.
- **Exhibitionistic disorder:** exposing one's genitals to an unsuspecting person in a public place.
- **Frotteuristic disorder:** touching or rubbing against a non-consenting person in crowded public places.
- **Voyeuristic disorder:** observing an unsuspecting person who is naked, getting undressed, or engaging in sexual activity.
- **Other paraphilic disorder involving non-consenting individuals:** includes animals (bestiality) and corpses (necrophilia).

Unwanted arousal may be extinguished by *covert sensitization:* learning to pair arousal with aversive images. During treatment, the person avoids activities which reinforce their paraphilia, e.g. fantasizing, viewing related pornography. Antiandrogen medications may be used in severe or dangerous situations but rely on the person's motivation and cooperation, outside of a forensic setting.

Gender incongruence

Gender terminology continues to evolve (**Box 17.2**). Currently, male/masculine, female/feminine, and non-binary—when the person doesn't feel their gender fits neatly into traditional boxes—are distinguished. Other terms include:

- Gender *identity*: how you experience your own gender.
- Gender *dysphoria*: unhappiness/discomfort about your assigned gender.
- Gender *incongruence*: persistent incompatibility between your gender identity and the gender you were assigned at birth. You may identify as *transgender*.

> **BOX 17.2** Gender and sexuality terminology
>
> - *Sexuality/sexual orientation*: who you find attractive, i.e. same sex (homosexual/lesbian/gay), opposite sex (heterosexual/straight), both sexes (bisexual), all gender identities (pansexual), nobody (asexual).
> - *LGBT:* Lesbian, Gay, Bisexual, Transgender.
>   - Extra letters are sometimes added, e.g. Q (queer/questioning), I (intersex), A (asexual or ally: friend or supporter).
> - *Cis*: the gender you were assigned matches your gender identity.
> - *Trans*: your assigned gender doesn't match your gender identity.
> - *Queer*: anyone who doesn't identify as straight or cis.

- *'Transsexual'*: an older term previously used for transgender people living as a member of the opposite sex, usually after receiving medical intervention (hormones, surgery).
- *Transvestism*: dressing/acting in a way traditionally associated with the opposite sex, e.g. for cultural reasons, to express gender identity, or to experience another gender identity (*dual-role transvestism*). Cross-dressing for sexual arousal is *transvestic fetishism*.

Gender incongruence is commoner in people assigned male at birth and usually starts before puberty, although it's only diagnosed in childhood after at least 2 years of symptoms. Children engage in make-believe and play with toys, games, activities, and playmates typical of their experienced gender. Adolescents and adults experience at least two of:

- A strong dislike/discomfort with their primary or secondary sexual characteristics *due to* incongruity with their experienced gender.
- A strong desire to *lose* some or all of these.
- A strong desire to *gain* the primary and/or secondary sexual characteristics of their experienced gender.

People with gender incongruence may seek help for associated distress or mental health problems (e.g. depression), sexual dysfunction, or gender reassignment. Treatment options include hormone therapy and gender reassignment surgery, following careful joint assessment by psychiatrists, surgeons and other specialists. The person must live in their experienced gender for an extended period before surgery is considered.

💡 **Unlike biological sex, gender is a *social construct*.** Some gender-related distress results from rigid societal 'norms' and expectations.

💡 **Homosexuality and bisexuality (Box 17.2) *aren't* disorders** but remain illegal in some countries. LGBTQ people often face stigma, bullying, and abuse, increasing their risk of mental health problems.

Prognosis

Many conditions related to sexual health respond well to therapy, although HSDD is difficult to treat and paraphilic disorders may show little improvement. Hormonal treatment for gender incongruence can improve well-being and quality of life, while surgery is associated with improved well-being and sexual functioning. Psychiatric morbidity, suicide, and overall mortality are elevated in transgender people, whether or not they've undergone surgical reassignment.

❗ **Always check the person's knowledge of safe sex and access to contraception**, providing education and information where needed. Even sexually experienced people may not be fully aware of risks posed by their sexual activities.

REALITY

General approach: tips, tricks, and cautionary tales

Ideally, see the person and their partner together *and* alone.

1. Confidentiality

People may feel shy or ashamed, especially if they've never discussed sex with anyone before. Explain confidentiality early on to reassure them and show that you take their privacy seriously.

❗ **If anything in the history sounds non-consensual, ask specifically about sexual assault, violence, and abuse (including coercive control).** If someone discloses non-consensual or abusive sexual activities (e.g. rape, child abuse), you can't always maintain confidentiality.

2. Assumptions

Never assume that someone's straight or cisgender—getting it wrong will make you both uncomfortable. Until sure, use *gender-neutral language* about sexual partners and check people's preferred pronouns:

- Use *they/them/their* instead of he/she, etc.
- Use *partner* instead of boyfriend/girlfriend/husband/wife.

Direct questions are fine, e.g. Who do you find attractive? Remember that someone's current relationship may not reflect their sexual history.

3. Don't judge

Regardless of your personal, cultural, or religious views, it's unprofessional to criticize or disapprove of another person's (consensual) sexual behaviour. As a doctor, you may offer advice about sexual health and safety, but otherwise, let them get on with it! It might not be *your* cup of tea, but other people can have a latte, espresso, or hot chocolate with whipped cream and marshmallows if they want to.

4. Jargon

People use different words for body parts and sex acts; ask the person to explain terms you don't recognize. Using your own slang may confuse or offend, so stick to everyday, factual language, e.g. *penis, vagina, having sex, oral sex*, or use the person's own words where appropriate.

5. Embarrassment

People engage in many kinds of sexual activities. Although it's natural to feel a little shy when talking about sex, you need to overcome this. Try not to show shock or embarrassment by fidgeting, changing the subject, or laughing; sit still, make eye contact, and keep asking the important questions.

Avoidance only increases discomfort, so:

- Learn more about sex, e.g. read novels, watch films/documentaries.
- Talk about sex with trusted friends or partners.

- Include sexual histories in general history taking *when relevant* (detailed sexual questioning without reason is intrusive and inappropriate).
- Sit in on sexual health clinics.
- If you don't know any LGBTQ people, broaden your horizons!

💡 **Don't assume that older people aren't sexually active! Many *are*, although loneliness, ED, and vaginal dryness are commoner in older age.**

Psychosexual history (15 minutes)

Candidate's instructions
You're a final year medical student, running a GP surgery clinic. Albert Irvine is a 48-year-old librarian, who's attended to discuss a 'private matter.' Take a history of his presenting complaint.

Patient's brief
Key characteristics
- I'm worried about confidentiality.
- I'm hesitant and shy, but open up to confident, compassionate students.
- I'll avoid details unless asked direct questions.

History
My partner, Annabel, suggested this appointment . . . I should start at the beginning . . . I married Natalie at 18 years old. She was my first partner and our sex life was great, initially. We hit a rocky patch in our marriage, 10 years ago, and Natalie lost interest in sex. I eventually gave up asking—I hated being rejected every night. Two years ago, she admitted to having an affair. She was cruel: told me how *he* satisfied her in ways I never had . . . I've been very lonely and depressed since she left.

I met Annabel 6 months ago, and it was love at first sight. It's exciting to feel wanted again! We waited 3 months, to make sure it was what we wanted, and I planned a romantic weekend in Venice. Everything was going well until . . . I just couldn't . . . keep my erection. She was very good about it, but we tried again and the same thing happened. It happens every time. We make do with oral sex, but I never . . . um . . . orgasm. Annabel knows I didn't have this problem before, so worries I don't find her attractive, or that I still have feelings for Natalie. Nothing could be further from the truth! I feel like a failure. I've been making excuses to avoid sex lately and I think I've hurt Annabel's feelings . . . *She's* now saying she's too tired for sex. It feels like my marriage all over again.

I'm not depressed, but if I lose Annabel I'll probably get very low again, antidepressants or not.

If specifically asked
- I don't get morning (or other) erections; nothing gives me a *full* erection, and I'm never hard enough for penetration.
- Before I was depressed, I could always maintain an erection and ejaculate.
- While I was depressed, I wasn't interested in masturbating, and until I met Annabel, I didn't realize it was a problem. Now, even masturbating doesn't work.
- During sex, I worry I'll fail again . . .

Other history
- I don't drink, smoke, or take drugs.
- My eczema's bad because I'm stressed. I use steroid creams.
- I started fluoxetine 20mg a year ago and never miss tablets. This is my third bout of depression, but I feel well now.
- I've no idea if relatives had sexual or psychiatric problems. We don't talk about those things!

Question
What's wrong with me?

Worries
If I can't satisfy Annabel, she'll leave me for someone who can.

💡 Albert's ED probably *started* with antidepressant use, but now has a secondary psychological element (performance anxiety). *Recurrent* depression may relapse if he stops the antidepressant (especially within 2 years of symptoms resolving) but his SSRI could be changed to something with fewer sexual side effects (e.g. mirtazapine or agomelatine).

220 17 Conditions Related to Sexual Health

Explaining that ED is a common medication side effect may relieve anxiety and help the couple restart sexual contact—potentially producing erections as SSRI side effects fade. Offer self-help materials (e.g. sensate focus therapy) and ensure he's had CBT or mindfulness before stopping his antidepressant, to prevent relapse.

NEXT STEPS

Psychosexual problems in primary care

You're an FY2 in general practice. Fran Coney, a 36-year-old woman, has come in for an overdue, routine smear test. She's quiet and nervous, and when you try to introduce the speculum she cries out in pain and bursts into tears. You abandon the test, and she explains that she's suffered pain ever since being raped several years ago; penetration is 'agony'. It's affecting her relationship with her partner, Tyler.

- How can you help today?
- What's her likely diagnosis? How could you explain this?
- What's your longer-term management plan?

Immediate management

Given time constraints, your main aim is to contain her distress by being compassionate and normalizing her emotions. Let her know this isn't her fault, and that you can and will help when she feels ready. Offer a double follow-up appointment, and suggest she brings Tyler for moral support. If you're male, offer for her to see a female colleague.

Diagnosis and explanation

Gently take a sexual and relationship history, letting her set the pace and being sensitive to areas that she feels uncomfortable discussing. Check the temporal relationship between the rape and onset of pain; the problem may have been pre-existing.

The most likely diagnosis, in the absence of a lesion or infection, is SPPD. You could say: 'Some women's vaginal muscles are extremely sensitive to touch. Smear tests, tampons, or having sex can all trigger sudden, painful spasms. Sometimes this happens for no obvious reason, but it may start after something painful or frightening, like an assault. You're not deliberately tensing up—it happens automatically—but it's common and curable.'

Further support and management

Self-help can be very effective, and will involve Fran exploring her body through touch, initially on the outside and then—when comfortable—inserting a finger into her vagina. She can gradually build up from there (e.g. using vaginal trainers), involving Tyler in the treatment at any stage.

If Fran feels able to discuss it, explore the issue of the rape. Find out whether she reported it or gained support at the time. She might still want to report the rape to the police, particularly if she knew her attacker, and can still benefit from rape support groups, or from psychological therapy. You shouldn't inform the police against her will: this is her decision. Screen for and treat psychological consequences, e.g. PTSD, depression, anxiety disorders, and substance use disorders.

Rape survivors often feel ashamed. Combined with SPPD, this may have stopped her from accessing sexual health checks. Sexually transmitted infections may be a source of discomfort and worry but can easily be identified and treated. If Fran wants to attend a sexual health clinic, you could write a brief referral, informing clinic staff of her situation with her consent.

💡 **Fran still needs a smear test. Delayed presentation is common for many intimate or embarrassing problems; empathy and sensitivity may be life-saving!**

Movie buff
LGBTQ
All About My Mother (1999)
Boys Don't Cry (1999)
Brokeback Mountain (2005)
Carol (2015)
Gentleman Jack (TV; 2019)
High Art (1998)
Milk (2008)
My Beautiful Laundrette (1985)
Moonlight (2016)

Philadelphia (1993)
Pride (2014)
The Danish Girl (2015)
Tomboy (2011)
Transamerica (2006)

CSBD:
Shame (2011)

Various sexual problems:
Sex Education (TV, 2019)

Book shelf

Boyle, T.C. (1999) *Riven Rock*: an exploration of CSBD at the turn of the century and early formulations of schizoaffective disorder as 'sexual mania'.

Byatt, A.S. (1990) *Possession: A Romance*: the lives of contemporary scholars researching two fictional Victorian poets become intertwined.

Ensler, E. (2001) *The Vagina Monologues*: this groundbreaking book addresses myths and misapprehensions about the vagina.

Lester, C.N. (2017) *Trans Like Me: a journey for all of us*. A collection of essays drawing on personal experiences and research challenging myths about trans identities.

Winterson, J. (1985) *Oranges Are Not The Only Fruit*. Semi-autobiographical account of growing up gay in a strict, religious family.

Note

1. Kinsey, A.C. et al. (1998) *Sexuality in the Human Male*. University of Indiana Press, Bloomington.

Journal club

Bancroft, J. (2008) *Human Sexuality and its Problems*. Edinburgh: Churchill Livingstone.

Kalamis, C., Brennan, S. (2007) *Women Without Sex: The Truth About Female Sexual Problems* (3rd ed.). London: Self-Help Direct.

Go to www.oup.com/uk/stringer2e for a wealth of additional resources, including an OCSE mark scheme, filmed scenarios, and self-assessment questions.

18 Perinatal Psychiatry

True or false?

Answers on p. 277

1. Pregnancy protects against mental health problems.
2. Bipolar affective disorder is eight times more likely to relapse in the 6 weeks after childbirth.
3. Postnatal blues usually respond to reassurance and explanation.
4. One in twenty women experiences postpartum depression in the year after childbirth.
5. Postpartum depression is usually treated in a mother and baby unit.
6. Electroconvulsive therapy is an effective treatment for postpartum psychosis.
7. Pre-eclampsia is the leading cause of maternal death in the UK.
8. Postpartum physiological changes alter pharmacodynamics.
9. It's always best to stop antidepressants when a woman becomes pregnant.
10. Postpartum psychosis runs in families.

Contents

Principles
Introduction
Epidemiology
Anxiety disorders
Baby blues
Postpartum depression
Postpartum psychosis

Reality
General approach: tips, tricks, and cautionary tales
The interview
- Perinatal history

Next steps
A tearful first-time parent
- Assessment
- Psychiatric referral
- Further management

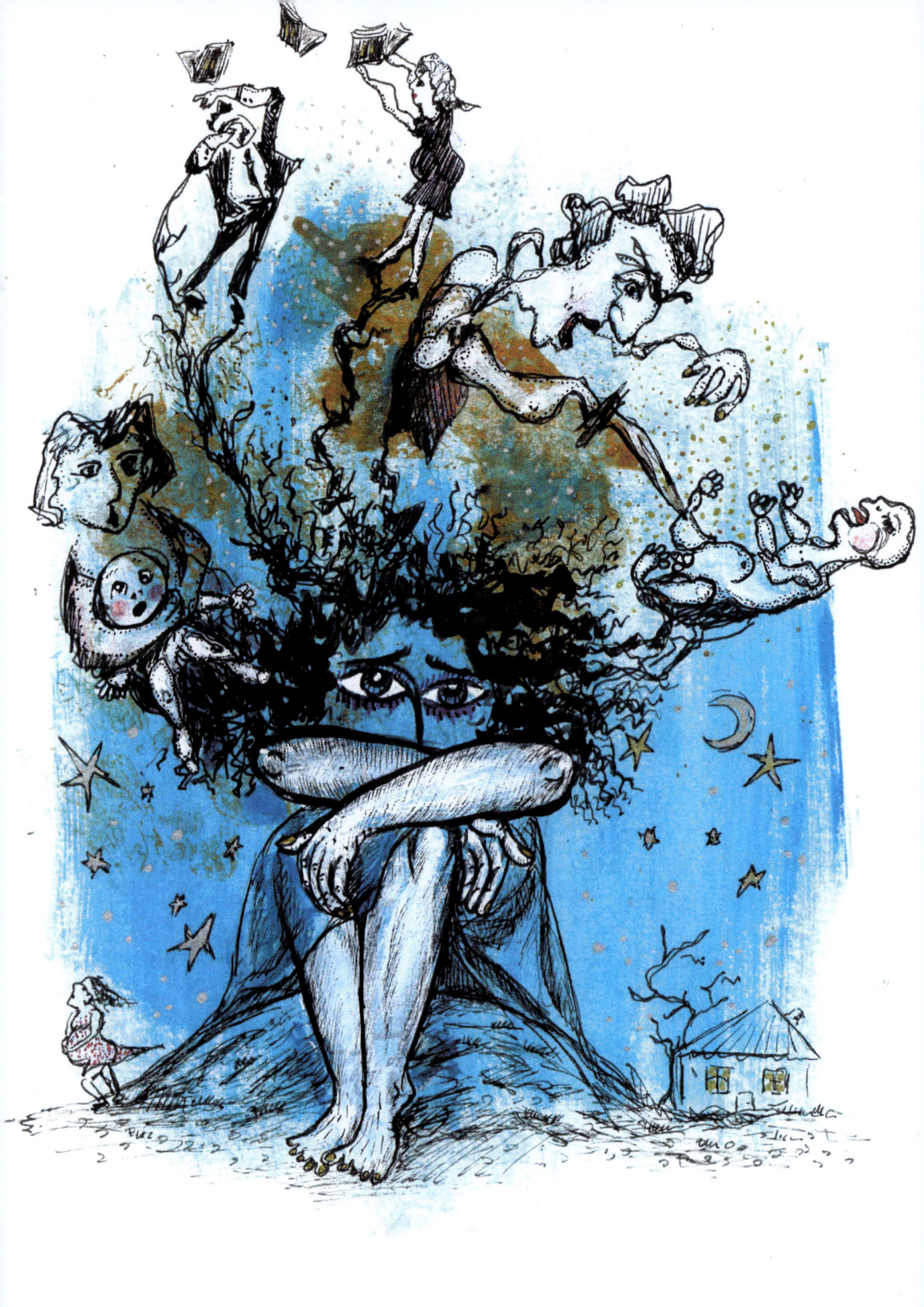

PRINCIPLES

She, and hence I, have not slept for many hours. For perhaps the twentieth time in ten hours I feed her and put her down in her cradle. I am not asking for a solid stretch: I merely require a few minutes to myself gluing parts of my face back on and saying things aloud in front of the mirror to see if I've actually gone mad. At this point I don't just want her to go to sleep. She has to go to sleep otherwise I don't know what will happen. My position is at once reasonable, utterly desperate, and non-negotiable.

Rachel Cusk, *A Life's Work: On Becoming a Mother*[1]

Introduction

The postpartum year, particularly the *puerperium* (from 0 to 6 weeks after childbirth) is associated with an increased risk of mental health problems. Perinatal mental health potentially affects *all* women of reproductive age (adolescence to menopause), whether under the care of a GP, physician, surgeon, or psychiatrist (**Box 18.1**). Decision-making is shared whenever possible, requiring a close working relationship with the woman and her partner/family, to build trust and understand attitudes towards pregnancy, mental health, and medication. Multiple services are often involved (e.g. midwifery, obstetrics, health visitors, psychiatric teams, GP), so multidisciplinary communication, information sharing, and meetings are essential to ensure care is 'joined up'.

BOX 18.1 Perinatal psychiatry services

Perinatal psychiatry services provide specialist advice, assessment, and management for women who need mental health input before, during, or after pregnancy. This includes:

- Prepregnancy planning for women with a history of mental health problems (especially regarding medication use).
- Care planning and monitoring of pregnant women at high risk of relapse of known mental health problems.
- Assessments of women on maternity wards with acute mental illness.
- Arranging admission to a MBU.
- Community follow-up after the birth (often up to a year).

Epidemiology

The estimated UK prevalence of common postpartum mental health problems is shown in **Table 18.1**.

Anxiety disorders

The postpartum period can trigger or exacerbate anxiety disorders, e.g. PTSD in response to traumatic labour or stillbirth. CBT is first line, and some women need an antidepressant.

💡 Western hospitals encourage parents to hold their baby following a stillbirth, to aid the grieving process. However, PTSD is actually *increased* in parents who hold their dead baby.

OCD is especially common in women with a history of OCD or anankastic personality traits (see p. 258).

Table 18.1 Prevalence of mental health problems postpartum

Problem	Rate, per 1000 maternities
Postpartum 'blues'	600
Mild–moderate postpartum depression	125
Severe postpartum depression	30
Post-traumatic stress disorder (PTSD)	30
Postpartum psychosis	2

Obsessions usually focus on a mother's greatest fear—of somehow harming her baby, e.g.:

- Thoughts—'What if I've contaminated my baby?'/ 'I'm a paedophile!'
- Images/urges—of hurling the baby downstairs.

Obsessions cause terrible anxiety, shame, and guilt, although the woman *doesn't* intend to act them out. She may develop compulsions to decrease anxiety (e.g. cleaning, checking the baby for injury).

Since nobody actually acts on OCD-related thoughts, the greatest risk is from the mother *avoiding* childcare (fearing she'll cause harm). A careful history differentiates these women from those who pose actual risks to their babies. Women with OCD need reassurance and support from relatives and/or CBT therapists to face their fears, e.g. to hold and wash their baby. An antidepressant may help, e.g. sertraline.

Baby blues

Postpartum blues are *normal,* starting a few days after the birth, and lasting around a week. New mothers may feel weepy, irritable, and muddled; their mood seems 'all over the place' (labile) and they may have trouble sleeping. Explanation and reassurance are usually all that's needed, although severe blues occasionally progress to postpartum depression.

Postpartum depression

Postpartum depression (PPD; previously called postnatal depression, PND) is depression in the year after birth. Women may avoid seeking help, or minimize symptoms, feeling they 'shouldn't' be depressed, or fearing negative consequences (e.g. judgement, social services involvement). Risk factors include a personal or family history of PPD, depression, or bipolar disorder; younger maternal age, stressful life events, marital discord, and poor social support. Symptoms are like any depressive episode (see p. 38), although fatigue, irritability, or anxiety may be particularly marked. Women may feel inadequate, or guilty that they're not doing or feeling 'enough' for the baby. Obsessional thoughts can arise, as seen in OCD.

Management is as for depression, although antidepressants are used cautiously in breastfeeding (**Box 18.2**). High risks may require hospital admission (e.g. not eating, suicidal, unable to care for the baby), ideally to a mother and baby unit (MBU) to keep the woman and her baby together, so bonding/attachment aren't interrupted. MBUs provide support with childcare, multidisciplinary treatment, and risk management.

BOX 18.2 Medication choices

In pregnancy

- Some psychotropic medications (e.g. mood stabilizers) can affect the development of the foetus (*teratogenicity*); risks are highest in the first trimester. Women with mental health problems who are planning pregnancy should be helped to weigh the risk of medication against the risk of relapse—to both themselves and the foetus/baby. They can then make an informed decision to stop, change, or continue medication.
- If pregnancy occurs *while* taking medication, discussions are more urgent.
- Doses should be regularly reviewed, as physiological changes during pregnancy/postpartum affect pharmacokinetics (absorption, distribution, metabolism, and excretion of medication).

In breastfeeding

- Psychotropics may affect the baby if secreted in breast milk (e.g. causing irritability, poor sleep/feeding).
- Medication is chosen carefully, and discussed fully beforehand:
  - Antidepressants: low-dose tricyclics/some SSRIs (e.g. sertraline) are safest.
  - Mood stabilizers: generally avoided (p. 49).
  - Antipsychotics: can cause lethargy; olanzapine is relatively safe.

Expert prescribing advice is available via:

- Perinatal psychiatrists and specialist pharmacists.
- The UK Teratology Information Service (UKTIS).
- UK Drugs in Lactation Advisory Service (UKDILAS).

Effective treatment is essential, as PPD can affect *attachment* and longer-term child and family health and well-being. Most women respond to treatment within a month, though some take much longer to recover. PPD increases a woman's risk of future PPD, but not of depression per se.

💡 **It would be strange for a new parent to report normal energy and sleep! When assessing depression, focus on *cognitive* symptoms (e.g. guilt, hopelessness), rather than parenthood 'symptoms'.**

💡 **Losing a baby—whether through miscarriage, stillbirth, or neonatal death—is terribly painful. Although both parents are understandably at increased risk of depression, they may struggle to discuss it or ask for help. Be alert to their need for support, including during subsequent pregnancies.**

Postpartum psychosis

Postpartum psychosis (PPP; also known as puerperal psychosis) may be a variant of bipolar affective disorder (BPAD) in which childbirth is the trigger, perhaps due to hormonal changes. Those at highest risk of PPP have a personal or family history of PPP or BPAD (BPAD is eight times more likely to relapse during the puerperium). Other risk factors include puerperal infection, obstetric complications (including Caesarean section), and first delivery. Aetiologically, psychosocial factors seem relatively unimportant.

Onset is usually rapid (within 2 weeks of delivery), often beginning with insomnia, restlessness, and perplexity. Clear psychotic symptoms then emerge, forming one of three clinical patterns:

- Affective (psychotic depression/mania, or mixed pattern, see p. 46).
- Schizophreniform (like schizophrenia, see p. 81).
- Delirious (see p. 130).

Symptoms can fluctuate dramatically and quickly; brief, symptom-free periods can be falsely reassuring. Organic causes and substance misuse (intoxication or withdrawal) must be excluded.

Depending on her presentation, the woman may need antipsychotics, antidepressants, or mood stabilizers; benzodiazepines may help with agitation. In severe cases, electroconvulsive therapy may be lifesaving. Inpatient admission is often required, preferably to an MBU. Recovery is usually within 6–12 weeks, but psychosis recurs in 50% of women having another baby, and in over 50% of women at another time (unrelated to childbirth).

> ❗ **Always assess risk.** Suicide is the commonest UK cause of direct maternal death in the first postpartum year. Risks to the baby include neglect or violence. Particularly serious signs are *command hallucinations* (instructing the woman to harm her baby), or *delusions about the baby* (e.g. that it's possessed/doomed). Women occasionally feel they must harm or kill their baby to protect it from a worse fate. Rates of infanticide in PPP are up to 4%.

REALITY

General approach: tips, tricks, and cautionary tales

1. Engage and assess

Don't patronize women by addressing them as 'Mum' or talking about 'Baby'—use their *names* to gain rapport. Be warm and friendly, without fussing over *or* ignoring the baby. Notice how the woman interacts with her infant, e.g. relaxed, anxious, warm, disinterested, hostile (ideally, judge her manner *after* looking after a baby yourself for at least 24 hours!). Try to interview her and her partner both together and alone, as their perspectives may differ.

2. Dispel myths

Important parenthood myths include:

- Babies are enchanting bundles of joy.
- 'Good mums' naturally know everything, and never need help.
- Social services take children away when parents struggle.

New parents are particularly vulnerable to these ideas, and can feel inadequate, especially when bombarded with social media 'evidence' of other families cuddling delightful babies.

Explain that *everyone* struggles and it's *normal* to feel overwhelmed sometimes (especially when sleep deprived). Babies are demanding and exhausting, and 'good parents' simply recognize their and their baby's needs, seeking help when needed. This normalizes stress and lets people admit problems. If social services are mentioned, explain that their role is primarily to *support* families and keep them together.

3. Stay

Although the risk of a woman harming her baby is very low, don't leave her alone with her baby if she's severely agitated, depressed, or experiencing psychotic symptoms. Be a calm, reassuring presence, and stay until help arrives.

The interview

• = Example question. * = Question linking to other parts of the history. X = The baby's name.

See relevant chapters for more general symptom exploration.

General screening

Baby

- **Tell me about X.** [Screen: sleep, feeding, temperament, development]

Stress

- **How are you coping?**
- It's often really stressful looking after a baby. Do you ever feel overwhelmed?
    * What do you do when you feel like that?
    * Do family/friends/partner know how you're feeling?
    * How are they helping you?
- How do you feel when X cries? Are there times he/she won't stop?
    * How do you handle that?

Illness

Depression

- **Do you feel sad or miserable?**
- Are you looking after *yourself*? [Screen: sleep, eat, energy]

- How does it feel to be a parent? [Screen: anhedonia, guilt, worthlessness]

Psychotic symptoms

- **Is X different to other babies in any way? How?** [Screen: special, abnormal]
- Some women worry that their baby's ill, abnormal, or bad in some way. Do you?
- What's your biggest worry?
- Do you worry for X's safety?
    * How do/will you protect X?

Self-harm/suicide

- Do you ever feel so bad that you wish you were dead?
- Have you had any thoughts of harming or killing yourself?

Harm to baby

- **Do you have thoughts about X that you're worried to tell people?**
    – Is it ever so stressful that you wish you hadn't had X?
    – Have you had any thoughts about harming X?
    – Thinking something is really different from doing it. Do you actually intend to harm X?

💡 **The Edinburgh Postnatal Depression Scale is a 5-minute screening test that helps health visitors identify depressed women during routine home visits.**

Perinatal history (15 minutes)

Candidate's instructions

Mona Chu is 26 years old and an audiologist. Her parents brought her to the ED because they're worried she's not coping with her 14-day-old baby, Polly. The triage nurse reports that Polly is healthy, but inexplicably wrapped in a runner's foil blanket.

You're a medical student on attachment in ED. The liaison psychiatrist asks you to interview Mona while he interviews her parents. Please take a history, and suggest a diagnosis.

Patient's brief

Key characteristics

- I'm frightened, restless, and suspicious.
- I won't let the student see or touch Polly under the foil blanket.
- I'm slightly distracted by noises and voices.

> *History*
> Polly was fine until a week ago, then strange things started happening. Clicking noises came from her room, but stopped when I went in. Then muffled conversations, gradually getting louder: men discussing *Project Torture*, e.g. 'Start with the little one.' David [Polly's dad] is a computer programmer, and a bad person. I realized he was using the baby monitors to spy on us and instruct his colleagues; I was hearing accidentally leaked audio.
>
> I broke the baby monitors but conversations started coming from all around, so I threw out the TV, laptop, and mobile. When it continued, I realized it came *from* Polly. It's *Intrinsic Tech*: microphones *inside* her, and cameras in her eyes to film me. They've said this bump on the back of her neck is a microchip, recording everything. This foil blanket interferes with frequencies, and prevents her filming and recording me.
>
> David's hacked my Facebook and mobile. 'Friends' kept sending weird emoticons and asking if I was *OK* (*Object Kill*—look it up, I can't talk about it here). I only trust my parents, but they think it's all in my head, so whose side are they *really* on?
>
> *Other history*
> - Polly was born by C-section.
> - We live alone since David beat me and hospitalized me. I've not seen him in 6 months.
> - No mental illness in my family. I was depressed with David, but never treated.
> - I'm physically fit. No medicines. I don't smoke, drink, or use drugs.
> - I'm not confused, depressed, or elated. I'm tired and scared to sleep, but eating normally.
>
> *Question*
> Can Polly have an MRI? It'll prove I'm right, and then doctors can remove the tech.
>
> *Worries*
> David wants to torture and kill us. I won't let that happen. I'd smother Polly with a pillow and hang myself if there was no other way.

💡 **This is PPP. The extreme risks to Polly and Mona require admission, ideally to an MBU for psychiatric assessment and treatment. The MHA may be needed if she refuses, or lacks capacity to consent to admission. She'll need an antipsychotic, CBT, nursing support to care for Polly, and social services input.**

NEXT STEPS

A tearful first-time parent

You're an obstetric FY2 in outpatients. Carmel Pritchard, 24, gave birth to her first child (Sam) 5 weeks ago by forceps-assisted vaginal delivery. She required an episiotomy and has struggled with poor wound healing. Today, Carmel tearfully admits she isn't coping.

- What are the important areas to cover today?
- When might you need to involve a psychiatrist?
- What's your management plan?

Assessment

The timing (5 weeks) is too late to be the 'blues'. Carmel may be suffering with PPD, *or* simply having a bad day, so don't jump to conclusions. Let her talk—empathically exploring her sense of 'not coping'. Find out *why* she feels she's struggling, and how it's affecting her mood, energy, and enjoyment of parenting. Decide whether she's clinically depressed and, if so, how severely (see p. 38). Assess for psychotic symptoms, especially abnormal thoughts about Sam. Check past psychiatric history (particularly depression/psychosis and any treatments), social support, and current alcohol or drug use. Observe Carmel's manner with Sam, e.g. whether she's interested, warm, responsive.

Fully assess the wound. Complications will exacerbate low mood and affect Carmel's ability to care for Sam, e.g. infection, bleeding, faecal incontinence, dyspareunia. Have a low threshold for gaining senior review.

Psychiatric referral

Contact the hospital liaison or perinatal psychiatrist for advice if you don't know how to proceed, or have identified severe symptoms or risk (e.g. depression/ psychotic symptoms, self-neglect, thoughts of suicide/ infanticide). They may advise community psychiatric follow-up, or facilitate urgent assessment and admission if risks are high.

Further management

Whether or not you involve the psychiatrist, liaise with Carmel's GP. A clinic letter may take a week to reach the GP, by which time Carmel may be in a more desperate state. Call her GP *now* to discuss options over the telephone. Seek Carmel's permission to discuss problems with her closest supporters, e.g. partner, parents.

Uncomplicated depression can often be managed at home with support from the family, GP, health visitor, and community psychiatric services (generic or perinatal team, depending on local resources). Social services may advise additional childcare support (e.g. via a UK Sure Start centre) and should be involved if Carmel's health could affect Sam's welfare.

Ensure Carmel has adequate analgesia if she's in pain from her episiotomy; give shorter prescriptions if worried about her suicide risk. Offer flexible reviews.

> Carmel could neglect her own health if depressed, so may need more assertive follow-up, e.g. appointment reminders, and extended community midwife input.

Movie buff
The Babadook (2014): horror film about a monster terrorizing a widow and her child is an allegory for bereavement, but also offers a powerfully imaginative depiction of how psychosis can interact with motherhood.

Tully (2018): this comedy starring Charlize Theron was inspired by writer Diablo Cody's own PPD after her third pregnancy. It's been praised as unsentimental about motherhood, and criticized as misleading—decide for yourself.

Book shelf
Martini, A. (2006) *Hillbilly Gothic*: this 'memoir of motherhood and madness' describes PPD, its effect on female relatives, inpatient treatment, and observations of PPP, first hand.

Perkins Gilman, C. (1892) *The Yellow Wallpaper*: an unnamed woman's diary entries narrate her experience of treatment for a 'temporary nervous depression—a slight hysterical tendency'.

Rogers, J. (1987) *The Ice is Singing*: Marion, a single parent of twins, drives aimlessly around the countryside, reflecting on PPD and the disintegration of her marriage. The cyclical passage of the seasons mirrors the course of her depression.

Note

1. Cusk, R. (2001) *A Life's Work: On Becoming a Mother*. London: Fourth Estate, p. 79.

Journal club

Chisolm, M. (2016) Management of psychotropic drugs during pregnancy. *BMJ*, **352**, h5918.

The Lancet (2014). Perinatal mental health series. www.thelancet.com/series/perinatal-mental-health

Resources

APNI—association for postnatal illness: www.apni.org/

PANDAS—pre- and postnatal depression advice and support: www.pandasfoundation.org.uk/

Go to www.oup.com/uk/stringer2e for a wealth of additional resources, including an OCSE mark scheme, filmed scenarios, and self-assessment questions.

19 Intellectual Disability

True or false?

Answers on p. 277

1. Intellectual disability (ID) affects more males than females.
2. The number of people with ID is rising.
3. An IQ score is essential to identify ID.
4. People with ID have higher rates of epilepsy.
5. People with mild ID have an increased risk of schizophrenia.
6. Down syndrome is associated with congenital heart abnormalities.
7. Fragile X is associated with expressive language deficits.
8. People with ID don't require more physical healthcare input than anyone else.
9. When talking to someone with an ID, use one idea per sentence to aid comprehension.
10. A 40-year-old man with Down syndrome begins to act in a sexualized manner at his residential home. Ideally, this should be managed in the home, rather than through hospital admission.

Contents

Principles
Introduction
Epidemiology
Aetiology
Clinical presentation
- Challenging behaviour
- Mental health
- Physical health

Differential diagnosis
Investigations

Management
- Biological interventions
- Psychological interventions
- Social interventions

Prognosis

Reality
General approach: tips, tricks, and cautionary tales
- ID/depression history

Next steps
Behavioural change
- Differential diagnosis
- Preparation
- Assessment
- Management

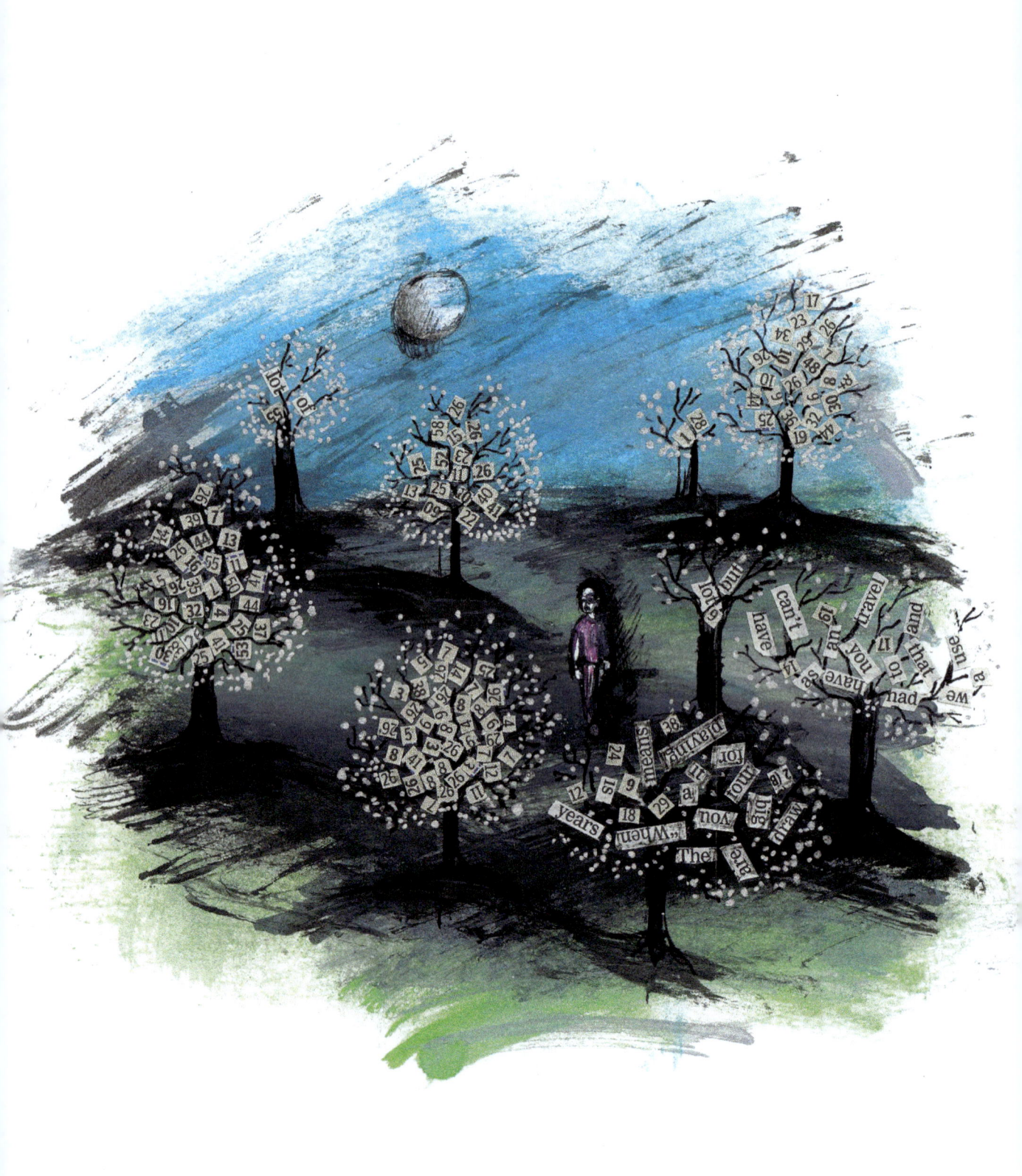

PRINCIPLES

I've learned that intelligence alone doesn't mean a damned thing. Here in your university, intelligence, education, knowledge, have all become great idols. But I know now there's one thing you've all overlooked: intelligence and education that hasn't been tempered by human affection isn't worth a damn.

Daniel Keyes, *Flowers for Algernon*[1]

Introduction

Intellectual disability (ID), or disorders of intellectual development (ICD-11 terminology), are a group of conditions in which intellectual functioning and adaptive behaviour are significantly below average. Diagnosis may be based upon appropriate standardized tests such as the intelligence quotient (IQ)—a normally distributed score with a mean of 100. Clinical assessment of day-to-day functioning and behaviour may, however, be equally valid where tests aren't available. Onset is before adulthood (usually counted as 18 years), while the brain is still developing.

ID isn't necessarily a mental health problem, and most people with ID never see a psychiatrist. Try to remember the *social model* of disability: that people with impairments are disabled by the way society is organized, rather than by what makes them different. However, ID is associated with comorbid mental and physical health difficulties, and whatever area of medicine you end up working in, you'll meet people with ID.

💡 Many older words for ID are now considered stigmatizing and offensive (e.g. *mental retardation* isn't used now). *Learning disability* (LD) is an acceptable term, but increasingly being replaced by ID.

Epidemiology

ID affects slightly more males than females (3:2). **Table 19.1** shows the prevalence of ID. It's thought that the number of people with severe and profound ID is rising, due to the increased survival of very premature babies.

Aetiology

Around 50% of people have no clear cause for their ID; this probably results from a combination of environmental and non-Mendelian polygenic factors. Chromosomal abnormalities account for 40% of severe ID, and up to 20% of mild ID. Genetic causes, in particular, may arise as *syndromes*, associated with recognized physical abnormalities (*dysmorphisms*). Specific causes of ID are listed in **Tables 19.2 and 19.3**; preventative measures are covered in **Box 19.1**.

Table 19.1 ID epidemiology

Intellectual disability	Standard deviations (SD) below mean[a]	Approximate equivalent IQ score	Approximate prevalence
Mild	2–3	55–69	2.5%
Moderate	3–4	35–54	0.4%
Severe	4 or more	<35	0.1% combined
Profound	4 or more	<35[b]	

[a] For intellectual functioning and adaptive behaviour.
[b] IQ scores cannot reliably distinguish amongst those below 4th SD.

Table 19.2 Causes of ID

Antenatal	Perinatal	Postnatal
Genetic: *Chromosomal disorders* (most '*de novo*'), e.g. Down syndrome, Turner syndrome *Mendelian inheritance*: • Autosomal recessive, e.g. phenylketonuria, Tay–Sachs disease • Autosomal dominant, e.g. tuberous sclerosis • Sex-linked, e.g. fragile X syndrome **During pregnancy:** • Teratogen exposure, e.g. alcohol, drugs, tobacco, medications • Infection, e.g. rubella	Prematurity Neonatal hypoxia Birth trauma Infection, e.g. syphilis, herpes simplex Hypoglycaemia	Social deprivation Malnutrition Iodine deficiency (especially in low-income countries) causing congenital hypothyroidism Toxins, e.g. lead Infections, e.g. meningitis Head injury Child abuse/neglect

The risk of autosomal recessive disorders is increased in populations affected by *stratification*, where—for historical, cultural, or geographical reasons—a subpopulation is genetically separated. For example, the autosomal recessive allele for Tay–Sachs disease is carried by around 25% of the Ashkenazi Jewish population; this community may routinely screen for the allele before marriage. *Consanguinity*, where partners are both descended from a common ancestor (i.e. second cousins or closer), further increases the risk of autosomal recessive disorders.

Clinical presentation

ID usually presents in childhood, but may be missed if mild. Early indications include delayed developmental milestones and needing more support at school. In

Table 19.3 Specific syndromes associated with ID

	Live birth rate	Cause	Physical characteristics	Associated problems
Down syndrome	1:700 Commonest genetic cause of ID	Trisomy 21 (commonest) Translocations or mosaicism[a] of chromosome 21 Risk increases in older mothers	Upward-slanting palpebral fissures Epicanthic folds Protruding tongue (due to small mouth) Single palmar crease Hypotonia Short stature	Congenital heart abnormalities Hypothyroidism Epilepsy Alzheimer disease[b] Leukaemia Gastrointestinal disorders Hearing/visual impairment
Fragile X	1:4000 boys 1:8000 girls	Mutation in *FMR1* gene on X chromosome	Elongated face Prominent ears High-arched palate Hyperextensible joints Large testes	Features of ASD Anxiety Hyperactivity Expressive language deficits (Female) carriers have milder challenges
Foetal alcohol syndrome	6:10,000 (9:1000 spectrum disorders)	Alcohol during pregnancy	Short palpebral fissure Smooth philtrum Thin top lip	Behavioural difficulties Foetal growth retardation Neurological abnormalities

[a] Only some cells have the abnormality.
[b] Due to the presence of the amyloid precursor protein gene (*APP*) on chromosome 21; onset is roughly 10–15 years earlier than the general population.

> **BOX 19.1** Prevention of ID
>
> - Education, e.g. risks of alcohol during pregnancy.
> - Improved antenatal/perinatal care, e.g. MMR vaccination for prospective mothers, iodine supplementation of water in areas of deficiency.
> - Genetic counselling for prospective parents carrying risk alleles.
> - Early detection and treatment of preventable causes, e.g. excluding dietary phenylalanine in babies with phenylketonuria.

general, the more severe the ID (**Table 19.4**), the greater the likelihood of comorbid problems, e.g. epilepsy, sensory impairment, autism spectrum disorder (ASD).

💡 IQ gives an idea of the level of support someone may need, but tells you nothing about their personality, abilities, or their potential.

Challenging behaviour

Behavioural difficulties increase in frequency as severity of ID increases, e.g. overactivity, withdrawal, aggression, disinhibition, stereotyped movements (e.g. hand-flapping, pirouetting), self-injury (e.g. self-biting, eye-poking). These may be a way of communicating distress or coping with discomfort or strong emotions. Some behaviours may relate to associated neurodevelopmental disorders, e.g. repetitive movements in ASD; restlessness in attention deficit hyperactivity disorder (ADHD). *Behavioural phenotypes* occur with particular syndromes, e.g. compulsive eating in Prader–Willi syndrome; self-injury in Lesch–Nyhan syndrome. Whether new or longstanding, the behaviour may disappear if you solve the underlying problem (**Table 19.5**).

Mental health

Up to 50% of people with ID have comorbid neurodevelopmental or psychiatric disorders. This is largely mediated via shared genetic susceptibility, obstetric complications, and psychosocial stressors. Compared with the general population:

- Schizophrenia and bipolar disorder are two to three times commoner.
- Dementia affects four times as many older adults with ID.
- ASD and ADHD are more prevalent, increasing as IQ falls, e.g. ASD occurs in 10% of people with mild ID, and 30% of those with severe ID.
- Mood and anxiety disorders are at least as prevalent as in the general population.

However, substance misuse and anorexia nervosa are *less* common in people with ID.

Table 19.4 Impact of ID

Severity	Effect on person
Mild	- Language skills usually good, but may have developed slowly; vocabulary somewhat limited - At school: struggles/needs extra help to master reading, writing, and arithmetic; may be labelled with 'behavioural problems' - Usually lives and works independently, with appropriate support
Moderate	- Less developed language and cognitive abilities, e.g. uses simple words or sentences - May not read/write fluently - May need support with self-care and motor skills - Often lives long term with family/in supported group housing - Can undertake simple, practical work in supported settings
Severe	- Little/no speech in early childhood, but may learn basic words or gestures to communicate - Motor skills may be markedly impaired - May perform simple tasks, with help - Usually needs a high level of support with everyday activities - Lives in their family home or 24-hour-staffed housing
Profound	- Usually non-verbal, with very limited understanding of language - Can't usually mobilize or self-care - Often significant motor, sensory, and medical problems - Needs extensive support

Table 19.5 Causes of changed or challenging behaviour

	Triggers
Biological	Delirium
	Pain, e.g. infection (ears, dental), constipation
	Epilepsy
	Dementia
	Medication, e.g. side effects, withdrawal
	Substance misuse
Psychological	Distress, frustration, sadness, boredom
	Adjustment disorder
	Depression, mania
	Psychosis
Social	Environmental changes, e.g. accommodation, residents, carers, routine
	Social stressors
	Communication difficulty, e.g. earwax, lost glasses
	Frustration, e.g. unable to communicate needs
	Under/overstimulation
	Bullying, abuse/neglect

The greater someone's ID, the harder it is for them to describe their experiences (e.g. guilt, hopelessness, hallucinations). Detective work and collateral histories are often needed to interpret signs of illness:

- Changes from usual ('baseline') level of function, e.g. loss of usual abilities in self-care, continence, communication.
- Changed behaviour or personality, e.g. withdrawal in depression, destructive behaviour in anxiety.
- Biological/non-verbal symptoms, e.g. sleep/appetite, crying, catatonia.

💡 ID can be confusing, e.g. someone's fantasies may resemble delusions; speaking to 'imaginary friends' may seem as if they're responding to hallucinations. A key diagnostic question is whether these are *new* issues.

Physical health

People with ID have higher rates of epilepsy (up to 25% prevalence), sensory impairment, mobility problems, respiratory disease, obesity, and vascular risk factors (except smoking). Life expectancy is reduced due to:

- Difficulties accessing preventative interventions, e.g. lower uptake of influenza vaccination (despite respiratory infections being the leading cause of death).
- A lack of assertive, coordinated services for people with ID.
- Delayed diagnosis, due to atypical physical presentations, and communication barriers.
- Stigma and value judgements by healthcare professionals, leading to discrimination or inadequate treatment, e.g. disproportionate use of 'do not resuscitate' notices.
- Staff overlooking medical conditions due to *diagnostic overshadowing* (attributing everything to the ID itself), e.g. someone with ID who cries and stops eating is assumed to 'just be that way'—when they actually have appendicitis.

💡 Never make assumptions about someone's quality of life. People can feel happy and fulfilled despite high levels of disability.

Differential diagnosis

- **ASD:** significant difficulties with reciprocal social interaction, communication, and repetitive behaviours/routines (see p. 247). IQ may be normal. Where ID and ASD are comorbid, ASD-related difficulties are greater than would be expected for the ID alone.
- **Epilepsy:** can cause transient cognitive impairment during or after seizures. Frequent, uncontrolled absence or focal seizures can mimic persistent cognitive impairment. Long-term, untreated epilepsy can cause neuronal damage, or traumatic brain injury (TBI) through seizure-related accidents.
- **Adult TBI or progressive neurological conditions:** IDs are neurodevelopmental disorders, starting before adulthood. If an adult presents with cognitive impairment, it's important to decide whether difficulties are new or longstanding, e.g. Alzheimer disease isn't ID.
- **Psychiatric disorder:** severe and enduring mental health problems (e.g. schizophrenia) can mimic ID by causing chronic cognitive impairment and reduced social functioning. A history of premorbid functioning and educational ability helps to distinguish the two.
- **Educational disadvantage/neglect:** childhood neglect, poor schooling, or social under-stimulation can cause a picture similar to mild ID (e.g. illiteracy, dependence on others). This is usually reversible to some extent.
- **Developmental learning/motor disorders:** dyslexia, dyspraxia, and dyscalculia are examples of isolated learning impairments, where overall intellectual function is normal.

Investigations

- **IQ testing:** by educational or clinical psychologists.
- **Functional assessment:** occupational therapists (OTs) and/or social workers assess the person's strengths and skills, as well as areas for development or support.
- **Detailed developmental history from parents**, e.g. pregnancy and birth, language and motor development, schooling, emotional development, relationships. School reports are helpful.
- **Full physical examination and investigations as appropriate:**
  - To identify specific cause/syndrome in children, e.g. micro-array/chromosome analysis, fragile X analysis, TFTs (congenital hypothyroidism), metabolic screening (e.g. amino acids, FBC, U&Es, bone profile). Referral to clinical geneticist if necessary.
  - Investigations for associated physical illnesses, e.g. EEG for epilepsy.
  - MRI brain, e.g. if there is neurological abnormality, micro- or macrocephaly.

Management

People with ID should be supported to access mainstream services, though those with complex presentations may see specialist ID teams of psychologists, OTs, nurses, psychiatrists, speech and language therapists, and educational specialists.

Biological interventions

Hearing and visual impairments must be addressed, and annual health checks are recommended in the UK. Health promotion can increase the uptake of vaccinations, dental checks, and screening programmes (e.g. cervical). People with ID may carry *Healthcare Passports*, containing information about their health and communication needs.

Physical and mental health problems are treated as usual. However, people with ID may be particularly sensitive to medication effects and side effects, so it's essential to try low doses and increase slowly, monitor closely, and consider interactions with other medications, e.g. antiepileptics. Dosette boxes, written or pictorial instructions, and carer involvement can all increase adherence.

> 💡 Never assume that someone with ID lacks capacity to make choices about their healthcare. Help them understand information, so they can make decisions, e.g. use 'easy read'/audible/pictorial explanatory materials, enlist carers and other professionals to assist.

Psychological interventions

Psychological therapy may include counselling, group therapy, and modified CBT.

Behavioural therapy uses an ABC approach to address challenging behaviour. This identifies the *Antecedents* (triggers), *Behaviours*, and *Consequences* (of behaviour). This informs the *behavioural management plan*, which might include:

- Avoiding triggers.
- Reinforcing positive behaviours, e.g. with praise/rewards.
- Preventing reinforcement of unwanted behaviours, e.g. carers giving attention when the person shouts may make the person shout more (ignoring it might reduce it).
- Helping the person understand the consequences of their actions.

Social interventions

Early detection and an Education, Health and Care (EHC) plan (formerly, 'statement of special educational needs') enables appropriate support in mainstream or special schools, to maximize a young person's potential.

Augmentative and alternative communication (AAC) supports people with ID to speak (augmentative), or provides alternatives to verbal communication. It includes:

- Adapted sign language, e.g. Makaton.
- Staff and family learning how to interpret expressions and gestures.
- Communication boards with symbols or pictures the person chooses by pointing or gazing.
- Talking computers.

The social model of disability promotes integrating AAC into mainstream life, e.g. teaching Makaton to all nursery pupils, or integrating sign language into inclusive theatre performances.

Social services assess the level of need for help with activities of daily living (see p. 152), housing, employment, finances, and social inclusion. Day centres, clubs, and vocational schemes (for voluntary or paid work) help people develop skills and social networks. Apps on tablets and smartphones can enhance participation in education and make socializing easier. Many organizations provide help, education, and support for people with ID and their carers, e.g. Mencap, Scope, British Institute of Learning Disabilities (BILD), Down's Syndrome Association.

Supporting someone with lifelong, complex needs places *carers* at risk of burnout (see p. 40). Carers' assessments, social services support, and respite care are often crucial.

💡 Focus on the person's *strengths* as well as areas of difficulty. This can transform your view of them and their potential.

Prognosis

On average, people with ID die 16 years earlier than the general population. Although ID is lifelong, people can continue to develop and learn new skills throughout their lives—given the chance, they can often surpass the expectations of carers and health professionals alike.

💡 People with ID are vulnerable to neglect, abuse, bullying, and exploitation. Their problems may then be compounded by communication difficulties, and behavioural change may be their only way of communicating distress.

REALITY

General approach: tips, tricks, and cautionary tales

1. Don't patronize

Don't treat adults with ID like children. Avoid:

- Calling them a *girl* or *boy*.
- Nicknaming without permission, e.g. changing Nicholas to 'Nicky'.
- Using language below their level of understanding.
- Assuming they can't understand or make decisions.
- Talking exclusively to carers, e.g. 'Does he take sugar?'
- Ignoring their sexuality.

2. Start with *them*

Always try to engage directly, first. Greet them, give plenty of time, and gauge their response. If they have communication problems, explain that you'll ask their carer how to help you talk to them better.

Ask the person's carer how they usually communicate, and if they have visual or hearing problems; there may be simple ways to improve communication, e.g. sitting closer. When the person's speech is unclear or you need specialized skills to communicate, carers can often interpret. Just beware the tendency for some carers to say what *they* think, rather than representing the views of the person.

3. Pitch and pace

Pitch your conversation at *their* level. Speak clearly and simply, using short words and sentences, with one idea per sentence. Don't overcomplicate, e.g.:

> You: Fortunately, we've excluded cancer and you're not going to die.
> Roxy: Cancer? Die!

Wait for a response: understanding the question, choosing an answer, finding the right words, and getting these words out may all take longer than usual. It's frustrating not to be given time to answer. If they don't respond at all, simplify your question, before moving on. Be patient with anyone who speaks slowly: it's rude to finish people's sentences.

4. Be understanding

Check you've understood what the person is saying, e.g. 'Your leg hurts? Is that right?' The harder they are to understand, the more often you must check—but they'll be patient if you explain you're checking because their views are important.

When someone *can't* communicate, don't assume they can't *understand*; they may be listening intently, so keep your conversation accessible and use their name to show you're discussing them.

5. Assume nothing

People rarely admit when they don't understand, due to embarrassment, wanting to please you, or because they don't realize they've misunderstood. Don't *assume* understanding because someone nods, echoes the last thing you said, or says 'yes' or 'no'.

When someone *only* gives yes/no answers, check for consistent responses by reversing the question's meaning, e.g.:

> You: Are you sad?
> Roxy: Yes.
> You: Are you happy?
> Roxy: Yes.

Otherwise, ask open questions, and keep checking for understanding, e.g. 'I've said a lot. What can you remember about this medicine?' If they're anxious or embarrassed, try normalizing, e.g.:

- Sometimes I don't explain things very well. Tell me what you've understood, so I know what I need to explain better.
- This is difficult, so I'll go over it one more time.

6. More than words

Speech is only a small part of communicating. *Total communication* uses whatever works to communicate when someone has limited language, e.g.:

- Are you sad? *[Make a sad expression/draw a sad face]*
- Does your arm hurt? *[Rub your arm while looking pained]*

It may help to draw simple pictures, narrating as you go, then asking them to explain what the pictures mean.

7. ASD tips

People with ASD often find eye contact or face-to-face interviews deeply uncomfortable; they may look or turn away, while still listening. Try avoiding direct eye contact, or sit to their side (but not too close or touching).

They often think literally, and find metaphors and abstract language confusing, e.g. 'I'll give you a ring later' could be deeply disappointing! Don't be offended if they sometimes seem rude (e.g. making personal comments); they struggle to understand social conventions. Plan plenty of time for assessments, as they may talk at length about their particular interests before answering your questions.

💡 Someone might be terrified about meeting you or coming to hospital. To reduce their anxiety, explain what will happen and offer choices, wherever possible.

ID/depression history (20 minutes)

Candidate's instructions

You're a medical student in general practice. Ms Mary Knight is 58, and a supermarket assistant; she has a mild ID. She presented last week with fatigue, but her blood tests were normal (FBC, TFTs, HbA1c, calcium, vitamins B_{12} and D). The GP suspects her tiredness may be due to depression, and asks you to assess her before his review.

Patient's brief

Key characteristics
- I speak slowly.
- I can't understand difficult words, but I don't ask what they mean.
- I'm sad, worried, and cry easily.

History

I've helped on the deli counter for 10 years. Tracy joined a year ago. I really liked her; she seemed so nice. She'd have lunch and walk home with me. It made me feel special because she was young and everyone liked her. A while ago (around Christmas), I came back from break and she was making fun of the way I say names of cheeses and meats ... I'd been getting them all wrong. Everyone laughed and I ran to the loo and cried. Tracy said we can't be friends if I can't take a joke.

I feel so sad and don't want to speak at work in case I get it wrong again. The deli ladies hold up foreign cheeses and meats and say, 'What's this, Mary?' They make me say it so I get it wrong in front of customers. I told my manager, but he said I should toughen up or go work the tills. But the tills are too hard for me. I used to love work and cheering up customers ... Now I don't want to go in, and spend all day waiting to go home.

I used to enjoy TV and sewing but I don't feel like it anymore. I tried to make a skirt last week, but my mind felt all jumpy-about and I couldn't work out what to do. I haven't tried since. I'm always thinking: *I'm stupid, I can't do anything right, it's all my fault.* I feel sad all day and cry a lot and can't see things getting better. I don't feel like eating much ... Tracy hasn't called me *chubby* for a while, so maybe I've lost weight. I sleep lots more, but I'm still so tired. I used to look after my grandsons (Alfie and Sam), but I got too tired, so my son got a *proper* babysitter. I really miss them.

My husband Mark was really angry and said he'd sort Tracy out, but I said he mustn't, so he didn't and now he says I need to *quit whining*. I can't tell my friends about it; I'll just cry and they'll think I'm stupid.

Other history

- I used to be friendly and happy and always laughing.
- I've never been so sad or stressed before.
- I take menopause tablets.

General approach: tips, tricks, and cautionary tales **239**

- I don't smoke. I have a glass of wine on birthdays.
- I'd never try to hurt or kill myself.
- I was never very good at school and needed special help.
- I've worked in the supermarket all my life: Mum got me the job when I was 16. I wouldn't know how to find a different job.

Question
Can you help me?

Worry
I want to quit but Mark says we need the money.

💡 Ms Knight's ID has made her vulnerable to bullying, triggering a moderate depressive episode. Management includes normalizing her distress (she's not being 'silly'; she's being *bullied*), and supporting her with this work situation, e.g. through her work union, Citizen's Advice, involving her family, manager, or an advocate. She should be offered CBT, plus an antidepressant (low dose, increased slowly).

NEXT STEPS

Behavioural change

You're an FY2 in general practice. A care home manager calls, requesting you visit a resident, Nathan Rowell. Nathan is 48 years old and has Down syndrome and moderate ID. He's lived happily at the home for 3 years, but over the past week has become irritable and sexually disinhibited, e.g. kissing and groping other residents. Last night, he tried to leave at midnight, and threw a cup when staff refused.

- What's the differential diagnosis?
- Describe your assessment and management.

Differential diagnosis
See **Table 19.5**. Specific issues in Down syndrome include sensory impairment (visual/hearing problems are common), early-onset Alzheimer disease, and hypo/hyperthyroidism.

💡 Changed behaviour can communicate any number of emotional or physical problems, which the person can't verbalize, from toothache to heartache.

Preparation
Review Nathan's notes and Healthcare Passport for communication needs, physical/psychiatric problems, and medication changes. If he's receiving psychiatric services, contact his care coordinator: suggest a joint visit, and ask about previous, similar episodes, and how these resolved.

Take a detailed history from placement staff, focusing on Nathan's:

- Usual level of functioning and any recent changes.
- Communication needs.
- Behaviour change:
  – Onset (sudden/gradual).
  – Possible triggers.
  – Details.
  – Staff response.
- Unusual responses to particular staff/residents, e.g. fear, crying, anger, silence.

As Nathan's been disinhibited, take a male chaperone, ideally someone he likes, who can facilitate communication. If able, speak to Nathan alone at some point, in case he's afraid to disclose worries with staff present.

Assessment
Your history and MSE should specifically consider mania (e.g. elation/irritability, restlessness, insomnia), and psychosis (e.g. distractedness, suspiciousness). Assess cognition, comparing Nathan's current and baseline ability, e.g. can he recognize staff and find his room, or is he confused? Check if he's happy at the home, who he likes/dislikes—and *why*. Who does he see outside the home? Is he frightened of anyone? Has anyone been unkind to him? Do he or his friends use alcohol or drugs?

Ask Nathan whether he feels well, checking specifically for pain. Perform a physical examination, remembering common comorbidities in Down syndrome, e.g. respiratory infections, thyroid dysfunction, cardiac problems (atrioventricular septal defects, infective endocarditis), constipation.

Risk assessment includes self-neglect, self-harm, and escalating aggression or sexual disinhibition. Nathan's behaviour may make him vulnerable to exploitation or retaliation. Additionally, his placement could break down if things don't improve.

Management

If possible, manage Nathan's presentation at home; relocation will remove familiar routines and environments, which could exacerbate challenging behaviour and confusion. Remind staff that Nathan usually isn't like this, and will probably settle once the underlying cause is addressed. Temporarily, they may need additional staff to safely manage his behaviour. Meanwhile:

- Investigate and treat physical illness or sensory impairment.
- If you suspect pain, consider regular analgesia, e.g. paracetamol.
- Encourage familiar routines and staff.
- Involve family and friends, to reassure Nathan and offer insight into his behaviour.

If you suspect an underlying mental health problem *or* can't resolve the problem easily, urgently refer Nathan to the CMHT (ideally, a specialist ID mental health team). They'll assess, advise on medication, and provide psychology input to help staff understand residual challenging behaviour with an ABC approach (see p. 237). Inpatient psychiatric admission is occasionally needed, but avoided wherever possible: specialist ID wards are scarce, general wards may lack specialist skills, and the change of environment may exacerbate Nathan's behaviour.

If Nathan can't be safely managed at home, consider alternatives, e.g. social services may organize an emergency placement. If you suspect serious physical illness, transfer Nathan to the emergency department. Beforehand, discuss thoroughly with the admitting doctor, and ensure that a carer accompanies him, to facilitate communication and provide reassurance. If you suspect abuse, raise this immediately with your GP safeguarding lead *and* Nathan's social worker.

> 💡 Nathan may be trying to express his sexuality or find a partner. His ID doesn't stop him being a sexual being, but he's particularly vulnerable to sexual exploitation. He needs clear boundaries at home, an appropriate level of sex education, and support to make choices and have relationships.

Movie buff

Flesh & Blood (2002): Joe (Christopher Ecclestone) was adopted at birth. When he finds his birth parents, he realizes they both have ID. Joe's parents are both played by people who have ID (Dorothy Cockin and Peter Kirkby).

Forrest Gump (1994): this six-Oscar-winning classic sanitizes Winston Groom's novel of the same name, but both showcase the abilities and adventures of a man with ID as his life passes through key twentieth-century historical events.

Marvellous (2014): this film tells the true story of Neil Baldwin, who worked as a clown, lay preacher, university welfare officer, and kit-man for Stoke City Football Club!

What's Eating Gilbert Grape (1993): a young Leonardo DiCaprio was Oscar-nominated for his performance as Arnie, a teenager with ID. Johnny Depp plays his brother, Gilbert, trying to hold the family together after their father's death.

Book shelf

Cook, D. (1980) *Walter*: set in the mid-twentieth century, this poignant and moving exploration of ID examines stigma, maternal love, social understanding, and the impact of developmental delay on behaviour and cognition.

Keyes, D. (1966) *Flowers for Algernon*: Charlie Gordon is a janitor with an IQ of 68, until he volunteers for an experiment which will *temporarily* boost his IQ.

Mardell, D. (2005) *Danny's Challenge: Learning to Love my Son*: this autobiography describes Mardell's heartbreak at his son's unexpected Down syndrome, and his long journey to love his son and raise awareness.

Note

1. Keyes, D. (1966) *Flowers for Algernon*. Harcourt, New York.

Journal club

Chiurazzi, P., Pirozzi, F. (2016) Advances in understanding—genetic basis of intellectual disability. *F1000Res*, **5**, 599.

Cooper, S.A., Smiley, E., Morrison, J., et al. (2007) Mental ill-health in adults with intellectual disabilities: prevalence and associated factors. *British Journal of Psychiatry*, **190**, 27–35.

Hemmings, C., Bouras, N. (2016) *Psychiatric and Behavioural Disorders in Intellectual and Developmental Disabilities* (3rd ed.). Cambridge: Cambridge University Press.

Resources

Mencap—*Treat Me Well* campaign and resources: aiming to transform how the NHS treats people with a learning disability in hospital. Mencap—'Communicating with people with a learning disability': www.mencap.org.uk/learning-disability-explained/communicating-people-learning-disability

Go to www.oup.com/uk/stringer2e for a wealth of additional resources, including an OCSE mark scheme, filmed scenarios, and self-assessment questions.

20 Child and Adolescent Psychiatry

True or false?

Answers on p. 277

1. Most babies smile by 2 months old.
2. Poor parenting style causes autism spectrum disorder.
3. All under 16s who self-harm must be seen by a child and adolescent mental health services (CAMHS) specialist before discharge.
4. First-line treatment for childhood depression is a selective serotonin reuptake inhibitor.
5. Girls are as likely to develop anxiety disorders as boys.
6. Encopresis is inappropriate defecation after 3 years old.
7. Conduct/dissocial disorder is commoner in boys than girls.
8. The main risk of stimulant medication for attention deficit hyperactivity disorder is dependence.
9. Using street slang usually improves rapport with teenagers.
10. If a child discloses physical abuse, the safeguarding lead must be informed.

Contents

Principles
Introduction
Normal development
Behavioural and emotional disorders
- Separation anxiety disorder
- School refusal
- Enuresis
- Encopresis
- Selective mutism

Neurodevelopmental disorders
- Autism spectrum disorder
- Attention deficit hyperactivity disorder

Disruptive behaviour or dissocial disorders
- Conduct/dissocial disorder

Tic disorders

Reality
General approach: tips, tricks, and cautionary tales
The interview
- Neurodevelopmental history

Next steps
Hyperactivity and non-accidental injury
- Response
- Interventions
- Effect of ADHD

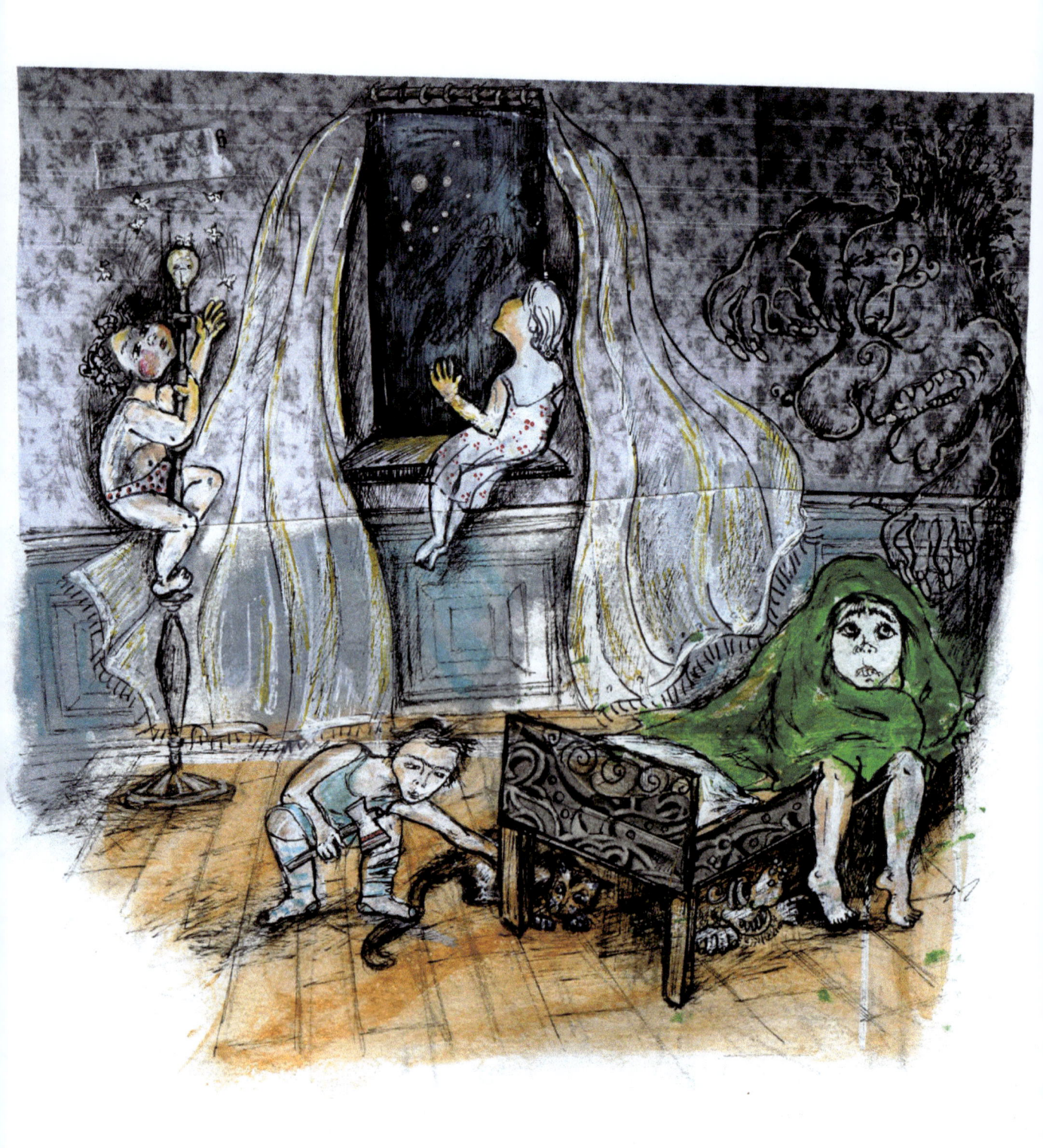

PRINCIPLES

I have quite a few worries. I have made a list of them in my notebook—it's a notebook for worst worries—because people say things aren't so bad if you make a list. And then you can tick things off when they are solved. So far I haven't ticked anything off.

Lauren Child, *Clarice Bean, Don't Look Now*[1]

Introduction

Up to 15% of children (younger than 12 years) and adolescents (12–18 years) are affected by mental health problems at any time, with potentially devastating effects on their health, development, and education. Early identification and intervention are crucial, although children rarely seek help from doctors, even when extremely distressed. Parents or teachers usually raise concerns first, and problems that can't be dealt with by their GP or school may be referred to child and adolescent mental health services (CAMHS). CAMHS teams usually include psychologists, specialist nurses, and psychiatrists.

Child and adolescent psychiatry concerns any mental health problem in people younger than 18 years at the time of referral. Depression, anxiety disorders, eating disorders, psychosis, and self-harm can all present in childhood or adolescence. They are comprehensively discussed in their own chapters; **Table 20.1** shows the main differences in young people. This chapter addresses problems which always start in childhood.

❗ **Child abuse doesn't always manifest in obvious behavioural problems or injuries. Inquiries have highlighted**

Table 20.1 Key differences in childhood/adolescent presentations of mental health problems

Disorder	Differences in childhood/adolescent presentation
Depression	• Affects 1–2% of children and 8% of adolescents • Sex ratio is equal before puberty, when girls begin to outnumber boys • Children often report somatic symptoms, e.g. headache, tummy ache • Teachers may note irritability or deteriorating school performance • First-line treatment for mild depression persisting after 4 weeks is CBT • Antidepressant medication is only offered in combination with psychological therapy • First-line medication is fluoxetine, prescribed by specialists following multidisciplinary discussion • Prognosis is generally good but severe episodes are likely to recur
Anxiety disorders	• Period prevalence: 9–32% during childhood and adolescence • Anxiety disorders affect boys and girls equally • Many anxiety disorders commence in adolescence • May present with somatic symptoms
Self-harm	• All under 16-year-olds who self-harm must be reviewed by a CAMHS specialist before discharge and admitted to a paediatric ward to facilitate this if necessary
Psychosis	• Very rare in children before puberty • Prognosis is poor, with disrupted social development • Important to exclude ASD and organic causes (e.g. autoimmune disorders)
Eating disorders	• May present with faltering growth or delayed puberty • Expected body weight calculations consider sex, age, and height on centile charts

missed opportunities to identify abuse and neglect prior to the high-profile deaths of Peter Connelly and Victoria Climbie. Child protection is everyone's job; any concerns are discussed immediately with seniors.

Normal development

A child who fails to meet normal developmental milestones may simply be a 'late developer' but could also have underlying problems requiring early intervention. For example, treating deafness can prevent speech delay and pronunciation difficulties. All children develop at different rates, and there's a wide range of normal development, though lengthy delays are concerning, e.g. not smiling responsively by 8 weeks, sitting unaided by 10 months, walking by 18 months, or saying their first word by 2 years. Parents may worry that their child has been slower to do things like smiling, sitting up, walking, and talking, compared with older siblings. Alternatively, their health visitor or GP may have noticed the delay and referred them to paediatrics or CAMHS. Further assessment is always needed when developmental milestone attainment is delayed beyond the upper limit, with consideration of risk factors (**Table 20.2**).

Behavioural and emotional disorders

Separation anxiety disorder

Children present with excessive fear of separation from specific attachment figures, usually parents or other caregivers, for at least several months, causing significant distress or functional impairment. Symptoms include thoughts of harm coming to their parent, reluctance to attend school or sleep apart, marked distress at separation, and nightmares about separation. Tactful exploration of the family history may reveal a threatened or unmourned loss, for which the family can be supported, while managing the child's anxiety with behavioural therapy, gradually increasing separation periods.

School refusal

Unlike truancy, this is unconcealed absence from school. It's common at times of transition, e.g. a new school or sibling. Bullying, fear of failure, or an unsympathetic teacher may be reported. It may occur in families with so-called precious children (following difficulty conceiving or a sibling's death) or vulnerable parents (e.g. experiencing life-threatening illness or agoraphobia). The child typically experiences tummy aches just before school, but never at weekends or holidays.

First, parents are supported to tackle the problem, enlisting the school's support to manage their child's anxiety. A rapid return to full attendance carries the best prognosis. If not, other problems (e.g. parental depression, separation anxiety) are likely.

> 💡 **Relevant problems may be missed unless young people are offered time to talk, separate from their parents. Always review young people with a chaperone.**

Enuresis

Enuresis is the repeated voiding of urine into clothing or bed by day or night above the age of expected urinary continence (5 years), in the absence of organic causes.

Table 20.2 Risk factors for childhood mental health problems

Child risks	Family risks	Environmental risks
• Genetic predisposition to specific disorders • Low birth weight • Developmental delay • Disorders of intellectual development • Sensory impairment • Physical illness • 'Difficult' temperament, e.g. easily frustrated, slow to adapt • Low self-esteem • Insecure attachment • Substance use • Trauma	• Parental psychiatric or physical illness • Substance use, including during pregnancy • Poor attachment, rejection, and lack of warmth • Parental loss • Family dysfunction including criminality • Parental conflict/hostility • Separation/divorce • Single-parent family • Child abuse/maltreatment • Poor parental supervision • Parenting styles: permissive/anxious childrearing/parental overcontrol	• Urban setting • Poverty • Social adversity including violence and criminality • Bullying • Stressful life events • Loss of close relationship/friends • Difficult experiences at school: poor academic achievement, poor attendance, peer rejection, unsafe school environment • Peer substance use

Poor bladder control affects up to 10% of 5-year-olds and 1% of adolescents. There's often a family history of similar problems. Enuresis can be primary (toilet training was never mastered) or secondary (dryness is lost after at least a year's continence). Nocturnal enuresis (bedwetting) is commoner in boys; diurnal enuresis affects girls more frequently.

Primary enuresis is usually due to delayed maturation of bladder innervation or neurodevelopmental disorders, although stress and excessively relaxed or strict toilet training can play a role. Secondary enuresis is usually stress related, e.g. starting a new school.

Management

- Reassure the family and child that the problem is common and nobody's fault.
- Refer organic causes to a paediatrician, e.g. epilepsy, urinary tract infection, constipation, diabetes.
- Address stressors and review toilet training received so far.
- Restrict fluids before bed.
- Use star charts to celebrate each dry night (positive reinforcement).
- Bell and pad 'underpants alarm': clips onto pyjamas, waking the child if moisture is detected, to retrain voiding.
- Medication, e.g. imipramine (tricyclic antidepressant) combined with desmopressin (synthetic antidiuretic hormone) may be considered when all other treatments have failed.

Encopresis

Encopresis is repeated defecation in inappropriate places above the age of expected faecal continence (4 years), in the absence of organic causes. It's commoner in boys and can be primary or secondary. Most cases result from constipation ('overflow incontinence'), due to:

- Dehydration.
- Painful defecation (e.g. anal fissure).
- Fear of punishment.
- Toilet fears (e.g. monsters in the toilet).
- Hirschsprung disease (rare: bowel obstruction due to an aganglionic section of the colon).

When constipation is absent, incontinence may result from diarrhoea, disorders of intellectual development, and, occasionally, hostility (e.g. angrily defecating in a parent's shoe). Some children feel defeated by the transition from potty to toilet, and punitive toilet training can compound this. Stress can trigger secondary incontinence.

Management

- Laxatives and stool softeners for constipation.
- Treat physical causes.
- Reassure, address stress, and review toilet training.
- Star charts to reinforce continence.

Prognosis is good: 60–90% of children become continent within a year.

Selective mutism

Selective mutism is consistent selective speech in specific social situations (e.g. home) but not others (e.g. school), lasting at least 1 month, not limited to the first month of school, to the extent of disrupting education. It affects 4 in 1000 children (girls slightly more than boys). Affected children are often talkative at home but painfully shy and silent elsewhere. Treatment involves reassurance; and stress and behavioural management.

Neurodevelopmental disorders

Disorders of intellectual development are discussed in Chapter 19.

Autism spectrum disorder

Terminology for ASD can be confusing: there have been a range of classifications. ASD includes Asperger syndrome and other, older terms. It affects over 1% of UK children, with a male-to-female ratio of 4:1. In girls, ASD may be better masked by imitating socially expected behaviours. It has a strong genetic basis via many alleles of small effect, with heritability of 90% supported by family and twin studies. Despite this, interest in environmental factors remains strong. The risk of ASD may be increased by older parental age, maternal infections in pregnancy, and obstetric complications leading to hypoxia. ASD is highly comorbid with other conditions including disorders of intellectual development, epilepsy, tuberous sclerosis, Down syndrome, Rett syndrome, and fragile X syndrome.

💡 **Neither parenting style nor measles–mumps–rubella (MMR) vaccination causes ASD but historical misinformation continues to adversely affect vaccination rates.**

Clinical presentation

People with ASD struggle to initiate and sustain reciprocal social interaction and social communication and show restricted, repetitive, inflexible interests and behaviour patterns. Symptoms are often identified in the first 3 years of life and are sufficiently severe to impair educational, occupational, and other functioning. ASD is associated with a range of intellectual and language abilities and its functional impact varies across the spectrum.

Reciprocal social interaction

Children with ASD struggle to express emotions and 'read' other people, to understand their feelings and intentions. This may be interpreted as insensitive or socially awkward, influencing their ability to make friends. People with ASD often prefer their own company, especially when surrounded by people; they may not seek comfort in the usual way.

Communication

Children with ASD have difficulty interpreting verbal and non-verbal communication, such as gestures (e.g. pointing), facial expressions, and tone of voice. They may interpret language literally (concrete thinking), including jokes and sarcasm. Speech onset is often delayed. Children may repeat sentences verbatim (echolalia) or speak continuously about their own interests without pausing to hear from others. Speech can be monotonous, with limited prosody and pronoun reversal (saying 'I'/'me' to mean 'you'/'she').

💡 **Children with ASD can struggle with eye contact. Staring intently at something else doesn't mean they're not listening.**

Repetitive behaviour

The world can feel confusing and unpredictable to a child with ASD. Daily routines, rigid food preferences, school, or transport habits can be comforting, but lead to distress or tantrums when they can't be accommodated. Children with ASD may play games repetitively or order toys by abstract properties (e.g. size, colour) rather than playing imaginatively. They may develop intense, focused interests from a young age, resulting in areas of specific ability despite marked functional impairment.

Associated symptoms

Sensitivity to sound, touch, taste, smell, light, colour, and temperature are common in ASD, causing anxiety and discomfort. Self-stimulating (e.g. hand flapping) and self-injuring behaviour (e.g. head-banging) are common. Around 50% of people with ASD have disorders of intellectual development.

Differential diagnosis

- Untreated deafness impairs language acquisition.
- Developmental language disorder causes persistent difficulties in language acquisition, understanding, production, or use, disproportionate to intellectual development.
- Disorders of intellectual development: significantly below-average (two to three standard deviations below the mean) intellectual functioning and adaptive behaviour, often associated with impairments of complex language acquisition and comprehension, academic skills, self-care, and domestic and practical activities.
- Developmental syndromes which cause ASD, e.g. Rett syndrome.
- Neglect can impair language acquisition and socialization (reversibly, unless it's particularly severe).

Investigations

- Hearing tests for deafness.
- Speech and language assessment.
- Neuropsychological cognitive assessment.
- Specialist ASD assessment incorporating nursery/school reports, detailed developmental and family history, observation in several settings, physical examination, and tailored assessment of the child's cognition, communication, behaviour, and mental state, e.g. Autism Diagnostic Interview (ADI), Autism Diagnostic Observation Schedule (ADOS).
- Genetic tests if dysmorphic features, congenital abnormalities, family history, or comorbid disorder of intellectual development.
- EEG if epilepsy is suspected.

Management

- Carer support and advice, e.g. National Autistic Society.
- Behavioural therapy (see p. 237) reinforces positive behaviours and discourages challenging ones.
- Speech and language therapy.
- School support via an education, health, and care (EHC) plan.
- Treatment for comorbid physical (e.g. epilepsy) and mental health problems (e.g. depression, anxiety disorders).
- Antipsychotics and mood stabilizers are occasionally prescribed for severe aggression or hyperactivity not responding to behavioural interventions.

Prognosis

ASD is a lifelong condition. Children and their families need skills and strategies to manage symptoms into adulthood. Comorbid disorders of intellectual development and functional language impairment reduce the person's chance of living independently in adulthood. People with less severe ASD without intellectual and language impairments may progress well academically and professionally but struggle with social interaction and adjusting to major life changes.

💡 **Autism without intellectual and language impairment was previously diagnosed as Asperger syndrome. However, it is no longer considered distinct from ASD.**

Attention deficit hyperactivity disorder

A persistent pattern (at least 6 months) of inattention and/or hyperactivity-impulsivity, starting in early to mid-childhood, outside the limits of normal variation expected for the child's age and intellectual functioning, which significantly interferes with his or her functioning, in more than one setting. The manifestations and balance of symptoms vary between children and across time.

ADHD is three times commoner in boys than girls and affects 2% of UK children. Although prevalence is thought to be stable worldwide, diagnoses are higher where DSM criteria are used (e.g. 6% of US children). It is 75% heritable but the cause is unknown. Environmental risk factors include prematurity, low birth weight, and prenatal tobacco and lead exposure. ADHD is associated with paternal dissocial behaviour, maternal depression, and lower socioeconomic status. Dopamine and noradrenaline deficiencies may impair regulation of frontal lobe executive function.

In children, 67% of ADHD is comorbid with other disorders, including oppositional defiant disorder (ODD) and conduct/dissocial disorder (CDD) (up to 50%), disorders of intellectual development (30%), and Tourette syndrome. In adolescents and adults, ADHD is often comorbid with mood, anxiety, substance use, or OCD.

Clinical presentation

Problems arise by 6 years old and are persistent and pervasive across different situations. A child who is calm at school but overexcited at home does not have ADHD.

Hyperactivity refers to excessive movement and difficulty keeping still, especially in situations requiring behavioural self-control. Children with ADHD are boisterous, with excessive energy. They can seem constantly on the move: running, jumping, climbing, unable to sit still for any length of time without fidgeting, squirming, or wandering about.

Inattention refers to distractibility, disorganization, and significant difficulty concentrating on tasks that aren't exceptionally stimulating, without frequent rewards. Children struggle to focus in class, flitting between activities, leaving tasks unfinished.

Impulsivity is the tendency to act in response to immediate stimuli without deliberating or considering the risks and consequences. This can place them in danger (e.g. road safety) and cause parental anxiety.

Associated features

Children with ADHD may be accident-prone or disobedient, through impulsivity rather than defiance. They may pay little attention to social conventions, interrupting others, and struggling to wait their turn.

Differential diagnosis

- Organic disorders e.g. hearing impairment, epilepsy.
- CDD.
- Agitation in depression or anxiety.
- Mania (rare in children).

Investigations

- Questionnaires, e.g. Conners Rating Scales, completed by the child, parents, and teacher.
- Clinician observation in a classroom setting.
- Educational psychologist assessment.

💡 **Teachers are important sources of information, because they see the child all day, every day and know the 'normal' range of behaviour for a particular age.**

Management

- Parent training and education programmes.
- Educational psychologist assessment of the child's classroom needs.
- Group CBT and social skills training.
- Social support and self-help for families, e.g. the national attention deficit disorder information and support service (ADDISS).
- Stimulant medications, which increase monoamine pathway activity, improve concentration, facilitating learning. These include methylphenidate, dexamfetamine and lisdexamfetamine, and are not addictive when used for ADHD. Adverse effects include nausea, diarrhoea, hypertension, tachycardia, appetite suppression, and insomnia. Drug-free weekends and school holidays limit the side effect of growth restriction. Non-stimulant medications for ADHD include atomoxetine and guanfacine.

💡 **Despite a lack of evidence, many parents report benefits to their child's ADHD from dietary changes.**

Prognosis

Children with ADHD may experience low self-esteem, peer rejection, educational underachievement, and harsh parenting. Although symptoms often improve in adolescence, they persist in up to 50% of adults; up to 30% retain the diagnosis. Untreated ADHD is a risk factor for later dissociality in personality disorder, criminal behaviour, and substance use.

Disruptive behaviour or dissocial disorders

Conduct/dissocial disorder

CDD is a repetitive and persistent pattern (1 year or more) of behaviour violating either the basic rights of others, or major age-appropriate societal norms, rules, or laws. Behaviour such as aggression towards people or animals, destruction of property, deceitfulness or theft, and serious rule violations is of sufficient severity to significantly impair the child's personal, family, social, educational, or occupational functioning.

CDD affects 10% of 10-year-olds and is four times commoner in boys than girls. It runs in families, with likely genetic and environmental components. Risk factors include urban upbringing, deprivation, parental criminal activity, harsh and inconsistent parenting, maternal depression, and a family history of substance use. Dissocial (antisocial) behaviour is often learned from parental or environmental exposure, and may be reinforced, e.g. by increased attention.

Clinical presentation

The behaviour of children with CDD is persistently dissocial, not merely 'rebellious', e.g. bullying, stealing, fighting, fire-setting, truancy, and cruelty to animals or people. In socialized CDD, dissocial behaviour is conducted within a peer group. Children with unsocialized CDD are rejected by other children, often making them more isolated and hostile.

Differential diagnosis

- ODD: a persistent pattern (6 months or more) of markedly defiant, disobedient, provocative, or spiteful behaviour, more frequently than is typical in children of comparable age and development, and not restricted to siblings. ODD can present with prevailing angry or irritable mood, with severe temper outbursts or headstrong, argumentative, and defiant behaviour sufficiently severe to impair the child's functioning.
- ADHD (comorbid with CDD in at least a third of cases).
- Depression: some children and young people externalize distress, presenting with dissocial behaviour.

Management

- Support to understand CDD and limit potentially reinforcing responses.
- Parent management training teaches caregivers to reward good behaviour and respond constructively to undesired behaviour.
- Family therapy: the family meets with a skilled therapist to discuss current problems. They are supported to collaborate on problem-solving.
- Educational support: close working with teachers is crucial, as children with CDD are at risk of exclusion.
- Anger management for the child or young person.
- Treatment of comorbid disorders, e.g. ADHD.

Prognosis

Up to 50% of children with CDD develop substance use or dissociality in adult life.

💡 **Psychiatric hospital admission is reserved for children and adolescents with complex, high-risk presentations which cannot be safely managed in the community. Diagnoses most commonly requiring inpatient treatment are eating disorders, affective disorders, psychosis, severe/complex neurodevelopmental disorders, and presentations with severe self-harm (Box 20.1).**

💡 **Heavy use (>2 hours per day) of social media may contribute towards low mood, increased anxiety, and poor sleep in adolescents. Over a third of young people report experiencing a high frequency of cyber-bullying.**

Tic disorders

Tics are sudden, rapid, non-rhythmic, recurrent movements or vocalizations. They're involuntary and may be simple (e.g. blinking, sniffing, tapping,

---

BOX 20.1 Self-harm

There was a 68% increase in self-harm among girls aged 16–18 years, between 2011 and 2014. Only 44% of those who self-harmed had a documented referral to mental health services. Referrals and prescriptions were lowest among those from the most deprived areas. While this dramatic increase is unexplained, poverty, negative effects of social media, and increasing sexualization (e.g. pornography exposure) may contribute.

Data from Morgan, C., et al. (2017) Incidence, clinical management, and mortality risk following self harm among children and adolescents: cohort study in primary care. *BMJ*, **359**, j4351.

throat-clearing) or complex (e.g. self-hitting, swearing). Transient motor tics affect 10% of children and are three times commoner in boys than girls. There is often a family history; OCD and ADHD can be comorbid. Stress and stimulant medications usually worsen tics, which recede when distracted. Tics can be voluntarily suppressed at the cost of internal tension, which is relieved by their expression. Reassurance and stress management are effective treatments, but clonidine (an adrenergic agonist) or antipsychotics can help.

💡 **(Gilles de la) Tourette syndrome is a chronic (at least 1 year) tic disorder featuring both motor and vocal tics (although not always concurrently or consistently), with onset in childhood. It tends to worsen in adolescence and persist into adulthood.**

REALITY

General approach: tips, tricks, and cautionary tales

1. Don't intimidate

New adults scare children. Even short adults are giants, so sit promptly and let them sit on their parent's lap (for safety), if preferred. Consider introducing yourself less formally, e.g. '(Dr) Juliet' rather than 'Dr Hurn'.

Although older children may speak immediately, younger children will feel overwhelmed if asked to explain what's wrong. Tell them you'll start by talking to their parents, but you'd like them to *listen*, to make sure their parents get everything right and don't forget anything important. Once they've got used to you talking to their parents, they'll usually feel more confident to speak. Pitch language for their age and developmental level and use simple words, checking for understanding.

💡 **A revealing question that children like is:** *If you could have three wishes, what would they be?*

2. Nervous children

The harder you try to befriend a shy or frightened child, the more they'll close down. Use graded exposure. After greetings, *ignore* them for a few minutes and talk to their parents. Consider placing an interesting toy/paper and pens near them (and away from you): children often eavesdrop as they play and may creep closer as they feel safer. Gradually include them, by intermittently nodding/smiling at them, or dropping their name into the conversation.

Gently draw them in, with easy, *closed* questions at first (e.g. 'Do *you* like Mummy's new car?'). Showing interest is your most powerful communication tool, and it's worth discussing non-clinical things, as this builds rapport and can tell you lots about the child. Start with non-threatening topics where they're the 'expert', e.g. a recent birthday, their best friend or pet. If they've drawn something, praise their drawing or choice of colours and ask them about the picture (e.g. 'The girl in your drawing looks happy. What makes *you* happpy?'). It's often easier for children to talk about an object (e.g. teddy's name/favourite food) before tackling harder topics (e.g. their worries).

A good first interview may *not* result in a completed assessment, but dispels fears, e.g. that doctors give painful injections or send 'bad' children to hospital. If the child thinks you're 'nice', they'll more happily attend and talk at follow-up appointments.

💡 **Avoid touch or direct eye contact with children who have ASD: they often find these deeply uncomfortable.**

3. Excitable children

Children have more energy than adults; with the added excitement or anxiety about seeing you, they may resemble little firecrackers. Forget this, and you'll greatly over-diagnose ADHD! Don't increase excitement by bouncing around, chasing or tickling them, or by raising your voice. Remember: *you* won't be taking them home in a worked-up state. Speak calmly and encourage them to settle with a (quiet) toy or task.

4. Don't infantilize

Children are often sensitive to being patronized or treated like babies, e.g. ruffling hair, pinching cheeks, or calling them 'champ', 'buddy', etc. If *you'd* find it patronizing, don't do it to them.

5. Ask the experts

Unless you have children, it's hard to judge what's typical for a child's age (like the first liver you palpated: Was that *normal*?). It's easier with experience, but always ask the experts (parents, teachers, colleagues): *How does s/he compare to other children of this age?*

6. Teenagers

Don't try speaking or acting like a teenager to gain rapport—you'll look ridiculous, as you're *old*. Instead, treat them as adults and be interested, understanding, and non-judgemental; this *will* build rapport and is actually quite cool.[2]

To fit in or avoid bullying, teens often put enormous effort into their image but this doesn't mean the inside matches the outside. Despite jeans halfway down their buttocks, the young person may harbour a secret passion for ornithology. Assume nothing and enjoy getting to know them.

If teenagers use slang that you don't understand, ask what they mean. *They* may not admit when they don't fully understand something (especially if trying to impress you), so avoid jargon and explain new terms.

7. Parents

Parents can feel guilty about their child's problems. Having a 'no-blame' attitude helps and once parents relax, children often follow suit. Sometimes parents are clearly part of the problem (e.g. abusive or neglectful). *Don't* become punitive or angry, since this can make them disengage or take their anger out on the child at home.

> Mentally perform two mental state examinations: one of the child and one of the family. These offer insight into family dynamics, parenting skills, personalities, and sociability.

The interview

For screening questions, think about how answers might differ for ASD, ADHD, and CDD.
 • = Example question. X = The child's name.

General screening questions

- *What are you most worried might be wrong with X?*
- If I observed X at home, what would I see?
- How's s/he doing at school? What do the teachers say?
- How does s/he get on with other children?
- What happens when X needs to share or take turns?
- What does X enjoy doing?
- Does X ever get into trouble? Why?
  – How does s/he react when told off?

Autism spectrum disorder

- *How does X get on with other children?*
- Can s/he take turns in a conversation?
- Can X understand how other people feel?
- Does s/he like cuddles? Would s/he seek comfort if hurt?
- Is there anything unusual about the way s/he speaks?
- Does s/he like to do things over and over in the same way?
- Does X like routines? Like what?
  – What happens if you have to *change* a routine?
- Does s/he understand and use gestures (e.g. waving, pointing)?

Attention deficit hyperactivity disorder

- *How energetic is s/he, compared with other children of the same age?*
  – How does that energy come out at home?
- Can s/he sit still? When? For how long?
- What's the longest X could concentrate on something? [*Not including computer games*]
- Does s/he tend to do things impulsively, without thinking? Such as?

Conduct/dissocial disorder

- *What's the most worrying/worst thing X has ever done?*
- How does s/he respond to rules?
- How does X react when s/he's hurt someone?
- Do you worry that X tells lies? What about?
- Have the police ever been involved? Why?

Neurodevelopmental history (15 minutes)

Candidate's instructions
You're a final year student in general practice. Michael McMahon has attended to discuss William, his 5-year-old son. Take a history to allow referral to a specialist if required.

Patient's brief

Key characteristics
- I'm not a 'touchy feely' person and see a lot of myself in Will.
- I'd *hate* to think there's anything wrong with him.

History
Will's teacher thinks he's a bit 'different'—she said I should talk to you. The pregnancy was easy but he was born by Caesarean after the placenta burst. Charlotte (my girlfriend) died from blood loss . . . Will needed the special care baby unit but was out the next day and he's been fine ever since. His baby checks were normal, he walked at 9 months—quite the athlete! His first word was 'cup', when he was 2. He's not chatty like his sister Lily, but he can speak if he wants to . . . He's never really got into sentences—mostly just names things and I know what he means . . . *cup* or *bread* or whatever. I can't remember him pointing or waving goodbye. He doesn't nod or shake his head but he says yes and no, so doesn't need to.

He's always been very independent—a man's man. Right from when he was little, he just got on with things. He doesn't mind if he's left alone (unlike Lily, who still cries, even at 7)—he's no wimp! Even when he's hurt he doesn't need mollycoddling—just cries and gets on with things. He's not cuddly, but there's nothing wrong with that. Lily's his biggest fan and very protective of him, even though, if the tables were turned, he doesn't really pay it back . . . Yesterday she fell over and was wailing her head off but Will just kept playing with his cars. I guess he's too little to realize she was hurt. He likes his own company— plays by himself all day if you let him. He's not interested in hanging out with the other boys yet.

Will's very single-minded. He'll play with toy cars for hours on end, just lining them up or holding them in the air and spinning the wheels around. Maybe he'll be a mechanic? He also has a real thing for yellow plastic forks and strokes the prongs along his arm, over and over. He's never liked soft toys or bedtime stories but give him a yellow plastic fork and he'll be no trouble for hours! He has tantrums if he can't find one, so I always carry a spare. He doesn't like red, so I keep red things away from him to prevent more tantrums. We both like routine: get up, breakfast, school, home, dinner, bed. We stick to that so nobody gets confused and Will reminds me if I get it wrong with a tantrum!

I was told children with autism don't make eye contact—but Will does: it's such a keen stare, it's like he's looking right through you . . .

Other history
- He's had all his vaccinations and never gets anything worse than a cold.
- His hearing is excellent. Actually, he's really sensitive to sound and I have to keep the TV volume low.
- Nobody in the family has mental health problems.

Questions
Could he have autism?

Worries
I shouldn't have let him have the MMR vaccination.

💡 **Will probably has ASD and needs referral to CAMHS. You couldn't *diagnose* ASD at first assessment but should reassure Michael that the vaccination hasn't caused** these symptoms. CAMHS will work with Will's family and school to clarify the diagnosis and advise on parenting and educational support.

NEXT STEPS

Hyperactivity and non-accidental injury

You're a paediatric FY2. Jack Rutherford is 12 years old and has needed three admissions in 6 months for asthma. He's very popular on the ward and has formed close relationships with staff. Jack is prescribed methylphenidate by CAMHS for ADHD. He's had a tough time recently: his parents divorced a year ago and he's often in trouble at school. You think his mother may be struggling to manage his behaviour.

On admission he had bruises on his back. He said they were from playground fights but on the day of discharge he's approached you asking if you can keep a secret. Before you can answer, he tells you the bruises were from his mother hitting him, which has been happening quite a lot recently.

- How will you respond to his disclosure?
- What longer-term interventions could help the family?
- How could Jack's ADHD affect his asthma? What could be done?

Response

Let Jack know that he's done the right thing in talking to you and he isn't in any trouble. Listen carefully, showing that you believe him and recording what he tells you without pushing him. Explain how you plan to help and that you have a duty to act to keep him safe. Jack may consent for you to share information, but if he still refuses after your best efforts to explore any reluctance, you should proceed, since he's at considerable risk of harm. Refer Jack to the hospital safeguarding team, following up any written forms with a telephone call. Inform your consultant, the nurse in charge, and the team's child protection lead.

As a rule, you should communicate openly and honestly with Jack's parents unless this might place Jack (or someone else, e.g. siblings) at increased risk of harm.

The initial assessment will take place urgently; Jack will stay in hospital until the lead social worker/safeguarding team recommends that he can be safely discharged. If Jack returns home, safeguards and a follow-up plan are needed. If the social worker considers Jack a 'child in need', a meeting will be arranged between social work, police, and other relevant agencies (e.g. CAMHS, GP). Further enquiries, a child protection conference, and a child protection plan may be necessary, depending on the risks to Jack.

Interventions

Help for the family is needed, regardless, since this incident shows that Jack and his family need support. Interventions include:

- **Jack:** referral to local CAMHS, who'll liaise with the school to ensure support is provided. CAMHS will also review Jack's medications.
- **Parents:** practical/emotional support, parenting skills groups tailored for ADHD, and referral for any untreated parental mental health problems.
- **Family:** family therapy, preferably with both parents via CAMHS, and referral for any sibling mental health problems.

Effect of ADHD

Jack's ADHD may affect his ability to take his asthma medication regularly, because of difficulties concentrating on tasks and impulsivity. He'll also be more likely to forget to carry his short-acting beta-2 agonist inhaler. You should check that he understands when he should take each inhaler and consider optimization strategies (e.g. phone reminders). His parents have a responsibility to ensure that he takes his medication and carries his inhalers; failure to do so could indicate neglect. Complicated prescribing regimens result in missed doses, so once- or twice-daily treatments will aid ADHD and asthma management.

> ❗ **Never offer unlimited confidentiality!** 'I can keep most secrets, unless you tell me something that makes me worry that you or someone else might be hurt. If I'm really worried I'll have to tell other people so that we can keep you safe.'

Movie buff

Kidulthood (2006).
Life, Animated (2016): ASD.
Pretty Persuasion (2005): CDD.
Rain Man (1988): ASD.
Temple Grandin (2010): ASD.
Thirteen (2003): self-harm and substance use in adolescence.

Book shelf

Haddon, M. (2003) *The Curious Incident of the Dog in the Night-Time*: Christopher, who has Asperger syndrome, unravels a mystery, sharing his perspective along the way.

Haden, T. (1988) *Just Another Kid*: a teacher's experience of working with children with selective mutism, ASD, disorders of intellectual development, schizophrenia, and CDD.

Ray, R. (1998) *A Certain Age*: sexuality, relationships, peer groups, and self-harm from a 13-year-old's perspective.

Notes

1. Child, L. (2006) *Clarice Bean, Don't Look Now*. Copyright Orchard Books, London.

2. Dr Stringer apologizes for the term 'cool'. She thought it was what all the kids were saying today.

Journal club

Morgan, C., Webb, R.T., Carr, M.J., et al. (2017). Incidence, clinical management, and mortality risk following self harm among children and adolescents: cohort study in primary care. *BMJ*, **359**, j4351.

Resources

Head Meds—information for young people about psychiatric medications: www.headmeds.org.uk/

Go to www.oup.com/uk/stringer2e for a wealth of additional resources, including an OCSE mark scheme, filmed scenarios, and self-assessment questions.

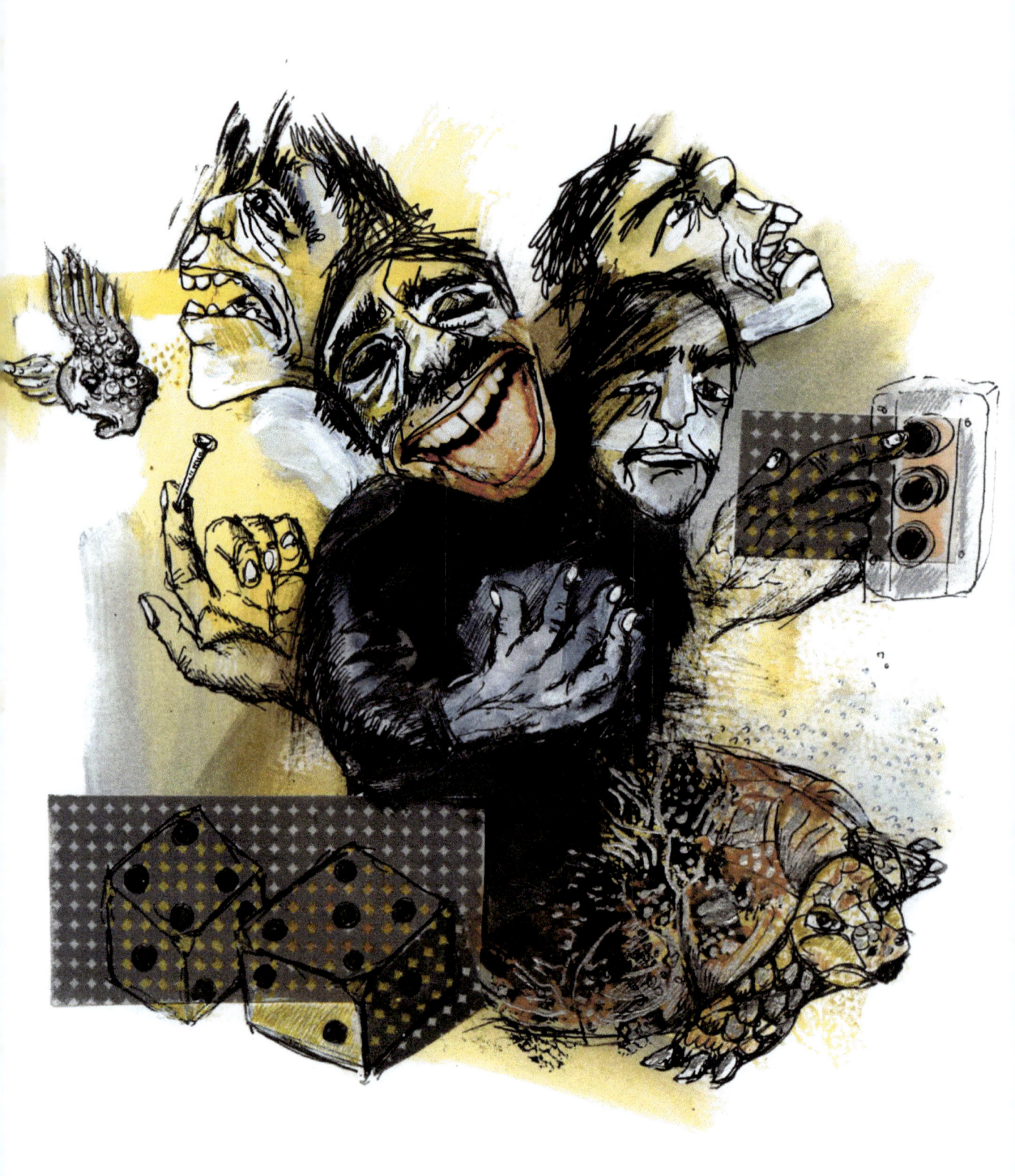

21 Personality Disorders

True or false?

Answers on p. 277

1. Personality disorders are more prevalent in general practice than psychiatric outpatient clinics.
2. Multiple personality disorder is the diagnosis given to people showing traits from each of the three personality clusters.
3. Overall, personality disorders are equally common in men and women.
4. Personality *difficulty* is less common than *no personality dysfunction*.
5. Anankastic traits are seen more commonly in people with eating disorders.
6. Splitting is an ego defence mechanism where a person behaves in a way opposite to their unacknowledged and unacceptable desires or impulses.
7. People with borderline pattern personality disorder are unlikely to be treatment seeking.
8. The severity of a personality disorder fluctuates over the course of a person's lifetime.
9. It is important to notice, but not react to, emotions that you feel when working with someone who has a personality disorder.
10. A diagnosis of severe personality disorder with prominent dissociality traits means that a person cannot be held responsible for their actions.

Contents

Principles
Introduction
Diagnosis
Epidemiology
Aetiology
- Genetics
- Childhood factors
- Psychological theories
- Neurochemical theories
- Neuroanatomical theories

Comorbidity
Clinical presentation
Investigations
Management
- Biological
- Psychological
- Social

Prognosis

Reality
General approach: tips, tricks, and cautionary tales

The interview
- PD history

Next steps
An angry husband in primary care
- Preparation
- Risk assessment
- Management

PRINCIPLES

'I know why I'm here. I'm here because I broke my hand, and because that's really just emblematic of a whole host of other things that are wrong with me, or that at least have been wrong with me in the past.' I throw the last out there, eager for her to ask what those other things might be. Starving, puking, binge drinking, sluttiness, pathological lying – did I mention those before? I don't mind talking about them.

Kristen Waterfield Duisberg, *The Good Patient*[1]

Introduction

Personality is who we are. It comprises ingrained, persistent *traits*: characteristics that determine how we think, feel, behave, and experience ourselves, the world, and other people. There are many personality traits and none are 'bad'; all have strengths and weaknesses, depending on the situation. For example, a doctor might be meticulous, but perfectionism would be unhelpful if they always double-checked protocols before attending crash calls.

When traits are persistently disabling or distressing, they might constitute a personality *disorder* (PD). Personality was once thought to be completely fixed, so people with PD were considered untreatable; we now know that personality *can* change and responds to various treatments. As PD causes interpersonal difficulties, people with PD can trigger strong emotions in others, leading professionals to dismiss, rather than work with them. An understanding approach is therefore essential to identify the support people need and ensure they can access it.

💡 ICD-11 replaces the specific personality disorders of ICD-10 with trait domains. We're including both, so you're not flummoxed by older diagnoses.

Diagnosis

PD is diagnosed when personality traits fulfil the '*3Ps*':

- *Persistent*: typically emerge in childhood/adolescence and endure into adulthood.
- *Pervasive*: occur in most (if not all) areas of life.
- *Pathological*: cause distress, affect relationships, and impair occupational/social functioning.

PD isn't diagnosed where other psychiatric disorders, substance use, or brain damage/disease explains the person's behaviour. Three broad clusters group specific PD types (**Table 21.1**).

💡 The American classification system, DSM-5 (see p. 27) adds *schizotypal* PD to cluster A, and *narcissistic* PD

Table 21.1 Personality clusters

Cluster	Cluster description	Specific PDs (ICD-10)	Trait domain qualifiers (ICD-11)
A	'Odd or eccentric'	Paranoid Schizoid	Detachment
B	'Dramatic or emotional'	Histrionic Emotionally unstable (EUPD) Dissocial	Negative affectivity Dissociality Disinhibition Borderline pattern
C	'Anxious or fussy'	Anxious (avoidant) Dependent Anankastic	Negative affectivity Anankastia

Data from Bach, B. and First, M.B. (2018) Application of the ICD-11 classification of personality disorders. *BMC Psychiatry*, **18**, 351.

to cluster B. While ICD-11 classifies schizotypal disorder (see p. 85) as a 'schizophrenia-like' disorder, it doesn't have a trait domain for narcissism (people who are grandiose, arrogant, exploitative, and preoccupied with power and success).

Epidemiology

The prevalence of PD varies with the setting and diagnostic criteria used (Table 21.2). Men have higher overall rates, particularly detachment, dissociality, and anankastic traits; disinhibited traits and borderline patterns are more common in women.

Aetiology

Genetics

Family, twin, and adoption studies all support a genetic contribution to PD, with heritability estimates ranging from 25% to 70%. PD is associated with a family history of PD, schizophrenia (cluster A), depression and anxiety (clusters B and C), and disorders due to substance use (cluster B).

Childhood factors

Temperament describes our innate characteristics, seen most clearly in infancy, e.g. activity pattern, attention span, response to new situations, and emotional responsiveness. The temperament of children as young as 3 years can predict adult personality traits. Children with 'difficult' temperaments have greater problems coping as adults, possibly because they find it harder to develop supportive relationships, and are more distressed by negative events; they're also at greater risk of developing PD.

PD is associated with inadequate or chaotic parenting and a child's insecure attachment to their parents. Those with PD (particularly borderline patterns) are more likely than the general population to have experienced childhood abuse (whether emotional, physical, sexual, or neglect). Abuse and neglect may mean that the child doesn't learn (through consistent and containing parenting) to validate and manage their own emotions. It's unclear why some people are unaffected long term by childhood abuse, while others develop PD or other mental health problems, including depression, eating disorders, or psychosis.

Psychological theories

Behaviour is motivated by a combination of beliefs and desires; cognitive theories favour beliefs and psychodynamic/analytic theories emphasize desire. Both agree that our expectations tend to be fulfilled and perpetuated. For example, warm people usually receive a friendly response, confirming to them that others are friendly, and reinforcing their warm approach. Aggressive people tend to spark hostility in others, 'proving' their view that people are threatening and deserve a heavy-handed approach.

Attachment theory

The quality of early relationships and the nature of the environment in which someone is raised influence their expectations about themselves and the world. For example, people feel lovable because they were first loved, feel fearful if others were unpredictable or frightening, and behave cruelly if first treated with cruelty.

Defence mechanisms

Ego defences are the unconscious strategies we all use to manage uncomfortable feelings, especially fear and guilt. They're problematic when people rely on them excessively, rather than addressing their underlying emotions—a common problem for people with PD. Examples include:

- *Acting out*: expressing impulses through actions, without conscious awareness of the underlying emotion (e.g. self-harming rather than *feeling* sad).
- *Splitting*: viewing people in polarized terms, either idealizing or denigrating them (e.g. dividing people into heroes and villains).
- *Projection*: 'putting' uncomfortable feelings onto someone else (e.g. feeling ashamed for hating colleagues, so believing that *they* hate *you*).
- *Passive aggression*: showing anger or disagreement through negativity or passive resistance, rather than verbalizing problems (e.g. 'forgetting' to attend a friend's party, rather than admitting anger).
- *Fantasizing*: using imagination to escape from painful reality (e.g. escaping loneliness through daydreams).

Table 21.2 Prevalence of personality disorders/clusters

Setting	Prevalence	Main cluster
General population	10%	–
Primary care	20%	C
Psychiatric outpatients	30%	B
Psychiatric inpatients	40%	B
Prison	50%	B

Neurochemical theories

Dysfunctional dopaminergic systems may be implicated in detached and anankastic trait domains. Serotonin has a role in regulating impulsivity and aggression; lower levels are linked to cluster B disorders. Dysfunctional noradrenergic systems have also been associated with PD.

Neuroanatomical theories

Cluster B personality disorders have been linked to functional underactivity in the prefrontal cortex, as well as volume reductions in the amygdala and hippocampus. These changes may be linked to traits such as lack of empathy in dissociality or difficulties regulating emotions in borderline patterns.

Comorbidity

People with PD have higher rates of depression, anxiety disorders, and substance use disorders. Cluster B disorders are associated with childhood conduct disorder, ADHD, bipolar disorder, and somatoform disorders; borderline patterns are associated with PTSD, eating disorders, substance use disorders, and dissociative disorders. People who have anankastic traits are more likely to experience OCD and eating disorders.

Clinical presentation

The ICD-11 recognizes that our personality characteristics are on a spectrum. For a specific PD diagnosis, people need to show the *3Ps* over an extended period (at least 2 years). The *severity* is then assigned (**Table 21.3**) according to the degree of impairment of self (identity, self-worth) and interpersonal (maintaining close and healthy relationships, empathizing and managing conflict) functioning.

> 💡 Most of us have *personality difficulties*: in certain situations our interpersonal functioning is less optimal. Imagine you're competing against another team to solve a challenge. Would you ever show your irritation with colleagues (dissociality), or withdraw and try to solve it yourself (detachment)?

One or more *trait domain qualifiers* (**Table 21.4**) may then be added, describing the prominent personality traits. In general, more severe PD is associated with multiple trait domain qualifiers (i.e. more complexity).

> 💡 The rare and controversial multiple personality disorder is classified within dissociative disorders (p. 192).

Investigations

Diagnosis requires multiple sources of information across multiple meetings.

- *Follow-up interview(s)*, including:
  – Screening questionnaires, e.g. Standardised Assessment of Personality Abbreviated Scale (SAPAS).
  – Diagnostic semi-structured interviews, e.g. International Personality Disorder Examination (IPDE).

Table 21.3 Severity of personality disorders

Severity	Estimated prevalence	Description
No personality dysfunction	35%	Shows no abnormalities of personality, even under pressure, across all domains in life
Personality difficulty	48%	Intermittent disturbance of social functioning and interpersonal relationships below the severity of mild PD, only seen in certain contexts
Mild personality disorder	12%	3Ps plus disturbance in some but not all areas of functioning; may be associated with distress and some impairment in discrete areas of work or social life. Typically no harm to self or others
Moderate personality disorder	4.5%	3Ps plus disturbances in multiple areas of personality functioning, marked problems in work and social life. History of harm to self or others, not to a fatal degree
Severe personality disorder	0.5%	3Ps plus profound personality dysfunction. Shallow or non-existent relationships, absence of expected social and work roles. Associated with serious harm to self or others causing long-term damage or endangering life

Data from Tyrer, P. (2018) *Taming the Beast Within: Shredding the Stereotypes of Personality Disorder*. London: Sheldon.

Table 21.4 Prominent personality traits

Negative affectivity

Features	Example
Also known as *neuroticism*: unpleasant emotions (anger, fear, misery) are experienced more often and out of proportion to the situation	I'd wanted to join the walking group for ages, but the idea of going alone terrified me: what if nobody liked me? You could hardly blame them! Nika agreed to come with me. I worried about it all week getting my clothing and backpack ready. I felt so sick and panicky on the morning of the walk that I dropped out. I felt so *stupid* and angry with myself

Differential: anxiety disorders, depression, ASD

Detachment

Features	Example
Avoidance of social interactions and emotionally distant (aloof, reserved)	I'm a night security guard: the solitude suits me. My manager said the day staff complained about a 'body odour smell' in the office. So what? Washing isn't essential. I don't care if people think I'm weird: I've never needed friends or girlfriends. I game online, but nothing makes me happy, sad or angry—that's my life and fine by me

Differential: ASD, social phobia, psychosis, depression

Dissociality

Features	Example
Disregard for rights and feelings of others. Lack of empathy, self-centred	I was really popular at my snooker club until Frank arrived. He really wound me up, acting like he owned the place. He 'borrowed' my cue while I was at the bar, so I broke his nose with it and beat him 'til he cried like a little girl! I'd happily do it again—he deserved it. I've been banned from the club and charged with grievous bodily harm. I'm not afraid of prison! I've been inside before: domestic violence, robbery, assault, drink-driving . . .

Differential: psychotic episode, mania, substance use disorder

Disinhibition

Features	Example
Acting rashly without thinking about the consequences: impulsive, reckless, distractible, irresponsible.	I was in a bar with my 'friend' Sally when a gorgeous guy started chatting me up. I'm a bit of a flirt, so we were quickly cuddling up . . . I popped to the loo to do my make-up, and when I returned, my new guy was chatting up Sally! I threw my drink over him, told Sally to find a new best mate, and stormed out

Differential: hypomania/mania, substance use disorder, ADHD, frontal lobe pathology

Anankastia

Features	Example
Narrowly focusing on rigid standards of perfection and of right or wrong. Controlling own and others' behaviour in order to keep to those standards	I'm an accountant. I'm in trouble for being 'too conscientious' and slow. I never cut corners or take shortcuts, in case I make mistakes and fraud slips through. I've developed my own system for checking each receipt and transaction before signing anything off. Yes, I've missed some deadlines, and yes, we've been fined, but that's the price you pay for principles. I don't do much beyond work: getting things right is more important than having fun. I had a girlfriend once, but she said I was 'too set in my ways' for her . . .

(continued)

Table 21.4 Continued

Differential: OCD, ASD	
Borderline pattern	
Features	Example
The core feature is *emotional dysregulation*: extreme, unstable emotions triggered by internal or external factors. Also, unstable and often intense relationships, impulsivity, fears of abandonment, unstable self-image, chronic feelings of emptiness, recurrent self-harm, intense anger which can be hard to control and transient dissociative or psychotic-like features when highly emotionally aroused	I wasn't sure if I was straight or gay, but after two dates with my *perfect* girlfriend [Louise], I knew I'd found my soulmate, I've never been so happy! Today she said she 'needed space'. I felt so alone and empty, just numb inside. Then suddenly, she left me, just like everyone else. I couldn't live without her. I started hearing voices again, so I took an overdose. I'm sure I 'blacked out' when I did it, I don't remember ringing Louise to say it was her fault I'd die. Louise rushed round and called the ambulance, and we're back together, loved up more than ever. I'm taking the week off work to be with her
Differential: adjustment disorder, depression, bipolar disorder, psychosis (occasional fleeting psychotic symptoms)	

- *Collateral history:* family/friends offer essential insights into traits and their impact.
- *Assessment of psychological mindedness*, i.e. whether someone's resilient and reflective enough to use therapy. People are sometimes described as *type R* (treatment-resisting) or *type S* (treatment-seeking) *personalities*. Typically, people with borderline pattern PD are more personally distressed by their symptoms and likely to seek treatment.

💡 You *can't* accurately assess personality when someone's acutely distressed from a life event (e.g. bereavement) or unwell with another mental disorder (e.g. mania, psychosis).

Management

PD is treatable. A long-term approach is needed, with non-judgemental, empathic therapeutic relationships that promote engagement. Boundaries (see p. 264) are essential, and all staff must clearly understand the plan and their respective roles. Comorbid problems (e.g. disorders of substance use, affective disorders) need treatment in their own right.

💡 Classifying the *severity* in PD helps inform prognosis and intensity of treatment and the *trait qualifiers* determine the focus and style of treatment.

Biological interventions

Medication

No medications are licensed for PD itself, and there's a limited evidence base. Nonetheless, medication is occasionally trialled for distressing symptoms, to facilitate psychosocial treatments, e.g.:

- *Antipsychotics* may reduce:
  - Auditory pseudohallucinations in borderline PD (e.g. voices instructing self-harm).
  - Impulsivity/aggression.
- *Antidepressants* may reduce impulsivity/anxiety.
- *Mood stabilizers* may help mood fluctuations.
- *Sedatives or anxiolytics* are sometimes used short term (e.g. 1 week), as part of a crisis plan.

Psychological interventions

Various approaches are used.

Cognitive behavioural therapy

CBT focuses on interactions between thoughts, feelings, and behaviours, here and now. It can be applied to different PD subtypes, in groups or individually.

Dialectical behavioural therapy

This reduces self-harm in borderline PD. It's based on CBT principles and teaches skills to manage intense emotional fluctuations through *interpersonal effectiveness, distress tolerance, emotion regulation*, and *mindfulness*. The learning from weekly group and individual sessions is reinforced through diaries and telephone support. Its use is being widened to other conditions such as disorders of substance use and eating disorders.

Cognitive analytical therapy

CAT promotes self-awareness. Current problems are understood by exploring past relationships and experiences; the therapist shares these in an early *reformulation letter*. Sessions then explore thought and behaviour patterns which hold the person back. At the end, ways in which future things could be done differently are summarized and shared in written material to promote ongoing change. CAT is a relatively short-term treatment, over an average of 16 individual sessions.

Mentalization-based therapy

MBT is offered for people with various PD subtypes. Mentalization is the ability to *think about thinking*: exploring thoughts and feelings in emotive situations and considering what's happening in someone else's mind. This reduces the 'acting out' of emotion and makes people aware of previously unconscious defence mechanisms. MBT is delivered to individuals and/or groups, and lasts 12–18 months.

Therapeutic communities

Therapeutic community residents are empowered to take collective responsibility for how their community runs, from preparing meals to responding to a struggling resident. There's a *flattened hierarchy* where residents share decision-making democratically, encouraging personal effectiveness and healthy relationships with others, while reducing dependence on professionals. Therapeutic communities help people with a variety of PDs and have also been adapted for addictions, forensic, and CAMHS settings.

Psychodynamic and psychoanalytic psychotherapy

Both use the relationship between therapist and patient to understand the past and how it relates to current interpersonal difficulties. Individual or group therapy is provided over months, or sometimes years.

Social interventions

Psychoeducation for the person with PD and their family improves autonomy, decision-making about treatment, and life choices. Peer support is an important part of many people's recovery.

People with cluster B conditions can present with recurrent crises, e.g. threats or acts of self-harm. Managing these safely and consistently is part of routine care planning and happens collaboratively outside of crisis periods.

Given the importance of attachment in the aetiology of PD, transitions into/out of services and across boundaries (e.g. CAMHS to adult, community to inpatient) are carefully planned.

Prognosis

PD disrupts relationships, education, and employment, and can be associated with domestic violence or child maltreatment. Treatment response for mental disorders such as depression and schizophrenia is also poorer in people who have comorbid PDs. However, the prevalence and severity of PD can reduce over time, e.g. cluster B disorders reduce with age, due to maturation, gradual 'burning out' of symptoms, and elevated mortality through suicide and accidents.

> ❗ **Self-harm and suicide are the commonest risks in borderline PD (10% die through suicide). Risk management is an important part of treatment, but needs to be thoughtful, e.g. although psychiatric admission may reduce someone's short-term risk of self-harm, it may be counter-productive, fostering dependence and preventing them from developing coping strategies.**

REALITY

General approach: tips, tricks, and cautionary tales

1. Wonder *why*

If you met someone covered in physical scars, you'd know they'd experienced trauma, and feel concern. People with PDs have often suffered early neglect, abuse, or trauma, but the resultant 'scar' of a challenging personality tends to rile those around them. By remembering this, you're more likely to respond compassionately.

2. *Notice* transference and counter-transference

People sometimes talk about *emotional baggage*: the idea that we carry feelings, thoughts, and issues from past relationships into our current relationships. Although the term's often used unkindly, it's a useful concept if we accept that it applies to *everyone*: good, bad, or ugly, our past relationships influence our responses to new people and situations. We're often unaware of this baggage (it's mostly subconscious), but its thoughts and feelings spring into action whenever we meet people, nudging (or sometimes shoving) us to react in particular ways.

Psychodynamically speaking, we *transfer* bits of past relationships onto new ones, re-enacting our experience of how relationships work (e.g. you might treat some consultants a little like your parents). Traditionally, the patient's emotional baggage is called *transference* and the health professional's is *counter-transference*. Transference and counter-transference interact in every clinical encounter, but most people only notice it when it's annoying, describing it as someone 'pushing' their 'buttons'.

By definition, people with PD relate to others in challenging ways, often because they're re-enacting past relationships. Something about you may (unconsciously) evoke someone who abused or disappointed them, triggering an unexpected response, e.g. anger. Your counter-transference might make you respond with an urge to protect, avoid, or blame them (depending on *your* past relationships).

The key message is: *neither ignore, nor react to these feelings; simply notice them*. Notice when people react unexpectedly, and how you feel in return. Remain neutral, see what happens next, and take time to think, rather than responding automatically. Your emotions offer insights into someone's past and how others might react to them. You may also begin to understand why their life's so difficult, even if they can't put it into words.

3. Know your limits

People with PD may struggle with *boundaries*, especially if these were abnormal in their early life. The onus is on *you* to be clear about boundaries, by being *reliable and fair*, as a student or a doctor. For example, don't say you'll 'be there' whenever someone needs you; instead, say you'll meet at 2pm for 30 minutes, and then do exactly that.

Care equally: spend your time, energy, and compassion at a rate that allows lifelong work with many people, rather than a few exhausting days with one.

4. Don't believe the hype

Beware compliments like, 'You'll be the *best* doctor, ever!' or 'You're the *only* one who understands'. Those who idealize quickly often denigrate at the slightest imperfection, without middle ground, e.g. 'You'll be a *terrible* doctor'/'You're just like all the rest'. *Don't* ride this emotional rollercoaster, reject the person, *or* work extra hard to regain their praise. Treat them the same as everyone else and take *none* of it to heart. Recognize how unstable and disappointing the world feels, when people seem so changeable.

5. Don't judge

Self-harm, fighting, drug-taking, or casual sex may not be *your* way of dealing with problems, but for some people, they seem the best—or only—option at the time. Consider what the behaviour *communicates*, e.g. drugs may suppress painful memories, and casual sex may indicate a longing for intimacy.

> 💡 It's easy to believe that challenging people don't deserve care. If likeability defined the role of the patient, we'd only treat delightful but completely healthy people! Even if you struggle to *like* someone, they still deserve your courtesy and professional care.

The interview

• = Example question. * = Question linking to other parts of the history.

Self

- *How would you describe yourself?*
- How would people who know you well describe you? [Screen: partner/family/friends/colleagues]
- What are your strengths?
- * What are your weaknesses?

Mood

- *What's your mood like, most of the time?*
  – Would you say you're an emotional person?
- What sorts of things make you angry?
  – What are you like when you're angry?
  * Has your temper ever got you into trouble?

Impulsivity

- *Do you make quick decisions or prefer to think things through?*
  * Has this ever caused problems?

Activities

- *What are you like at work?*
- *How do you spend your spare time?* Why do you like [activity]?
- Do you daydream? What about?

Coping/risk

- *What sorts of things do you find stressful?*
  – How do you cope under stress?
  * Have you ever harmed yourself?
  * Have you ever lashed out?

Relationships

Others
- *What do you think most people are like, deep down?*

Interpersonal
- *How do you generally get on with other people?*
- How close do you feel to your friends?
  - * Do your friendships last? Why do they end?
  - – Can you rely on other people when things get difficult?
  - – How much do you depend on others?
- * How do you react to criticism?
- * How do you handle disagreements?
  - – What would you argue about?
  - – Do certain types of people upset or annoy you?

Effect on life
- *Overall, do you think your personality's made life easier or harder for you?*
  - – Why?
- Does [trait] ever cause you difficulties? How? [Screen: work, relationships]
- * If you could change one thing about yourself, what would it be? Why?

PD history (30 minutes)

Candidate's instructions
Mrs Elsie Winters is 54. Her son, Michael, requested a GP home visit as she's 'taken to her bed'. You're a medical student with the GP. Interview Elsie and suggest a psychiatric diagnosis.

Patient's brief

Key characteristics
- I'm self-effacing and have low self-esteem.
- I feel like a burden but just want to be helped.

History
I'm sorry you had to come here, but Michael insisted; he knows best. I stopped coping when Steve died last year (stroke). We were married 35 years. We met when I was 15 and being bullied; he protected me, and promised he'd always look after me.

I'd always dreamed of running my mother's lovely bookshop—but Steve was keen to have children, and be closer to his parents, so we moved away, and I became a housewife. I had five miscarriages, but he kept me going, and we had Michael eventually. I knew nothing about parenting. Without Steve, I'd have been lost—I can't count the times I called him at work and he'd advise or reassure me. He sorted everything out: holidays, mortgages, parents' evenings... I never chose things like holidays or which house we bought—he was so clever and capable, he didn't need my silly ideas. My only worry was how I'd cope if he ever left me. Now he's gone, and everything's too much and my ankle's flared up again.

If it wasn't for Michael, I don't know what I'd do. Despite his A-Levels, he helps me with everything around the house. I never ask for a thing, but he's so caring, just like his dad. I get so anxious when he goes shopping—what if someone calls about something important and I don't know what to do? He's going to university in September and he's started house hunting for me so I can be close to him. I'll miss my friends, but it'll be for the best.

Other history
- My old ankle sprain flared 2 weeks ago. I have to rest and take herbal remedies.
- I can get out of bed with Michael's help. I'm happy and enjoy being with Michael.
- I had anxiety and depression for years, but Steve helped me recover.
- My father was depressed and killed himself when I was five. Mum always worried about me, in case she lost me too.
- I've never smoked or used alcohol or drugs.

Question
How can you help?

Worry
I'm not clever or strong enough to cope alone.

> 💡 Elsie probably has a moderate PD, with prominent traits of negative affectivity but *low* dissociality (previously 'dependent PD'). Introducing the diagnosis this early may alienate her. Exclude or treat other problems contributing to her dependence on Michael (e.g. ankle fracture, early-onset dementia, depression, agoraphobia). Then focus on practical problems, e.g. low confidence disables her and pressurizes Michael; treatment would let Michael go to university knowing that she's coping (independently, at home, near her friends). Family therapy would help them talk this through, while social treatments could reduce Elsie's reliance on Michael, e.g. a support worker could foster her capable side, building confidence while working towards goals, like volunteering in a charity bookshop or library, before gradually moving on to paid employment.

NEXT STEPS

An angry husband in primary care

You're an FY2 in general practice. Last week, you saw Samantha Charlton, who'd experienced domestic violence for years. She finally moved into a women's refuge, whose location is a secret from her husband, Gavin. He's booked an appointment to see you this afternoon. Although he's always been charming towards staff, you're aware he's been to prison for assaults, and repeatedly needed ED treatment after drunken fights. The practice manager said that they were briefly friends at college, but fell out because of Gavin's reckless and impulsive behaviour. You're concerned that Gavin may demand to know Samantha's whereabouts.

- What precautions will you take before seeing Gavin?
- Highlight the main points of your risk assessment.
- How might you help him, longer term?

Preparation

Discuss your concerns with a senior GP and gain their advice and support. Speak with reception staff as they need to know about foreseeable problems. They should let you know as soon as he arrives—keeping Gavin waiting won't help matters.

Arrange to see Gavin in a room with clear exits, close to reception. Ensure that it has a panic alarm or at least a telephone, to access assistance. If available, wear a personal alarm and check that it works. Remove clutter from the room, since objects may obstruct your exit or be used as weapons. Arrange the seats in advance (see 'Safety', p. 17). Finally, ensure that reception and the practice manager know where and when you're seeing Gavin, and ask them to check on you.

Risk assessment

Make sure you have a clear idea of Gavin's agenda before conducting your risk assessment. He may be attending for purely physical concerns and simply need treatment. If Gavin came to find out where Samantha is, be clear about your duty of confidentiality—you *can't* tell him, but as his doctor, you want to address his problems.

You must assess the risk that Gavin poses to himself and others (e.g. you, Samantha, other staff and patients in the surgery, Samantha's family, children). This requires a brief history and MSE, focusing on evidence of mood disturbance, psychosis, and risks of harming himself or others. Ask about drug and alcohol use, whether he carries weapons, and how he intends to resolve the situation. Ask about previous violence or self-harm and discuss details of criminal offences if possible, e.g. why he thinks they happened and whether he feels any remorse.

Longer-term management

People with PD are responsible for their actions. Nonetheless, risk modification is an important part of management. Always discuss risky individuals with seniors. If you identify risk to a specific person (e.g. Samantha), you may need to involve the police. Consider referral to psychiatry, if there's evidence of comorbid mental illness.

If Gavin recognizes that he has a problem managing his emotions and aggression, he may want to undertake *anger management* therapy. A referral to a Multi-Agency Risk Assessment Conference (MARAC) may well be appropriate. At a MARAC, information would be shared between local police, Independent Domestic Violence Advisors (IDVAs), health, child protection, probation, housing, and others in order to ensure

Samantha's safety as a victim of domestic violence and consider how to help Gavin change his behaviour.

💡 **Gavin has at least a moderate PD and prominent traits of disinhibition and dissociality (previously 'dissocial PD'): consistent patterns of violent behaviour, which are impulsive, irresponsible, and a lack of remorse or empathy towards the victim. He's legally responsible for his actions, even when drunk. To argue diminished capacity, a mental illness must substantially impair cognition and volition.**

Movie buff

Girl, Interrupted (1999): Oscar-winning film, adapted from Susanna Kaysen's autobiography, contrasting PD with other diagnoses in an inpatient setting, through the interactions and relationships between characters played memorably by Winona Ryder, Angelina Jolie, and Brittany Murphy.

Book shelf

Boyle, J. (1977) *A Sense of Freedom*: an autobiographical account of extreme violence, dissocial personality disorder, and recovery, within its social context.

Duisberg, K.W. (2003) *The Good Patient*: this ambitious novel follows a woman with borderline PD as she travels through psychotherapy, gaining understanding of herself and her relationships. The protagonist's self-harm, risk-taking, and interactions with others are sensitively narrated, becoming more understandable as her journey unfolds.

Shriver, L. (2003) *We Need to Talk About Kevin*: examines extreme dissociality through a series of poignant letters from Kevin's mother to her husband, detailing Kevin's birth and childhood in a desperate search for answers and reasons behind his crimes. An immensely readable, disquieting exploration of nature versus nurture in antisocial behaviour.

Note

1. Waterfield Duisberg, K. (2003) *The Good Patient*. St Martin's Press, New York.

Journal club

Bach, B., First, M.B. (2018) Application of the ICD-11 classification of personality disorders. *BMC Psychiatry*, **18**, 351.

Balint, M. (1957) *The Doctor, His Patient and the Illness*. London: Tavistock Press.

Caspi, A., Silva, P.A. (1995) Temperamental qualities at age 3 predict personality traits in young adulthood. *Child Development*, **66**, 486–98.

Main, T. (1987) *The Ailment and Other Psychoanalytic Essays*. London: Free Association Books.

Ryle, A., Kerr, I.B. (2002) *Introducing Cognitive Analytic Therapy: Principles and Practice*. Chichester: John Wiley.

Tyrer, P. (2018) *Taming the Beast Within: Shredding the Stereotypes of Personality Disorder*. London: Sheldon.

Go to www.oup.com/uk/stringer2e for a wealth of additional resources, including an OCSE mark scheme, filmed scenarios, and self-assessment questions.

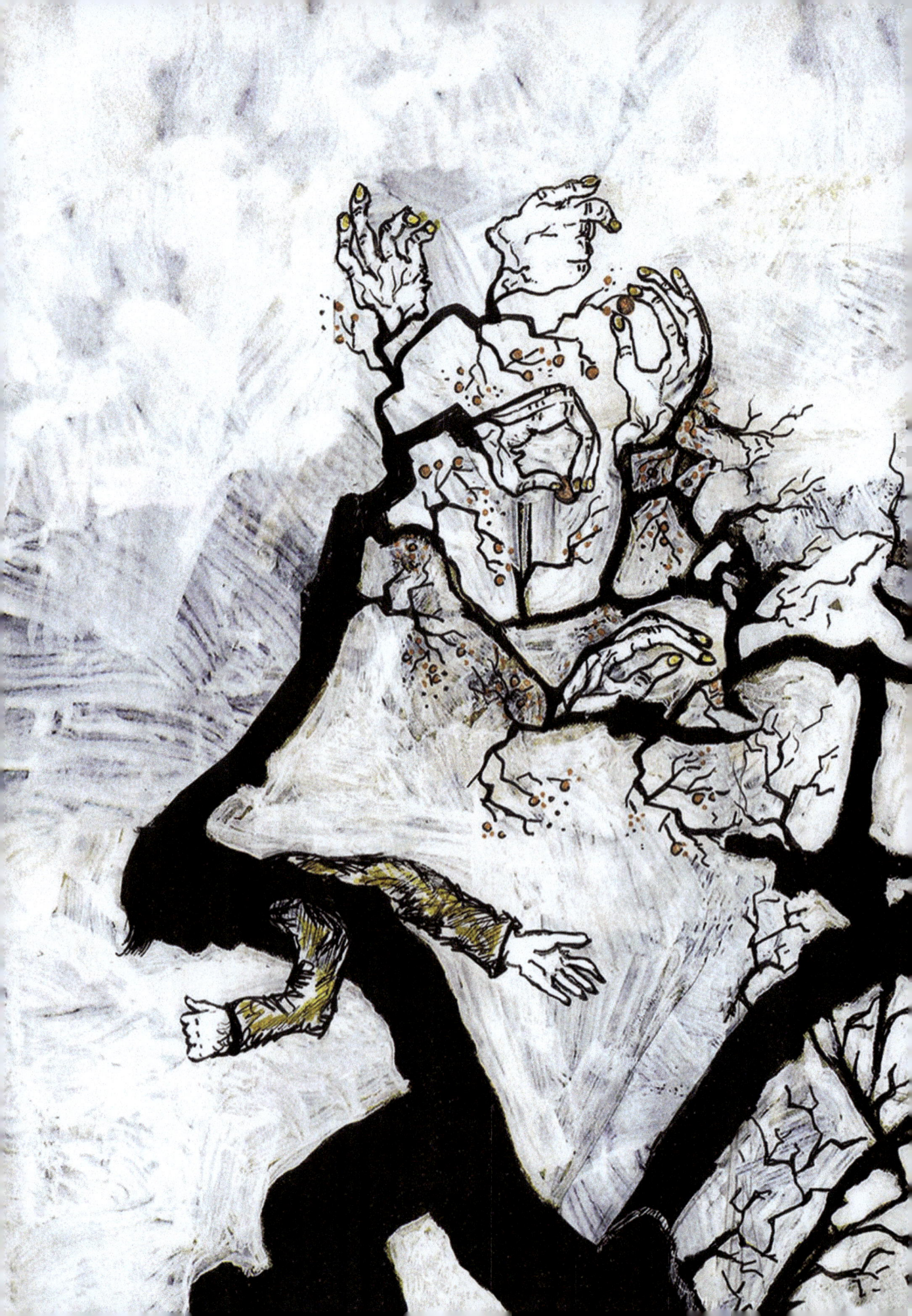

22 Forensic Psychiatry

True or false?

Answers on p. 277

1. A psychiatric diagnosis is associated with an increased risk of violent offending.
2. Forensic psychiatry is the branch of psychiatry based in prisons.
3. Threat/control override delusions are associated with violent offending.
4. Command hallucinations are not associated with increased offending.
5. A dizygotic twin is more likely to engage in bullying if his or her twin does, than a monozygotic twin.
6. English secure hospitals are low, medium, or high secure.
7. The greatest predictor of violent offending is past violent offending.
8. Offending behaviour does not run in families.
9. The Mental Health Act is used in prison health wings.
10. People with mental health problems with a criminal conviction are treated by forensic psychiatric services.

Contents

Principles
Introduction
Epidemiology
- Offending and mental health
- Mental health of offenders
- Mental health in prisons

Aetiology
- Genetics
- Childhood and life events
- Organic causes

Main theories
- Behavioural and cognitive theories
- Attachment theory
- Psychoanalytic theories
- Neurochemical and neuroendocrine theories

Clinical presentation
- Diagnoses
- Presentation
- Assessment

Management
- Community treatment
- Inpatient treatment

Reality
General approach: tips, tricks, and cautionary tales
- Forensic history

Next steps
A young man at risk of radicalization
- Differential diagnosis
- Risk assessment
- Further resources

PRINCIPLES

I have reflected on the fact that for most of us, there is a hard, impassable barrier between the most imaginatively detailed depravity and its real-life execution. It's the same solid steel wall that inserts itself between a knife and my wrist even when I'm at my most disconsolate. So how was Kevin able to raise that crossbow . . . and then really, actually, in time and space, squeeze the release? I can only assume that he discovered what I never wish to. That there is no barrier.

Lionel Shriver, *We Need to Talk About Kevin*[1]

Introduction

Forensic psychiatry operates at the interface between mental health and law. While many people receiving care from forensic psychiatric services have had contact with the criminal justice system (CJS), not all have convictions. People receiving forensic care will at some time have presented a significant risk to others, but the boundaries of 'forensic' psychiatry aren't always clear. To be managed by forensic teams in the UK (community and inpatient), the person usually needs to present an *immediate* risk to others, and usually has (or is awaiting) a conviction for a severe offence, ranging from grievous bodily harm to the most serious sexual and violent offences. In some cases, people referred to forensic services show a worsening pattern of risk behaviour, attributed to their psychiatric diagnosis. Forensic mental health teams are expert in assessing and managing risk and liaising with different organizations in the CJS. They work across all stages of the CJS and mental health services, including police stations, courts, prisons, secure units (low, medium, and high) and the community.

Epidemiology

Mental health problems have historically been conflated with dangerousness, perpetuating the stigma associated with them. Whether psychiatric diagnoses actually increase a person's chance of being violent or committing crimes isn't clear cut. People with mental health problems are actually much more likely to be *victims* of crime than people without them. It's clear that mental health problems are highly over-represented in the CJS. Remember though most offenders don't suffer from severe, enduring mental health problems, and most people with a psychiatric diagnosis don't offend.

Offending and mental health

The risk of violent offending in people with 'severe' mental health problems like schizophrenia, bipolar affective disorder, and recurrent depression may be up to seven times higher than in the general population. However, a lot of this risk results from comorbid substance misuse, and personality disorder. Further factors such as poverty, living in deprived communities, younger age, male sex, and poor treatment response or compliance also play important roles. People with schizophrenia have a three times higher risk of conviction than people without it. However, most people with schizophrenia don't commit violent crimes.

> Contrary to some media and film portrayals, only 5–7% of people convicted of homicide have a psychiatric diagnosis.

Certain symptoms are associated with a greater risk of violence, due to their nature. For example, delusions grouped as '*threat/control override*' entail believing that one is at risk of harm and being controlled by outside forces. You can imagine how these may lead someone to feel they need to defend themselves *and* believe they aren't responsible for their actions.

Hallucinations, especially command hallucinations, predict violent behaviour, but this seems to be because they indicate illness severity and poor prognosis rather than a direct causal effect.

Mental health of offenders

There's increasing concern that people with mental health problems are over-represented throughout the CJS *and* that CJS involvement adversely affects defendants' mental health. The UK CJS pathway (**Figure 22.1**) starts with arrest and, sometimes, police cell custody. If there's enough evidence, the arrested person is charged with an offence and attends court. All cases are heard initially in a Magistrates' Court; more serious

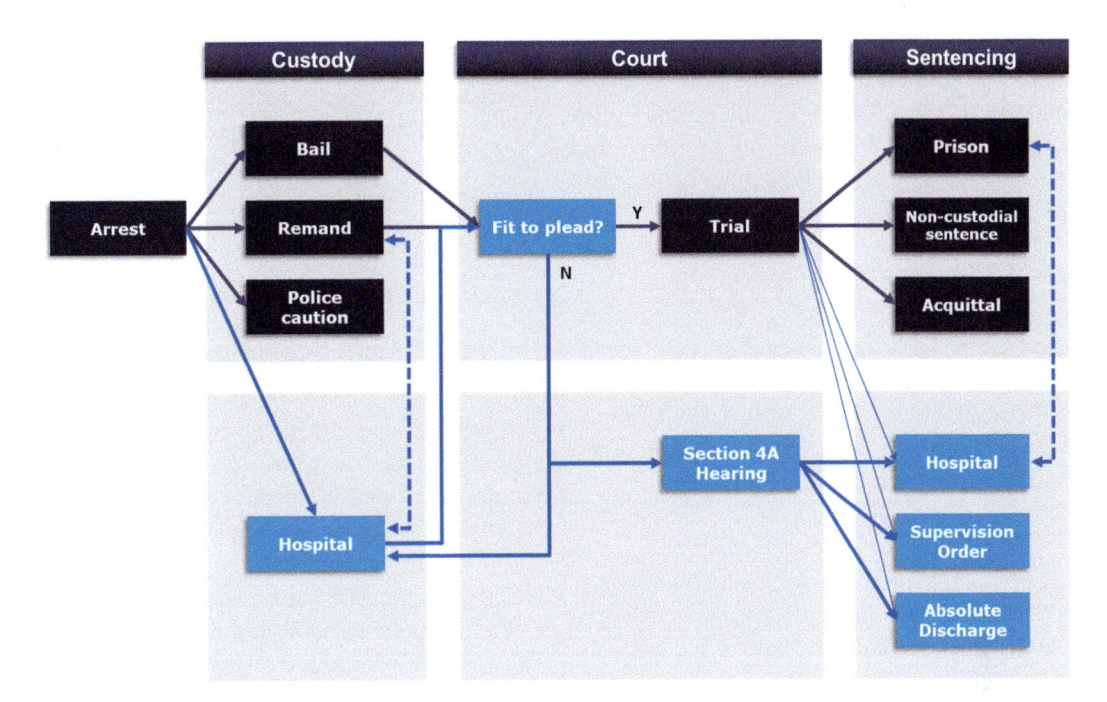

FIGURE 22.1 The criminal justice pathway and diversion into mental health services

cases move to a Crown Court. If found guilty, offenders receive custodial (prison) or community-based sentences. Diversion into mental health services can happen at *any* CJS stage.

Compared to prisons, there's little research into mental health in police custody and courts. UK studies suggest about 40% of people detained in police custody have a mental health problem, such as depression (5–8%), psychosis (8%) and intellectual disabilities (3%). Rates are higher in studies outside the UK. In Australia, over 50% of people detained by police have substance misuse. These figures are important because people in custody have a high risk of self-harm, suicide, and drug or alcohol withdrawal.

Mental health in prisons

Out of 10 million prisoners worldwide, 86,000 are in the UK; less than 5% are female. **Table 22.1** shows the prevalence of common psychiatric diagnoses in prisoners. Other disorders such as ADHD (11–26%) and dissocial personality disorder (47% in men, 21% in women) are also over-represented.

Suicide in prisoners

The risk of suicide is particularly high in prisoners and people recently released from prison. Internationally, men and women in prison are three and nine times more likely, respectively, to commit suicide than the general population. In England and Wales, suicide rates are five times (men) and over 20 times (women) higher in prisoners than the population rate.

Aetiology

Forensic psychiatric services treat a diverse group of people: men and women of all ages, from various backgrounds, with a range of diagnoses.

Genetics

Violence runs in families, although the role of genetics is unclear. While no single gene underpins violent and aggressive behaviour, several genes are associated with hostility (catechol O-methyltransferase on chromosome 22q) and aggression (tryptophan hydroxylase). Bullying behaviour is more commonly perpetrated by both

Table 22.1 Prevalence of psychiatric diagnoses in adult prisoners

Disorder	Prevalence (%)	
	Men	Women
Psychosis	3.6	3.9
Depression	10.2	14.1
Alcohol misuse	18–30	10–24
Drug misuse	10–48	30–60

Reprinted from *The Lancet Psychiatry*, **3**, 9, Fazel S et al., Mental health of prisoners: prevalence, adverse outcomes, and interventions, pp. 871–881, Copyright © 2016 Elsevier Ltd. All rights reserved. https://doi.org/10.1016/S2215-0366(16)30142-0.

identical (monozygotic) than non-identical (dizygotic) twins, suggesting a genetic component. Twin studies of *psychopathy* (an extreme subtype of dissociality) show a strong genetic component, especially in callous and unemotional personality traits, which are particularly associated with aggression and violence.

Childhood and life experiences

A tendency to commit violence can't be explained by genetics alone. Early life experiences play significant roles in the development of aggressive behaviour. Childhood risk factors for antisocial behaviour include negative parenting, abuse, witnessing violence, truancy, and limited social support.

Organic causes

Traumatic brain injuries, space-occupying lesions (e.g. tumours), intracerebral infections (e.g. encephalitis), strokes, and dementia can cause aggressive and violent behaviour. Metabolic and endocrine irregularities and seizures can also be associated with aggression. Acute intoxication and withdrawal of drugs and alcohol are important factors associated with violent and non-violent offending. Medical assessment is therefore essential for anyone presenting with unusual or changed behaviour.

Main theories

Behavioural and cognitive theories

Antisocial beliefs and attitudes and poor social problem-solving skills contribute to offending. *Operant conditioning* models explain repeated offending despite negative consequences: some people experience positive reinforcement, including pleasure (e.g. sexual offences), relief from stress (sexual or violent offences), and material rewards (acquisitive offences). As a result, the greatest risk factor for future violence is past violence.

Functional analysis considers the *antecedents* (e.g. alcohol, sexual fantasies, boredom) and *consequences* (e.g. negative reinforcements such as punishment, imprisonment, loss of employment) which might affect the chances of someone reoffending, to inform risk assessment and treatment targets.

Attachment theory

Influential thinkers like Bowlby have argued that an absent 'senior attachment figure' could cause 'affectionless psychopathy'. The Cambridge Delinquency Study confirmed that offenders were more likely to have experienced authoritarian discipline, parental conflict, and poor parental supervision than non-offenders.

Psychoanalytic theories

Psychoanalytic theories are controversial in forensic psychiatry. Freudian theorists argue that criminal behaviour arises from abnormal development of the psyche. They propose that individuals with underdeveloped egos and superegos may seek instant gratification, while struggling to differentiate right from wrong. Early childhood adversity again plays a significant role.

Neurochemical and neuroendocrine theories

Testosterone levels positively correlate with violence and aggression in both males and females; testosterone is thought to activate subcortical structures in the amygdala and hypothalamus which regulate aggression. Cortisol and serotonin are inversely related to aggression. High testosterone:cortisol ratios are associated with aggression and low serotonin levels are associated with impulsivity. People with low serotonin and cortisol and high testosterone levels are more likely to show 'instrumental aggression' (premeditated and goal-directed), rather than impulsive aggression (a 'heat of the moment' reaction).

Clinical presentation

Diagnoses

The commonest diagnoses of people receiving forensic psychiatric support are psychosis, bipolar affective disorder, and neurodevelopmental disorders (including ASD, intellectual disabilities, and ADHD), often with comorbid substance misuse and/or personality disorders. PTSD is increasingly being identified in offenders and depression, anxiety, and cognitive impairment may also be treated by forensic teams. The risk of self-harm and suicide is especially high in women treated by forensic psychiatric services.

Presentation

While prisons and secure hospitals may support the most acute forensic presentations, offending behaviour often presents in other settings. If police are concerned that a person needs mental health assessment or treatment, they can arrange this in police custody, in the emergency department, or in a designated 'place of safety'—usually attached to a psychiatric hospital.

Assessment

The clinical assessment of a person under the CJS is the same as for a person seen in a health setting, with additional attention paid to risks. Forensic specialists take care when seeking collateral risk history. They liaise closely with CJS staff to avoid influencing defendant and witness police statements.

Management

The management of people treated by forensic psychiatric services depends on the level of risk at that point in time.

Community treatment

UK forensic community mental health teams (FCMHTs) are sometimes integrated into general teams. They support and treat people with a history of offending, who have previously been treated in secure hospitals or prisons, and are now living in the community. FCMHTs may also treat people deemed to require higher levels of risk management than general CMHTs can provide.

Some people are managed under a *restriction order* (Section 41 of the MHA). This occurs if a Crown Court orders a hospital order (Section 37) with restrictions which are deemed necessary to protect the public from serious harm due to the antecedents of the offender. At the time of discharge into the community, restriction orders specify conditions, e.g. avoiding substances, taking medication and living in a particular place. Changes to these conditions must be approved by the Ministry of Justice. If the person breaches these conditions, they may be recalled to hospital, usually a psychiatric intensive care unit or secure hospital, depending on the reasons for recall.

Inpatient treatment

Hospital admission may be to a general or secure ward. In the UK, secure hospitals are classed as low, medium, or high secure. In England, three high-secure hospitals treat about 800 people in total. Criteria for high security include presenting a grave and immediate danger to the public; many people admitted to high-secure hospitals are treated under hospital orders imposed by the court. Some are transferred from prison after developing symptoms which can't be managed there.

In England, medium-secure hospitals treat about 3000 people assessed as presenting a significant danger (usually to the public but sometimes also to themselves). Admissions usually last 2–5 years, for a combination of medication and psychological treatment aimed at reducing reoffending.

Low-secure hospitals treat about 3500 people, who have often been transferred from medium-secure hospitals as they recover, before discharge.

Many prisoners with mental health problems are treated in prison by GPs and psychiatrists. Many prisons have healthcare wings but as they are not hospitals, the MHA cannot be used. If a prisoner becomes severely psychiatrically unwell, they can be transferred to hospital under the MHA, with permission from the Ministry of Justice. Specialist secure units exist to meet the needs of women, adolescents, older adults, and people with intellectual disabilities.

Biological interventions

Clinical management is as for the person's diagnosis. However, due to the severe and complex nature of presentations, higher doses of antipsychotic medication and specialist combinations of medication may be required. In cases of sex offending, *anti-libidinal* medication is sometimes used (see p. 218).

Psychological interventions

Secure forensic settings provide a range of specialist psychological therapies which aim to reduce reoffending. These include CBT-based groups (e.g. 'reasoning and rehabilitation') and psychological therapy tailored to person's particular diagnosis. Therapy for substance misuse is also commonly provided.

Social interventions

Social interventions are provided in line with the person's diagnosis and needs. Occupational therapy is particularly important in engaging the person with education, courses and routes into employment after discharge.

REALITY

General approach: tips, tricks, and cautionary tales

1. Risk assessment quick tips

Full forensic risk assessment is beyond the remit of this book or your role as a medical student. Nevertheless, these are sensible, basic tips:

- Read about general safety (see p. 17) and boundaries (see p. 55, 264).
- Review the person's risk with staff before interviewing.
- Never see someone with a history of violence alone.
- Avoid looking shocked; calmness helps people disclose risk information.

- Keep exploring risk, while safe to do so. Fully explore their pattern of violence, triggers, victim profile, and future plans (when, where, why, how, who?).
- Document and share your findings with the team and expect them to share information with other agencies, e.g. police, social services. If anyone (e.g. a relative/partner/acquaintance/enemy) is at risk, teams may need to break confidentiality to contact them directly.

2. Humanize

Avoid an 'us and them' mentality. Society labels people who offend as though their crimes define them (e.g. murderer, thief) or dehumanize them (e.g. animal, evil). People who've committed crimes are still people. Let police, judges, and juries determine their culpability and punishment; your focus is their healthcare.

Empathy helps you see the person behind the offence. It doesn't mean you approve of their crime but makes compassion and rapport easier. These help people to open up: essential for short-term risk assessment and longer-term treatment. Taking a personal history can help you to empathize: many offenders have experienced childhood adversity which influences how they react to feeling threatened in adulthood.

3. Notice emotions

Meeting people who've been accused or convicted of certain crimes might make you feel upset, scared, angry, or disgusted. Ignoring these feelings can mean they leak out during interviews, e.g. accidental abruptness/dismissiveness. Noticing your emotional response lets you rein it in, keeping you safe and the assessment on track by not offending them. Noticing your emotions also:

- Highlights risk, e.g. a nagging 'gut feeling' that you've missed something or you're in danger.
- Reflects how other people may react to the person.
- Shows the importance of protecting yourself, emotionally.

It's OK to step away from distressing interviews, e.g. if you've suffered abuse, you might struggle to interview someone accused of rape. This might mean avoiding details or ending an interview early, asking someone else to complete the full assessment. Discuss how you feel with a trusted senior and consider accessing longer-term support or talking therapy; medical training often reactivates upsetting past experiences.

4. Contextualize

Don't jump to diagnose simply because someone's behaviour violates social norms. Context is essential: acceptable language, vocal tone/volume and gestures vary by age, culture, ethnicity, and social background. Don't mistake these differences for symptoms.

Where delusional beliefs seem to underpin offending, use collateral information to clarify what's real: there can be a surprising amount of truth in the most unusual stories. Conversely, someone with dissocial personality traits isn't necessarily paranoid for thinking 'everyone hates' them: they might provoke hostility wherever they go.

Finally, remember that you may represent an authority figure (yes, you!). People with negative experiences of authority may therefore be irritable or mistrustful of you. This doesn't necessarily reflect their baseline, so comparing assessments (e.g. by ambulance, nursing, CJS, and medical staff) can be informative.

Forensic history (15 minutes)

Candidate's instructions

Michael Martin is a 30-year-old carpenter, known to the local CMHT with a diagnosis of paranoid schizophrenia. He has engaged poorly over the past year. Michael was admitted to hospital under Section 2 from police cells after breaking into an elderly woman's house (Rose, 83 years old). The police report that Michael was carrying a knife and duct tape. Rose had locked herself in the bathroom and was terrified. She alleges that Michael has been following her, staring through her windows and pushing threatening notes under her door, despite a restraining order.

Michael has been calm on the ward but often talks to himself. The consultant asks you to interview Michael and suggest possible management.

Patient's brief
Key characteristics

- I'm an important man and angry that I've been treated so badly.
- I'm disgusted that Rose is seen as the victim and don't believe she's scared.
- I won't explain my future plans. These are between Interpol and me.

History

Rose isn't a sweet old lady. It's a clever disguise; she's *much* younger and extremely dangerous. I passed her house about a year ago and heard a weird noise, like a circular saw. Soon after, Interpol contacted me and explained everything: Rose is people trafficking and trading in organs. Kidneys especially, but she says everything sells and people pay big money. Her gang brings in men, women, and children using a secret tunnel under the house. She enjoys cutting them into pieces and although she's two streets away, I hear terrible screaming, day and night. There's no point calling the police: she always fools them with her old lady act. She got me put on a restraining order for smashing a window.

Commander H3A gives me my orders through eardrum vibrations: 'Follow the bitch . . . Film that!' I follow Rose when she goes out and photograph her contacts. I've written letters to stop her but she ignores them. That's why I was in her house: Interpol ordered me to cut the victims free and tie Rose up. The police ruined the whole operation and fell for Rose's lies. Fortunately, Interpol will clear my name and protect me, whatever happens . . .

Other history

- Dad was a drinker. He beat me and my mum until I was 15 and fought back.
- I worked as a carpenter until Interpol recruited me.
- Another 'elderly lady' was using kids to run drugs on my estate, 7 years ago. She stopped after I broke her arm, but I did 4 years for that (grievous bodily harm): mostly in prison but some in psychiatric hospital.
- I've always been physically and mentally well but psychiatrists think I have schizophrenia. They want to drug me with olanzapine but I rarely take it.
- Most evenings I drink beer (4 × 500mL cans, ABV 5%).
- I have flatmates but don't trust them.
- I'm not depressed or suicidal, just angry.
- I don't know what will happen with Rose. I just follow Interpol's instructions . . .

Question

What would *you* do about someone like Rose?

Worries

While I'm here, nobody's monitoring her.

💡 Michael's offending behaviour is in the context of untreated paranoid schizophrenia. He has a forensic history (grievous bodily harm) and his risk to a specific victim is escalating: breaching the restraining order with stalking and harassment, carrying weapons, and obeying command hallucinations. His substance use, medication non-adherence, and poor engagement are risk factors. Ward staff will clarify with police about charges, bail conditions, and plans to interview Michael about the alleged crime. A forensic psychiatric referral would be beneficial, while he receives inpatient biopsychosocial treatment for psychosis.

NEXT STEPS

A young man at risk of radicalization

You're a psychiatry FY1 in a CMHT. You and a colleague visit 21-year-old Adam Hutton, following GP referral of recent behaviour change and concern about his risk to others. Adam has ASD and was recently made redundant by an electronics manufacturer; his job was outsourced to India. His mother told the GP that Adam was 'ranting about Asians, Blacks, and Jews,' had drawn swastikas on his bedroom walls, and become secretive at home. He has few friends and little social life but has been called a lot by 'an old colleague' lately. Ms Hutton worries that they're attending right-wing extremist meetings.

- What's the differential diagnosis?
- Who is at risk?
- What resources might be considered?

Differential diagnosis

Review the evidence for ASD. If accurate, also consider:

1. Psychotic episode: change in behaviour with delusions and hallucinations.
2. Manic episode: change in behaviour, euphoria, irritability, increased energy, etc.

3. Depressive episode ± psychotic symptoms.
4. Dissociality in personality disorder: extreme views and aggression would have persisted over an extended period (2 years or more) across a range of personal and social situations.
5. ASD: Adam may be vulnerable to radicalization, e.g. limited social skills could make him more impressionable than his peers. More concrete thinking could impair his understanding of the effects of his actions on others, or lead him to bear grudges.

Risk assessment

As Adam's mother raised concerns with his GP, Adam may not anticipate your visit. Be aware that he may feel angry, placing you and your colleague at risk. You need to take a collateral history but take care: Ms Hutton may be at risk of violence if Adam thinks she is 'telling on him'. She has the right to give third-party information in confidence but using this information without him realizing the source takes skill.

Ascertain *who* is most at risk from Adam and his associates' extremist behaviour, *where* (targets, e.g. places of worship), and *when* (e.g. specific events, rallies). As far as possible, take a history of Adam's involvement with the group, his beliefs about their activity, and any criminal behaviour, extremist views, or less serious offending. Discuss the case and document your assessment with the consultant and team colleagues as soon as possible.

! Because of Adam's ASD he may be vulnerable to radicalization by the extremist group. Risks they pose to Adam also need to be considered.

Further resources

'Prevent' is part of the UK Government's counter-terrorism strategy. Individuals considered at risk of radicalization are discussed with the local Prevent lead, much like a safeguarding concern. If the lead identifies vulnerability to radicalization, they make a referral to the local authority or police. Ideally, Adam should be told about the concerns and the Prevent referral, and kept informed of progress. However, if this would increase risks to him or others, this would be documented and the referral made without his knowledge. Otherwise, he will be kept informed of the process.

The police run background checks and gather information. If they deem Adam to be at risk of radicalization, they will refer him to the 'Channel Panel', a multidisciplinary panel chaired by the local authority, with representation from police, social care, health, education, immigration, probation, and housing services. If Adam is experiencing psychosis or affective symptoms, mental health services will offer treatment immediately. The panel considers risks and agrees a support plan which may involve other organizations, e.g. vocational support for training/employment, National Autistic Society for social support and inclusion.

Movie buff
Enduring Love (2004): psychological thriller based on Ian McEwan's best-selling novel. Two strangers witness an accident. Erotomanic delusions (De Clérambault's syndrome) ensue.
Spider (2002): directed by David Cronenberg, a man with schizophrenia revisits traumatic childhood memories of domestic violence and murder.
We Need to Talk About Kevin (2011): a mother's perspective after her son commits a terrible crime.

Book shelf
Fowles, J. (1963) *The Collector*: a withdrawn young lepidopterist expands his collection.
McGrath, P. (1998) *Asylum*: Stella Raphael joins her husband at his new job in a high-secure forensic hospital.
Nabokov, V. (1955) *Lolita*: Humbert Humbert falls in love with his landlady's 12-year-old daughter.
The Secret Barrister (2018). *The Secret Barrister: Stories of the Law and How it's Broken*: not mental health focused but an excellent introduction to the reality of the CJS today.

Note

1. Shriver, L. (2005) *We Need to Talk About Kevin*. London: Serpent's Tail.

Journal club

Fazel, S., Ramesh, T., Hawton, K. (2017) Suicide in prisons: an international study of prevalence and contributory factors. *Lancet Psychiatry*, **4**, 946–52.

Link, B.G., Stueve, A., Phelan, J. (1998) Psychotic symptoms and violent behaviors: probing the components of "threat/control-override" symptoms. *Social Psychiatry and Psychiatric Epidemiology*, **33**(Suppl 1), S55–60.

Morgan, V., Morgan, F., Valuri, G., et al. (2013) A whole-of-population study of the prevalence and patterns of criminal offending in people with schizophrenia and other mental illness. *Psychological Medicine*, **43**, 1869–80.

Go to www.oup.com/uk/stringer2e for a wealth of additional resources, including an OCSE mark scheme, filmed scenarios, and self-assessment questions.

TRUE/FALSE QUESTION ANSWERS

Chapter	Q1	2	3	4	5	6	7	8	9	10
8. Affective disorders	F	T	F	T	T	F	T	F	F	F
9. Self-harm and suicide	F	T	T	F	T	F	F	T	F	F
10. Psychotic disorders	F	T	T	F	F	F	F	F	F	T
11. Substance use disorders	F	F	T	F	F	F	T	F	F	F
12. Organic psychiatry	T	T	F	F	T	F	F	T	F	T
13. Old age psychiatry	F	F	T	F	T	F	T	F	F	F
14. Anxiety disorders	T	F	T	T	T	F	T	F	F	F
15. Medically unexplained symptoms	F	F	F	F	T	T	T	F	F	T
16. Eating disorders	F	F	T	F	F	T	T	F	T	T
17. Conditions related to sexual health	T	T	F	T	T	T	F	T	T	F
18. Perinatal psychiatry	F	T	T	F	F	T	F	T	F	T
19. Intellectual disability	T	T	F	T	T	T	T	F	T	T
20. Child and adolescent psychiatry	T	F	T	F	T	F	T	F	F	T
21. Personality disorders	F	F	F	F	T	F	F	T	T	F
22. Forensic psychiatry	T	F	T	F	F	T	T	F	F	F

INDEX

1,4-BD (1,4-butanediol) 112, 117

A

ABC approach 237
aberrant salience 87
abstract reasoning test 146–7
acamprosate 118
acetylcholinesterase inhibitors (AChEIs) 159
acting out 259
active listening 19–20
activities of daily living (ADL) 152
acute confusional state *see* delirium
acute stress reaction 175
Addenbrooke's Cognitive Examination III (ACE-III) 143
Addison disease 141
adjustment disorders 176
aetiology
  affective disorders 35–6
  Alzheimer disease 152–3
  anxiety disorders 168–9
  bipolar affective disorder 35–6
  delirium 129–30
  depression 35–6
  early-onset dementias 133–6
  eating disorders 201–2
  forensic psychiatry 271–2
  intellectual disability 233–4
  Lewy body dementia 153
  medically unexplained symptoms 190–1
  personality disorders 259–60
  schizophrenia 79–80
  self-harm and suicide 63–4
  substance use disorders 103–5
  vascular dementia 153
affective disorders 33–60, 204
agnosia 155
agomelatine 42
agoraphobia 172, 182
  case history 184–5
  clinical presentation 171–2
  differential diagnosis 174, 175
  epidemiology 168
  management 179
AIDS dementia complex (ADC) 135
akathisia 88
Al-Anon 120
alcohol misuse 84, 106–8, 117, 120–2
  anxiety 176
  case history 122–3

delirium tremens 106
detoxification 118
intoxication 106
management 118, 119, 120
rehabilitation 120
relapse prevention 118
units 106
withdrawal 106, 118
Alcohol Use Disorders Identification Test (AUDIT) 122
alcoholic hallucinosis 108
Alcoholics Anonymous 120
Alzheimer disease 157
  aetiology 152–3
  clinical presentation 155, 157
  pathology 153
American Psychiatric Association (APA) 27
amisulpride 87, 88
amitriptyline 41
amnesia 136–7, 139, 154, 162–3
  psychogenic 192
amnestic disorder 136–7
amorous delusions 9
amphetamine (speed) 109, 116
amyl nitrite 115
amyloid precursor protein (APP) 153
anankastic personality disorder 176, 261
anorexia nervosa (AN) 201–2, 204–7, 208
anorgasmia 217
antiandrogens 218
anticonvulsants *see* mood stabilizers
antidepressants
  action 40
  in anxiety disorders 177
  in bipolar affective disorder 49
  in bulimia nervosa 207
  comparison table 41–2
  in depression 40–2, 151
  discontinuation symptoms 42
  in epilepsy 141
  in personality disorders 262
antihypertensives 141
antipsychotics 86–7, 159
  in mania and bipolar affective disorder 47–8
  in personality disorders 262
  side effects 88–9
anxiety
  hierarchy 178
  organic causes 141, 176
anxiety disorders 167–98
  body dysmorphic disorder 173

case histories 183–5
in childhood and adolescence 245, 246
differential diagnosis 174–6, 204
generalized anxiety disorder 169
obsessive–compulsive disorder 173
in old age 151–2
panic disorder 169–70
perinatal 225–6
phobias 170–2
post-traumatic stress disorder 173–4
risk of suicide 64
theories 169
anxiolytics 177, 262
aphonia 192
apolipoprotein E4 153
appearance *see* assessment
apraxia 155
arcuate fasciculus 131
aripiprazole 87, 88
arrhythmia 176
arts therapies 90
Asperger syndrome 247
assault 18
assessment
  appearance and behaviour 7
  capacity 164
  case study 1–4
  collateral history 6
  delusions 8–9
  formulation 11–12
  mental state examination 4, 6–11
  mood 8
  premorbid personality 6
  risk of suicide or self-harm 67, 73–4
  speech 8–9
  'Take me with you' guide to 16
  thought 9–10, 94, 95
at-risk mental state (ARM), psychotic disorders 81
atomoxetine 249
attachment theory 169, 259, 272
attention deficit hyperactivity disorder (ADHD) 235, 249–50, 251, 254
auditory hallucinations 82, 94
augmentative and alternative communication (AAC) 237
autism spectrum disorder (ASD) 235, 236, 239, 247–9, 252
  case history 253
  differential diagnosis 204
  in OCD 176
autoimmune encephalitis 141–2
automatic obedience 85

autoprosopagnosia 155
avoidance 174, 183
avoidant/restrictive food intake disorder (ARFID) 201

B

baby blues 226
barbiturates 112, 117
Beck Anxiety Inventory (BAI) 177
behavioural and cognitive theories
  affective disorders 36
  anxiety 169
  forensic psychiatry 272
  medically unexplained symptoms 191
behavioural and psychological symptoms of dementia (BPSD) 155, 159
behavioural difficulties 235, 236
  in childhood 246–7, 249
behavioural therapy 237
benzodiazepines
  anxiety disorders 177
  delirium 133
  dementia 159
  substance use disorders 112, 117, 118, 119
bereavement 40
  suicide 69
bestiality 218
beta-blockers 141, 177
Bethlem Hospital 84
binge eating disorder (BED) 201, 204
biological interventions
  bulimia nervosa 207–8
  forensic psychiatry 273
  intellectual disability 237
  personality disorders 262
biological models, medically unexplained symptoms 191
bipolar affective disorder (BPAD) 44–50
  aetiology 35–6
  antidepressants 42
  epidemiology 35
  risk of suicide 64
  see also affective disorders; mania
bisexuality 219
bodily distress disorder 191
body dysmorphic disorder (BDD) 172, 183
  clinical presentation 173
  differential diagnosis 174, 176, 204
  epidemiology 168
  management 179
body language 7, 20
body mass index (BMI) 202
borderline personality disorder 85, 262

bradykinesia 133, 140
bradyphrenia 133, 140
brain 105, 129, 130, 131
breastfeeding and drugs 226
brief interventions, substance use disorders 119
Broca's area 131
bulimia nervosa (BN) 201–2, 203–6, 207–8, 210–11
buprenorphine 118–19
butyl nitrite 115

C

caffeine 176
CAGE screening questionnaire 121–2
cannabinoids 109, 112, 115
cannabis (delta-9-tetrahydrocannabinol) 109, 112, 116
  risk of schizophrenia 80
capacity 29, 164–5
carbamazepine 48, 49
care homes 160
career in psychiatry 31–2
carers 90, 160
carpopedal spasm 173
case histories
  agoraphobia 184–5
  alcohol misuse 122–3
  autism spectrum disorder 253
  cognitive assessment 145
  dementia 163–4
  depression 53–5
  eating disorder 210–11
  erectile dysfunction 220–1
  intellectual disability 239–40
  mania 57–8
  medically unexplained symptoms 195–6
  memory loss 162–3
  neurodevelopmental history 253
  obsessive–compulsive disorder 183–4
  opioid dependency 123–4
  overdose 74
  paranoid schizophrenia 274–5
  personality disorders 265–6
  postpartum psychosis 228–9
  psychotic depression 54–5
  psychotic disorders 95–7
  self-harm 73–4
  subdural haematoma 143–7
  suspected malignancy 196–7
  van Gogh 1–4
catastrophizing 178
catatonia 86
catatonic schizophrenia 85
cerebral atrophy 153
cerebral function localization 130, 131

challenging behaviour 235, 236
cheese reaction 41
child abuse 245–6
child and adolescent mental health services (CAMHS) 245
child and adolescent psychiatry 243–55
childhood and life experiences
  affective disorders 36
  anxiety disorders 168–9
  forensic psychiatry 272
  personality disorder 259
  schizophrenia 80
  self-harm and suicide 63
  substance use disorders 104
chlordiazepoxide 118
chlorpromazine 87, 89
cholinergic pathways 153
chorea in Huntington disease 134, 135
chromosomal abnormalities 234
chronic fatigue syndrome (CFS) 191, 192, 196
circumstantial speech 8
citalopram 41
clang associations 8
classical conditioning (Pavlovian) 105, 169
classification and diagnosis 27–8
clinical presentation
  Alzheimer disease 155, 157
  amnestic disorder 137
  anorexia nervosa 202
  attention deficit hyperactivity disorder 249
  autism spectrum disorder 247–8
  body dysmorphic disorder 173
  conduct/dissocial disorder 250
  delirium 130, 132
  dementia 154–7
  depression 38–40
  forensic psychiatry 272–3
  generalized anxiety disorder 169
  intellectual disability 234–6
  Lewy body dementia 157
  mania and bipolar affective disorder 44–7
  medically unexplained symptoms 191–2
  obsessive–compulsive disorder 173
  panic disorder 169–70
  Parkinson disease 140
  personality disorders 260
  phobias 170–2
  post-traumatic stress disorder 173–4
  schizophrenia 81–2
  self-harm 65–7
  traumatic brain injury 139
  vascular dementia 155, 157
clomipramine 41, 177

clouding of consciousness 130
clozapine 86, 87
   side effects 88, 89, 98–9
cocaine 109, 111, 113, 116
Cocaine Anonymous 120
cockroach phobia 178
codeine 108, 116
coercive sexual sadism disorder 218
cognition 11
   assessment 145
cognitive analytical therapy (CAT) 262–3
cognitive behavioural therapy (CBT)
   affective disorders 36
   anxiety disorders 177–9
   depression 43–4
   eating disorders 207
   forensic psychiatry 273
   mania and bipolar affective disorder 49
   medically unexplained symptoms 192
   personality disorders 262
   schizophrenia 87–90
   self-harm 69
   substance use disorders 119
cognitive remediation therapy (CRT) 90
cognitive stimulation therapy 159
cognitive test score, causes of low 158
cognitive theories *see* behavioural and cognitive theories
cognitive triad 36, 37
coma 139
command hallucinations 270
compulsions 7, 10, 173, 182–3
compulsive sexual behaviour disorder (CSBD) 216
concussion 139
conduct/dissocial disorder 250, 251
Conners Rating Scale 249
control, delusions of 9, 82
conversion disorder 191–2
cortical atrophy 153
cortical dementia 133
corticosteroids 141
counselling 159
counter-transference 263–4
covert sensitization 218
crack cocaine 109, 113, 116
Creutzfeldt–Jakob disease 135–6
criminal justice system (CJS) 270–1, 272
Cushing syndrome 141
cyclothymia 47

D

de-escalation 18
defence mechanisms 259
deliberate self-harm *see* self-harm
delirium (acute confusional state) 129–33, 142–7, 158
delirium tremens 84, 106
delusional disorder 85
delusional perception 82, 94
delusions 8–9, 79, 81, 93–4
   depression 39–40
   forensic psychiatry 270
dementia
   AIDS dementia complex 135
   case history 163–4
   comparison with delirium 132
   cortical vs subcortical 133
   early-onset 133–6
   frontotemporal (FTD) 133–4
   HIV-associated 135
   with Lewy bodies (DLB) 153, 154, 157, 157
   in older adults 152–60
   in organic conditions 141
   in Parkinson disease 140
   prevention 158
   prognosis 160
   psychological therapies 159
   psychotropic medication 159
   social interventions 159–60
   vascular 153, 154, 155, 157
depersonalization 11
depression 35–44, 51–3
   case histories 53–5
   in childhood and adolescence 245
   comparison with mania 46
   differential diagnosis 40, 174, 204
   in old age 151
   in organic conditions 139, 140, 141
   in Parkinson disease 140
   pseudodementia 158
   psychoanalytic theory 37
   risk of suicide 64
Deprivation of Liberty Safeguards (DoLS) 30
derailment 8
derealization 11
desensitization 178
detachment 261
detoxification 118
developmental milestones 246
dexamfetamine 249
diabetes 204
diagnostic overshadowing 236
dialectical behavioural therapy 262
diamorphine 119
diazepam 118, 177
differential diagnosis
   anxiety disorders 174–6
   attention deficit hyperactivity disorder 249
   autism spectrum disorder 248
   conduct/dissocial disorder 250
   dementia 157–8
   depression 40
   eating disorders 204
   formulation 11
   intellectual disability 236
   mania and bipolar affective disorder 47
   medically unexplained symptoms 192
   psychotic disorders 82–6
   substance use disorders 117
dihydrocodeine 108, 116
disinhibition 261
disruptive behaviour in childhood 250
dissocial personality disorder 250, 251, 261
dissociative neurological symptoms disorder 191–2
disulfiram 118
domestic violence 266–7
donepezil 159
L-dopa 141
dopamine hypothesis 80–1
dopaminergic reward pathway 103–4, 105
Down syndrome (trisomy 21) 234, 240–1
drug misuse 108–18, 120–4
   anxiety 176
DSM-5 (Diagnostic and Statistical Manual-5) 27
duloxetine 41
duration of untreated psychosis (DUP) 86
dysarthria 8
dyscalculia 155
dyspareunia 217
dysphasia 8, 154
dystonia 88

E

early intervention services in schizophrenia 86
eating disorders 199–212, 245
ecstasy (3,4-methylenedioxy-methamphetamine) 109–11, 113, 116, 120
Edinburgh Postnatal Depression Scale 228
ego defences 259
ejaculatory dysfunctions 215, 217
elder abuse 160
electroconvulsive therapy (ECT) 42, 151
emotional disorders in childhood 246–7
empathy 21–2
encephalitis 141
   autoimmune 141–2

encopresis 247
enuresis 246–7
epidemiology
　affective disorders 35
　anxiety disorders 168
　dementia 152
　eating disorders 201
　forensic psychiatry 270–1
　intellectual disability 233
　medically unexplained symptoms 190
　perinatal psychiatry 225
　personality disorder 259
　schizophrenia 79
　self-harm and suicide 63
　substance use disorders 103, 104
epilepsy 141, 236
erectile dysfunction (ED) 216–17, 220–1
erotomanic delusions 9, 10
escitalopram 41
ethnicity, and schizophrenia 80
excitement 85
exercise, in depression 43
exhibitionistic disorder 218
exposure therapy 177–8, 179
expressed emotion 90
extrapyramidal side effects (EPSEs) 7, 88
eye movement desensitization and reprocessing (EMDR) 179–80

F

factitious disorder 192
family theories, of eating disorders 202
family therapy
　eating disorders 207, 208
　mania and bipolar affective disorder 49
　psychotic disorders 90
fantasizing 259
female sexual arousal dysfunction (FSAD) 216
fetal alcohol syndrome 234
fetishism 218
first-generation antipsychotics (FGAs) 87, 88, 89
first-rank symptoms (schizophrenia) 81, 82
fitness to drive 147–8
flashbacks 183
flight of ideas 8
flooding 178
flumazenil 119
fluoxetine 41
flupentixol 87
fluphenazine 87
fluvoxamine 41

focal psychodynamic therapy (FPT) 207
folate 141
forensic psychiatry 269–76
formal thought disorder 8, 79, 81, 95
formulation 11–15
fragile X syndrome 234
frontal lobe
　functions 131
　syndrome 137–9
　testing 143–7
frontotemporal dementia (FTD) 133–4
frotteuristic disorder 218
fugue 192
functional neurological symptom disorder 191–2
functional psychosis 84–5

G

Gage, Phineas 137, 138
GBL (gamma butyrolactone) 112, 114, 117
gender incongruence 218–19
gender terminology 218
generalized anxiety disorder (GAD) 172, 182
　clinical presentation 169
　cognitive behavioural therapy 178, 179
　differential diagnosis 175
　epidemiology 168
　genetics
affective disorders 35–6
Alzheimer disease 153
anxiety disorders 168
eating disorders 201
forensic psychiatry 271–2
intellectual disability 233, 234
personality disorder 259
schizophrenia 79–80
self-harm and suicide 63
substance use disorders 103–4
genogram 2
GHB (gamma hydroxybutyrate) 112, 114, 117, 118
Gilles de la Tourette syndrome 251
glue sniffing see solvent abuse
grandiose delusions 9, 10, 94
guanfacine 249
guilt, delusions of 9, 94
gustatory hallucinations 95

H

habituation 178
hallucinations 10–11, 79, 81, 82, 94–5, 108, 140
　depression 39–40
　forensic psychiatry 270

hallucinogens 111–12
haloperidol 87, 89
harm reduction 69, 119–20
head injury 139
hebephrenic schizophrenia 85
heroin 108, 109, 116, 118, 119
hierarchy of fears 178
history
　collateral 6
　personal 5–6
　psychiatric 4–6
HIV-associated neurocognitive disorder (HAND) 135
homosexuality 219
Hospital Anxiety and Depression scale (HAD) 177, 192
Huntington disease (HD) 134–5
hyperactivity 249
hyperadrenalism 141
hyperarousal 183
hyperkinetic disorder
　see attention deficit hyperactivity disorder (ADHD)
hyperparathyroidism 141
hyperphagia 39
hyperprolactinaemia 86, 88
hypersomnia 39
hyperthyroidism 141, 176
hyperventilation 173
hypoactive sexual desire dysfunction (HSDD) 215–16
hypoadrenalism 141
hypochondriacal delusions 9
hypochondriasis 191
hypoglycaemia 141, 176
hypomania 45, 47
hypoparathyroidism 141
hypothyroidism 141

I

illusions 10
imipramine 41
impotence see erectile dysfunction
impulsivity 249
inattention 249
infidelity, delusions of 9
inhalants 114–15
insight 11
insomnia 38
intellectual disability (ID) 231–42
interferon 141
International Classification of Diseases (ICD-11) 27
interpersonal and social rhythm therapy (IPSRT) 49
interpersonal therapy 44
interview skills 19–23
intravenous drug use 108–9
　complications 111

introductions 19
intrusive memories 183
investigations
   anxiety disorder 176–7
   attention deficit hyperactivity disorder 249
   autism spectrum disorder 248
   delirium 130–2
   dementia 158
   depression 40
   eating disorders 204–6
   intellectual disability 237
   mania and bipolar affective disorder 47
   personality disorders 260–2
   schizophrenia 86
   substance use disorders 117–18

J

jealousy, delusions of 10

K

ketamine 112, 113, 116
khat (chat, qat) 111, 113, 116
knight's move thinking 8
Korsakoff syndrome (KS) 108, 136, 137

L

lamotrigine 48
lanugo hair 204
law 29–30
learned helplessness 36
learning theories, substance use disorders 105
Lesch–Nyhan syndrome 235
levetiracetam 141
levothyroxine 141
Lewy bodies 154
Lewy body dementia 153, 154, 157
LGBT terminology 218
liaison psychiatry 129
libido (sexual drive) 215–16
life experiences *see* childhood and life experiences
light therapy 43
limbic system 105
lisdexamfetamine 249
lithium toxicity 49, 50
lofepramine 41
loosening of associations 8
lurasidone 87
Luria test 146
lysergic acid diethylamide (LSD) 111, 112, 113, 116

M

magic mushrooms 112
malingering 192
management
   anxiety disorders 177–80
   attention deficit hyperactivity disorder 249
   autism spectrum disorder 248
   conduct/dissocial disorder 250
   delirium 133
   dementia 158–60
   depression 40–4
   eating disorders 206–8
   encopresis 247
   enuresis 247
   forensic psychiatry 273
   intellectual disability 237–8
   mania and bipolar affective disorder 47–9
   medically unexplained symptoms 192–3
   personality disorders 262–3
   schizophrenia 86–91
   self-harm and suicide 67–9
   substance use disorders 118–20
mania 44–50, 55–8
   differential diagnosis 47, 204
   neurochemical theory 37
   in organic conditions 141
   see also bipolar affective disorder
mannerisms 7
Matthews, James Tilley 84
medical school 31
medically unexplained symptoms (MUS) 189–98
melanosis coli 205
melatonergic antidepressants 42
memantine 159
memory 137
   loss *see* amnesia
meningovascular syphilis 142
Mental Capacity Act 2005 29–30
Mental Health Act 2007 29
mental health in childhood 245, 246
   see also child and adolescent psychiatry
mental health of older adults (MHOA) 151, 159
   see also old age psychiatry
mental state examination (MSE)
   assessment 6–11
   delirium 132
   eating disorders 208
   van Gogh 3–4
mentalization 64, 263
mephedrone 115, 116
metabolic syndrome 86
methadone 118–19, 124
methamphetamine 109, 111, 113, 116

methylphenidate 249
migration, and schizophrenia 80
mild cognitive impairment (MCI) 158
mindfulness 180
mindfulness-based cognitive therapy (MBCT) 44
Mini-Addenbrooke's Cognitive Examination (M-ACE) 143, 144
mirror sign (autoprosopagnosia) 155
mirtazapine 41, 151
Misuse of Drugs Act 1971 115
moclobemide 41
monoamine hypothesis 36–7
monoamine oxidase inhibitors (MAOIs) 41
mood 8
   disorders *see* affective disorders
mood stabilizers 47–8, 49, 262
morbid jealousy 108
morphine 108, 116
motivational interviewing (MI) 119, 207
motivational theory, substance use disorders 105
motor cortex 131
multiple personality disorder 192, 260
multiple sclerosis (MS) 140, 147–8
multisensory therapy 159
Munchausen-by-proxy 192
Munchausen syndrome 192
myxoedema madness 47, 141

N

naloxone 119
naltrexone 118
Nar-Anon 120
Narcotics Anonymous 120
necrophilia 218
negative affectivity 261
negative automatic thoughts (NATS) 43, 179
negative reinforcement 169
negative symptoms (in schizophrenia) 81–2
neologisms 8
neonatal abstinence syndrome (opioids) 111
neuroanatomical/neurobiological theories
   affective disorders 38
   anxiety disorders 169
   eating disorders 201
   organic psychiatry 129
   personality disorders 260
   substance use disorders 105
neurochemical theories
   affective disorders 36–7
   forensic psychiatry 272
   personality disorders 260

neurodevelopmental disorders in childhood 247–50
neurodevelopmental history 253
neurodevelopmental theories of schizophrenia 80
neuroendocrine theories in forensic psychiatry 272
neurofibrillary tangles 153
neuroleptic malignant syndrome (NMS) 89
neuropsychiatry 129
neurosyphilis 141, 142
neurotic disorders *see* anxiety disorders
neuroticism 169
neurotransmitter theories
  anxiety disorders 169
  schizophrenia 80–1
neutropenia 98
next steps
  alcohol-induced aggression 124–5
  anxious colleague 185–6
  behavioural change in a woman with Down syndrome 240–1
  capacity and risk at 78 years 164–5
  domestic violence 266–7
  heart attack with complications 58–9
  infertility and amenorrhoea 211–12
  non-accidental injury in ADHD 254
  postpartum depression 229–30
  radicalization risk 275–6
  refusal of treatment following self-harm 75
  seizures on clozapine 98–9
  steroid induced hypomania 147–8
  suspected malignancy 196–7
  vaginismus 221
nihilistic delusions 9, 94
nitrites 114, 115, 117
nitrous oxide 114–15, 117
noids 115
non-accidental injury in childhood 254
non-steroidal anti-inflammatory drugs (NSAIDs), overdose 65–7
noradrenergic and specific serotonin antidepressants (NASSAs) 41
normal pressure hydrocephalus (NPH) 135
novel psychoactive substances (NPS) 108, 115, 116, 117
nucleus accumbens 105
nursing homes 160

O

objective structured clinical examinations (OSCEs) 24–6
obsessions 10, 173, 182
obsessive–compulsive disorder (OCD) 168, 172, 182–4
  clinical presentation 173
  differential diagnosis 174, 175–6
  management 179, 180
  neuroanatomical theories 169
  perinatal 225–6
  prognosis 180
obstetric complications, and schizophrenia 80
occipital lobe functions 131
occupational factors
  alcohol use disorders 105
  self-harm and suicide 64
olanzapine 48, 87
  side effects 88, 89
old age psychiatry 149–65
olfactory hallucinations 95
Open Dialogue 90
operant conditioning (Skinnerian) 105, 272
opioids 108–9, 116
  case history 123–4
  neonatal abstinence syndrome 111
  overdose 119
  substitute prescribing 118–19
  withdrawal 109, 110, 118
organic psychiatry 127–48
  affective disorders 36
  differential diagnosis 174, 204
  forensic psychiatry 272
organic psychosis 84
orgasmic dysfunctions 215, 217
other specified feeding or eating disorder (OSFED) 204
overdose 65–7, 68, 69
  case history 74
  substance misuse 109, 111, 112, 114, 119
over-inclusive thinking 8
overvalued ideas 10

P

paedophilia 218
paliperidone 87
panic attacks 181, 182
  differential diagnosis 174, 175
panic disorder 172, 182
  biochemistry 173
  clinical presentation 169–70
  differential diagnosis 174, 175
  epidemiology 168
  management 178–9
paracetamol overdose 65, 67, 68
paranoia 10
paranoid personality disorder 85
paranoid schizophrenia 85, 274–5
paraphilic disorders 218
paraphrenia (late-onset schizophrenia) 152

parasuicide *see* self-harm
parietal lobe functions 131
Parkinson disease (PD) 139–40
Parkinson plus syndromes 140
parkinsonism 88
  secondary 140
paroxetine 41
partial delusions 10
passive aggression 259
passivity 9, 82, 94, 95
  delusions of 9
pathology
  Alzheimer disease 153
  Lewy body dementia 154
  vascular dementia 154
peer support, in substance use disorders 120
perception 10–11
perinatal psychiatry 223–30
persecutory delusions 9, 10, 93–4
perseveration 8, 85
perseveration 8, 85
perseveration 8, 85
personality change, and traumatic brain injury 139
personality clusters 258, 259, 263
personality disorders 257–67
  differential diagnosis 85, 175
  risk of suicide 64
personality traits 258, 260, 261–2
pethidine 108, 116
phaeochromocytoma 141, 176
phenelzine 41
phenylcyclidine (PCP) 112, 116
phobia 168, 170–2
  agoraphobia 171–2
  social 170
physical illness, and self-harm/suicide 64
Pick disease 134
plaque formation in Alzheimer disease 153
polypharmacy, and dementia 159
porphyria 141
positive symptoms (in schizophrenia) 80–1, 82
post-concussion syndrome 139
postpartum depression 226, 229–30
postpartum psychosis (PPP) 85, 227, 228–9
post-traumatic amnesia 139
post-traumatic stress disorder (PTSD) 172, 183
  aetiology 169
  clinical presentation 173–4
  differential diagnosis 174, 176
  epidemiology 168
  management 179–80
  neuroanatomical theories 169
  perinatal 225
  prognosis 180

posturing 85
poverty of speech 8
Prader–Willi syndrome 235
prefrontal cortex 105, 131
pregabalin 177
pregnancy and drugs 49, 226
premotor cortex 131
presenilin genes 153
pressure of speech 8
primary delusions 9
primitive reflexes 147
prion diseases 135–6
prisoners, mental health of 271
prognosis
  anxiety disorders 180
  attention deficit hyperactivity disorder 249–50
  autism spectrum disorder 248–9
  conduct/dissocial disorder 250
  delirium 133
  dementia 160
  depression 44
  eating disorders 208
  intellectual disability 238
  mania and bipolar affective disorder 49
  medically unexplained symptoms 193
  personality disorders 263
  psychotic disorders 91–2
  self-harm 69
  sexual health conditions 219
  substance use disorders 120
  van Gogh 14–15
projection 259
pseudodementia 151, 158
psilocybin 111–12, 116
psychiatric factors
  eating disorders 202
  intellectual disability 235–6
  self-harm and suicide 64
  substance use disorders 105
psychoactive drugs – summary 116
Psychoactive Substances Act 2016 115
psychoanalytic psychotherapy 263
psychoanalytic theories
  forensic psychiatry 272
  medically unexplained symptoms 190–1
psychodynamic psychotherapy 44, 263
psychoeducation
  anxiety disorders 177, 180
  bulimia nervosa 208
  dementia 159
  mania and bipolar affective disorder 49
  personality disorders 263
  psychotic disorders 90
psychological defences 259

psychological interventions
  anxiety disorders 177–80
  dementia 159
  eating disorders 207, 208
  forensic psychiatry 273
  intellectual disability 237
  personality disorders 262–3
  psychotic disorders 87–90
  substance use disorders 119
psychological theories
  anxiety disorders 169
  eating disorders 202
  personality disorders 259
  schizophrenia 81
psychopathy 272
psychosis
  in childhood and adolescence 245
  differential diagnosis 174, 204
  in old age 152
  organic causes 140, 141
  in Parkinson disease 140
  postpartum 227, 228–9
  in substance use disorders 109
psychosocial models, of medically unexplained symptoms 191
psychotherapy 208
psychotic depression 54–5
psychotic disorders 77–100
  see also schizophrenia
puerperal psychosis 85

Q

question funnel 20–1
quetiapine 87, 88, 89

R

radicalization risk 275–6
rape 221
rapport 7, 21–3
reattribution model 193
recovery model, psychotic disorders 91
re-experiencing phenomena 183
refeeding syndrome 207
reference, delusions of 9, 94
reflection 22
rehabilitation 91
religious delusions 94
reminiscence therapy 159
repetitive transcranial magnetic stimulation (rTMS) 43
residential care 160
residual schizophrenia 85
restriction orders 273
retrograde amnesia 139
reversible inhibitors of monoamine oxidase A (RIMAs) 41

rigidity 85
risk assessment
  perinatal psychiatry 227
  schizophrenia 86
  self-harm and suicide 67, 73–4
risk management, self-harm/suicide 67
risperidone 86, 87, 88
rivastigmine 159
Royal College of Psychiatrists (MRCPsych) 31–2
Russell's sign 205

S

sadism 218
safety 17–18
safety-seeking behaviours (SSBs) 169
salience hypothesis 81
schizoaffective disorder 47, 85
  see also affective disorders
schizoid personality disorder 80, 85
schizophrenia 77–100
  forensic psychiatry 270
  late-onset 152
  risk of suicide 64, 91
  subtypes 85
schizotypal disorder 80, 85
Schneider's first rank symptoms 82
school refusal 246
seasonal depressive disorder 43
second-generation antipsychotics (SGAs) 42, 87, 88
secondary delusions 9
sections of the Mental Health Act (MHA) 2007 30
sedatives 112–14, 117, 262
seizures, non-epileptic 192
selective attention 191
selective mutism 247
selective serotonin reuptake inhibitors (SSRIs)
  in affective disorders 40, 41, 151
  in anxiety disorders 177
  in bulimia nervosa 207
  overdose 69
self-cutting 65, 67, 73
self-harm 63–76
  in childhood and adolescence 245
  personality disorders 263
Self-Management and Recovery Training (SMART) 120
self-preservation theory 64
sensate focus therapy 216
separation anxiety disorder 246
serotonin and noradrenaline reuptake inhibitors (SNRIs) 41
serotonin antagonist and reuptake inhibitors (SARIs) 42
serotonin syndrome 42

Index   **285**

sertraline 41
sexual and relationship history 6
sexual arousal
    dysfunctions 215, 216–17
sexual desire problems 215–16
sexual dysfunctions 215–17
sexual health conditions 213–22
sexual pain disorders 215, 217
sexual pain-penetration disorder
    (SPDD) 215, 217, 221
silence 20
simple schizophrenia 85
sleep hygiene 44
social anxiety disorder 172, 182
    clinical presentation 170
    differential diagnosis 174, 175
    epidemiology 168
    management 179
social disadvantage, and
    schizophrenia 80
social interventions
    anxiety disorders 180
    dementia 159–60
    depression 44
    eating disorders 207, 208
    forensic psychiatry 273
    intellectual disability 237–8
    personality disorders 263
    psychotic disorders 90–1
    substance use disorders 119–20
social isolation, and self-harm/
    suicide 64
social learning theory 105
social model of disability 233, 237
social skills training 90
sociocultural theories, eating
    disorders 202
solvent abuse 114, 117
somatic hallucinations 95
somatization 190
somatoform disorders 190
speech 8–9
spice 115
splitting 259
St John's Wort 42
Stages of Change model 105
startle reflex 174
stereotypies 7
stimulants 109–11, 113, 115, 116
stress, extreme 175
stroke 140–1
stupor 85
subcortical dementia 133

substance use disorders 101–26
    intoxication 103, 106, 109, 111,
        112, 115
    risk of suicide 64
    schizophrenia 80
    withdrawal 106, 109, 111, 112–14,
        115, 118
suicide 63–76
    bereaved people 69
    postpartum 227
    prevention strategies 64
    in prisoners 271
    risk factors 66
    in schizophrenia 91
sulpiride 87
supplementary motor area 131
synthetic cannabinoid receptor
    agonists (SCRAs) 115, 116
syphilis 142
systematized delusions 10
systemic lupus erythematosus
    (SLE) 141

T

tactile hallucinations 95
tardive dyskinesia 88
tau protein 153
Tay–Sachs disease 234
temperament 259
temporal lobe functions 131
tertiary neurosyphilis 142
therapeutic communities 263
thiamine 118, 137
thought
    block 8
    broadcast 9, 94
    disorder 79, 81, 95
    insertion 9, 94, 95
    interference 82, 94
    withdrawal 9, 94
thought–action fusing 173
tic disorders 250–1
tics 7
Tourette syndrome 251
training 31–2
transference 44, 263–4
transient global amnesia (TGA) 137
transmissible spongiform
    encephalopathies (TSEs) 135–6
transsexualism 218
transvestism 218

tranylcypromine 41
traumatic brain injury (TBI) 139
trazodone 42
treatment-resistant schizophrenia 87
tricyclic antidepressants
    (TCAs) 41, 177
    overdose 69
trifluoperazine 87, 89
tri-iodothyronine 42
trisomy 21 *see* Down syndrome

U

urbanicity and schizophrenia 80
urine drug screen (UDS) 117, 118

V

vaginismus 221
validation 22–3
validation therapy 159
valproate (sodium) 48, 49
van Gogh, Vincent 1–4, 12–15
vascular dementia 153, 154,
    155, 157
venlafaxine 41
verbal fluency test 146
vestibulodynia 217
visual hallucinations 94–5
vitamin B deficiencies 141
volatile anaesthetics 114–15
volatile solvents 114
voyeuristic disorder 218
vulnerability factors, depression 36
vulvodynia 217

W

waxy flexibility 85
Wernicke encephalopathy 108, 137
Wernicke–Korsakoff syndrome 108
Wernicke's area 131
word salad 8
World Health Organization
    (WHO) 27

Z

zuclopenthixol 87